Operating Department Practice A-Z
Second Edition

Operating Department Practice A–Z

Second Edition

Tom Williams and Brian Smith

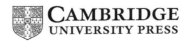
CAMBRIDGE UNIVERSITY PRESS

CAMBRIDGE UNIVERSITY PRESS

Cambridge, New York, Melbourne, Madrid, Cape Town, Singapore, São Paulo, Delhi

Cambridge University Press

The Edinburgh Building, Cambridge CB2 8RU, UK

Published in the United States of America by Cambridge University Press, New York

www.cambridge.org
Information on this title: www.cambridge.org/9780521710213

© T. Williams and B. Smith 2008

This publication is in copyright. Subject to statutory exception and to the provisions
of relevant collective licensing agreements, no reproduction of any part may take
place without the written permission of Cambridge University Press.

First edition © B. Smith and T. Williams 2004
Second edition © T. Williams and B. Smith 2008

Printed in the United Kingdom at the University Press, Cambridge

A catalogue record for this publication is available from the British Library

Library of Congress Cataloguing in Publication data
Williams, Tom, 1948 Sept. 16-
  Operating department practice A-Z / Tom Williams, Brian Smith.
    p. ; cm.
  Rev. ed. of: Operating department practice A-Z / edited by Brian Smith,
Tom Williams. 2004.
  Includes bibliographical references and index.
  ISBN 978-0-521-71021-3 (pbk. : alk. paper)
1. Operations, Surgical – Terminology. 2. Operations, Surgical – Dictionaries.
I. Smith, Brian, 1965- II. Title.
  [DNLM: 1. Surgery – Abbreviations. 2. Surgery – Dictionary – English.
3. Surgical Equipment – Abbreviations. 4. Surgical Equipment – Dictionary –
English. 5. Surgical Procedures, Operative – Abbreviations. 6. Surgical Procedures,
Operative – Dictionary–English. WO 13 W727o 2008]
  RD16.O626 2008
  617′.003–dc22
2007050654

ISBN 978-0-521-71021-3 paperback

Cambridge University Press has no responsibility for the persistence or
accuracy of URLs for external or third-party internet websites referred to
in this publication, and does not guarantee that any content on such
websites is, or will remain, accurate or appropriate.

Every effort has been made in preparing this publication to provide accurate and
up-to-date information which is in accord with accepted standards and practice at
the time of publication. Although case histories are drawn from actual cases, every
effort has been made to disguise the identities of the individuals involved. Neverthe-
less, the authors, editors and publishers can make no warranties that the information
contained herein is totally free from error, not least because clinical standards are
constantly changing through research and regulation. The authors, editors and publishers therefore disclaim all liability for direct or consequential damages resulting
from the use of material contained in this publication. Readers are strongly advised to
pay careful attention to information provided by the manufacturer of any drugs or
equipment that they plan to use.

Contents

Foreword

Liverpool has led the way in recognising and furthering the status of operating department assistants and practitioners (ODA/Ps). Two young men, Jack Probert and Bill Kehoe, were theatre technicians in the armed forces during the Second World War. After the war they came to Walton Hospital, Liverpool, and provided for the anaesthetists there a service that was virtually unknown elsewhere. They were instrumental in founding a Society for Anaesthetic Technicians, with its journal '*Technic*', which has become the *Journal of Operating Department Practice*. The anaesthetic trainees from Walton (and I was fortunate to be one of them) became consultants elsewhere and were then able to insist on properly trained assistants in the anaesthetic room. The concept that anaesthetists required skilled assistance was gradually and eventually accepted by the UK Department of Health and local administrators. By the mid 1980s, via insistence and persistence, anaesthetists in many hospitals had achieved suitable levels of assistance at the standards that were deemed to be essential by the Association of Anaesthetists and the Faculty of Anaesthetists. Sad that the achievement of this had to be confrontational.

Although the necessity of trained help for anaesthetists was accepted, there were still limitations in the training available for ODAs. What was needed was an energetic impetus and leadership from among the ODAs (later to be called ODPs) who would enhance academic credibility by acquisition of higher academic qualifications and then help to establish higher educational facilities for the profession. Two such influences have been Tom Williams and Brian Smith.

Tom's career has spanned the years since the first recognition and certification of ODAs right through to the present professional and academic status of ODPs.

Operating department practitioner training has moved into the realm of Higher Education with courses offering a Diploma in Higher Education or in some centres a bachelor's degree in operating department practice.

There has been little material written by and for ODA/ODPs. *Operating Department Practice A–Z*, which Tom and Brian have written with input from colleagues, has run to a second edition. It is very satisfying when the publishers agree to a second edition of a book and is tangible evidence that the first edition has been well received. Tom, Brian and their colleagues write with authority born of experience. It is an excellent book and I wish it had been available when

I was a teacher. Jack Probert and Bill Kehoe would have been very proud of their 'progeny', Tom Williams, Brian Smith and their associate authors.

Dr A. A. Gilbertson

Emeritus Consultant in Anaesthesia & Intensive Care Medicine,
Royal Liverpool University Hospital
Member of Court of Examiners, Royal College of Anaesthetists
Visiting Professor, Intensive Care Medicine,
McGill University, Montreal Canada
Academic Sub-Dean & Vice President, Royal Society of Medicine,
London

Preface

The first edition of *Operating Department Practice A–Z* was something of a trial run to assess demand, and the favourable response combined with positive feedback has been encouraging. The first edition was intentionally specialised, and focused narrowly on theatre practice and processes; however, the second edition has been expanded to include more medical, scientific and technical terms, in particular more anatomy and physiology. The inclusion of illustrations and expansion of the support sections will also be of value to the reader.

The modern Operating Department Practitioner (ODP) requires enhanced and broad knowledge in order to fulfil the diverse and differing requirements of the patients in their care, and this book was written with this in mind.

The curriculum for ODP learners, both before and after qualification, has broadened over the years to match the need to keep up to date with advancements in technology and knowledge, particularly of the healthcare and life sciences. By expanding the content of this book we are meeting that need and providing a companion to research and learning. The dictionary style of the first edition has been maintained but its nature does limit the detail of the explanation in the Quick Reference that can be provided. By reading the Advanced Reference and following the cross-references to the highlighted key words, the reader is guided to a more complete explanation.

Some may consider the range too broad and certain content a little obscure, but it is felt that the speed of change, advancements in health care and the anticipated requirements of the readers justify this.

In addition to the factual and standard input, we have continued to include terms, colloquialisms and even related slang that the learners may encounter. In spite of opposition and changing views over the years, abbreviations and acronyms continue to be part of healthcare vocabulary, and with this in mind the list of abbreviations has been expanded. Readers should be aware that sometimes acronyms and abbreviations may have more than one meaning, and that one interpretation may be favoured over another by a particular speciality or country. As an ODP working across many specialities and in different countries, it is important to recognise the appropriate context and interpret the abbreviation accurately.

Historically ODPs have relied on texts written for and by members of other professional groups. This book was written to go some way towards correcting this anomaly and will serve the ODP of the future, perhaps instigating similar projects within the profession.

While this book is broad in its content, it is far from a one-stop shop in terms of required knowledge for the ODP learner. Also, it is not intended to be used solely by theatre personnel, and the hope is that fellow health-care professionals and interested parties will find it of value as well.

Tom Williams
Brian Smith

Acknowledgements

We would like to thank the following for their comments, advice, contributions and support:

First Edition:
Professor J. Hunter, Rita Hehir, Jean Hinton, Jill McKeen, Cheryl Wayne, Paul Wicker, Josie Williams, Sandra Fox, Neil Herbert and Robert Mitchell.

Second Edition:
Dr. A. A. Gilbertson, Jerry Barrett, Robert Mitchell and Josie Williams.

Illustration acknowledgements:

- BUPA Hospitals group (www.bupa.co.uk) for the hiatus hernia illustration.
- Elsevier Ltd (www.elsevier.com) for illustrations relating to: Mercedes incision, volvulus, stereotaxy, skin tunnelling, rule of nines, pulmonary artery catheter.
- Dr. Edwin Liem (http://vam.anest.ufl.edu) for the Bullard laryngoscope illustration.
- *Update in Anaesthesia* (www.world-anaesthesia.org) for the intraosseus, dermatome illustrations.

Abbreviations

AAA	(triple-A) – abdominal aortic aneurysm
AACP	advanced anaesthetic & critical care practitioner
AAE	arterial air embolus
AAI	allergy, anaphylaxis and immunology
AAP	advanced anaesthetic practitioner
ABG	arterial blood gases
ABS	antibacterial substance
ABV	alcohol by volume
ACADs	ambulatory care and diagnostic units
ACE	angiotensin-converting enzyme
ACE	applied clinical ethics
ACh	acetylcholine
ACL	anterior cruciate ligament
ACLS	advanced cardiac life support
ACP	anaesthetic care practitioner
ACT	activated clotting time
ACTH	adrenocorticotrophic hormone
ADC	apparent diffusion coefficient
ADH	antidiuretic hormone
ADHD	attention deficit hyperactivity disorder
ADI	acceptable daily intake
ADP	accidental dural puncture
AEP	auditory evoked potential
AER	auditory evoked response
AFP	alpha fetoprotein
AHTR	acute haemolytic transfusion reaction
AIC	adverse incident centre
AIDS	acquired immuno deficiency syndrome
AIH	artificial insemination
AIHA	autoimmune haemolytic anaemia
AKPS	anterior knee pain score
AKU	artificial kidney unit
ALA	alpha-linolenic acid
ALBC	antibiotic loader bone cement
ALD	adrenoleukodystrophy
ALERT™	Acute Life-threatening Events Recognition & Treatment
ALI	acute lung injury

Abbreviations

AMD	age-related macular disease
AML	acute myelogenous leukaemia
AMV	assisted mechanical ventilation
ANH	acute normovolaemic haemodilution
ANH	artificial nutrition & hydration
AP	action potential
APH	antepartum haemorrhage
APLS	Advanced Paediatric Life Support
APOs	anaesthetic paramedical officers
APPT	activated partial prothrombin time
APRV	airway pressure release ventilation
ARC	aids-related complex
ARDS	adult respiratory distress syndrome
ARM	artificial rupture of membranes
ASA	American Society of Anesthesiologists
ASB	assisted spontaneous breaths
ASD	atrial septal defect
ASP	advanced scrub practitioner
ATACC	anaesthesia trauma & critical care
ATC	automatic tube compensation
ATG	antithymocyte globulin
ATLS	Advanced Trauma Life Support
ATP	adenosine triphosphate
ATS	antitetanus serum
AV	atrioventricular
AvMA	action against medical accidents
AVN	avascular necrosis
AWG	American Wire Gauge
BAAPS	British Association of Aesthetic Plastic Surgeons
BAHA	bone anchored hearing aid
BAL	broncho-alveolar lavage
BAN	British Approved Name
BAWO	bilateral antrum washout
BBV	blood-borne viruses
BCC	basal cell carcinoma
BCLS	Basic Cardiac Life Support
BD	base deficit
BD	twice daily
BE	bacterial endocarditis
BEIR	biological effects of ionising radiation
BEST	basic electronic surgical training
BGL	blood glucose level

BHP	British Horse Power
BHP	brake horse power
BHR	Birmingham Hip Resurfacing
BID	brought in dead
BIM	bispectral index monitor
BiPAP	bilevel positive airway pressure
BIPP	bisthmus iodine paraffin paste
BKA	below knee amputation
BMD	bone mineral density
BMI	body mass index
BMR	basic metabolic rate
BMT	bone marrow transplant
BP	blood pressure
BPH	benign prostatic hyperplasia
BRMs	biologic response modifiers
BSA	body surface area
BSI	bispectral index
BSO	bilateral salpingo-oophorectomy
BUN	blood urea nitrogen
BW	birth weight
Bx	biopsy
CABG	coronary artery bypass graft
CABPM	continuous ambulatory blood pressure monitoring
CAD	computer-aided detection
CAD	coronary artery disease
CAE	continuous ambulatory electrocardiography
CAH	congenital adrenal hyperplasia
CA-MRSA	community-associated methicillin-resistant *Staphylococcus aureus*
CAOS	computer-assisted orthopaedic system
CAPD	continuous ambulatory peritoneal dialysis
CAT	computerised axial tomography
CATS	clinical assessment treatment & support
CAVH	continuous arteriovenous haemofiltration
CBC	complete blood count
CBD	common bile duct
CBF	cerebral blood flow
CBI	combined behavioural intervention
CBT	cognitive behavioural therapy
CCF	congestive cardiac failure
CCU	Coronary Care Unit
C&D	cleaning & disinfection

CDH	congenital dislocation of hip
C-Dif	*Clostridium difficile*
CDP	Clinical Development Partnership
CE	clinical effectiveness
CELLO	columnar-endothelium-lined lower oesophagus
CF	cystic fibrosis
CFAM	cerebral function analysis monitor
CFC	chlorofluorocarbons
CFS	chronic fatigue syndrome
CGI	computer-generated imaging
CGS	centimeter-gram-seconds
CHD	coronary heart disease
CHD	congenital hip dysplasia
CHF	congestive heart failure
CHT	closed head trauma
CICU	Coronary Intensive Care Unit
CLL	chronic lymphocytic leukaemia
CMC	carboxymethyl cellulose
CML	chronic myeloid leukaemia
CMV	controlled mechanical ventilation
CMV	cytomegalovirus
CNS	central nervous system
CO	cardiac output
COAD	chronic obstructive airway disease
COMA	Committee on Medical Aspects on Food & Nutrition Policy
COPA	cuffed oropharyngeal airway
COPD	chronic obstructive pulmonary disease
COSHH	Control of Substances Hazardous to Health
CPAP	continuous positive airway pressure
CPB	cardiopulmonary bypass
CPD	citratephosphate dextrose
CPD	chronic papillomatous dermatitis
CPK	creatine phosphokinase
CPP	cerebral perfusion pressure
CPR	cardiopulmonary resuscitation
CQI	continuous quality improvement
CRF	chronic renal failure
CRNA	certified registered nurse anaesthetist
CRP	complex regional pain
CRP	c-reactive protein
CRTAP	cartilage associated protein
CS	Caesarean section

CSA	central sleep apnoea
CSA	compressed spectral array
CSEA	combined spinal epidural analgesia
CSF	cerebrospinal fluid
CSSD	Central Sterile Supply Department
CSU	catheter specimen of urine
CT	computerised tomography
CTG	cardiotocography
CTS	Carpal Tunnel Syndrome
CTZ	chemoreceptor trigger zone
CVA	cerebrovascular accident
CVD	cardiovascular disease
CVD	cerebrovascular disease
CVP	central venous pressure
CVS	cardiovascular system
CVS	chorionic villus sampling
CVVH	continuous veno-venous haemofiltration
CXR	chest X-ray
DAD	doctor-assisted suicide
DARE	database of abstracts and reviews of effectiveness
DASH	disabilities of the arm shoulder and hand
DBAC	deep bleeder acoustic coagulation
DBP	diastolic blood pressure
D&C	dilatation & curettage
DCIA	deep circumflex iliac artery
DCIS	ductal carcinoma in situ
DCM	dilated cardiomyopathy
DCP	dynamic compression plate
DCS	dynamic compression screw
DDT	dichlorodiphenyltrichloroethane
DES	drug eluting stent
DES	diethylstilbestrol
DEXA (scan)	dual-energy X-ray absorpiometry
DHS	dynamic hip screw
DHT	dihydrotestosterone
DIC	disseminated intravascular coagulation
DIS	drug infusion systems
DK	diabetic ketoacidosis
DLT	double lumen tube
DM	diabetes mellitus
DMARDs	disease-modifying antirheumatic drugs
DMT	disease-modifying therapy

DMV	difficult mask ventilation
DNA	did not arrive
DNA	deoxyribonucleic acid
DNAR	do not attempt resuscitation
DNR	do not resuscitate
DOA	dead on arrival
DPLD	diffuse parenchymal lung disease
DPT	diphtheria, tetanus, pertussis (triple vaccine)
DRE	digital rectal examination
DSS	discharge scoring system
DSST	digit-symbol substitution test
DTB	*Drug & Therapeutics Bulletin*
DTC	Drug & Therapeutics Committee
DTCs	diagnostic & treatment centres
DTI	diffusion tensor imaging
DU	duodenal ulcer
D&V	diarrhoea & vomiting
DVT	deep vein thrombosis
DWMRI	diffusion-weighted magnetic resonance imaging
EAE	experimental autoimmune encephalitis
EAP	equine-assisted psychotherapy
EBCT	electron beam computed tomography
EBM	evidence-based medicine
EBME	Electrical Biomedical Engineering
EBP	epidural blood patch
EBP	evidence-based practice
ECF	extracellular fluid
ECG	electrocardiography
ECMO	extracorporeal membrane oxygenation
ECP	external counter pulsation
ECT	electroconvulsive therapy
ED	erectile dysfunction
ED	effective dose
EDD	expected date of delivery
EDR	extreme drug resistance
EDTA	ethylenediamine tetra-acetic acid
EEG	electroencephalograph
EERP	extended endocardial resection procedure
EFA	elbow functional assessment scale
EFM	electronic fetal monitoring
EM	event monitoring
EMA	early medical abortion

EMU	early morning urine
ENT	ear nose & throat
EPR	electron paramagnetic resonance
ERCP	endoscopic retrograde cholangiopancreatography
ERPC	evacuation of retained products of conception
ERV	expiratory reserve volume
ESBL	extended spectrum beta lactamase
ESLD	end-stage liver disease
ESR	erythrocyte sedimentation rate
ESRD(F)	end-stage renal disease (failure)
ESU	electrosurgical unit
ESWL	extracorporeal shock wave lithotripsy
ETT	endotracheal tube
EUA	examination under anaesthesia
EWA	examination without anaesthetic
EWS	early warning score
FAS	fetal alcohol syndrome
FASD	fetal alcohol spectrum disorder
FB	foreign body
FBC	full blood count
FBS	failed back syndrome
FBS	fasting blood sugar
FBS	fetal blood sampling
FDA	Food & Drug Administration (USA)
FDP	fibrin degradation products
FDT	forced duction test
FESS	functional endoscopic sinus surgery
FEV	forced expiratory volume
FFP	fresh frozen plasma
FG	French gauge
FGF	fresh gas flow
FGM	female genital mutilation
FHH	fetal heart heard
FHNH	fetal heart not heard
FHR	fetal heart rate
FHS	food hypersensitivity syndrome
FID	faecal incontinence device
FMF	fetal movements felt
fMRI	functional magnetic resonance imaging
FNA	fine needle aspiration
FNAB	fine needle aspiration biopsy
FOB	fibre-optic bronchoscope

FRC	functional residual capacity
FRT	fluid replacement therapy
FS	frozen section
FSH	follicle-stimulating hormone
FVC	forced vital capacity
G&A	gas & air
GA	general anaesthesia
GABA	gamma-aminobutyric acid
GAF	global assessment functioning
GBM	glioblastoma multiforme with oligodendroglial component
GCS	Glasgow Coma Scale
GDM	gestational diabetes mellitus
GDT	goal-directed therapy
GERD	gastro-oesophageal reflux disease
GFR	glomerular filtration rate
GH	growth hormone
GI	gastrointestinal
GI	glycaemic index
GIFT	gamete intrafallopian transfer
GISTs	gastrointestinal stromal tumours
GIT	gastrointestinal tract
GKI	glucose potassium insulin (infusion)
GPH	gestational proteinuria hypertension
GPI	general paralysis of the insane
Grav (1, 11, 111)	number of pregnancies
GSS	group and save serum
GTN	glyceryl trinitrate
GTT	glucose tolerance test
GU	genitourinary
GUM	genitourinary medicine
GWP	global warming potential
HAART	highly active antiretroviral therapy
HAD	health anxiety disorder
HAI	hospital-acquired infection
HA-MRSA	hospital-associated methicillin-resistant *Staphylococcus aureus*
HART	hazardous area response teams
HAS	human albumin solution
HASAWA	Health and Safety at Work Act
HAV	hepatitis A
Hb	haemoglobin
HBD	heart beating donor

HBOCS	haemoglobin-based oxygen carrying solution
hBoV	human bocavirus
HBV	hepatitis B virus
HCA	health-care assistant
HCAI	health-care-associated infection
HCC	halothane-caffeine-contracture
hCG	human chorionic gonadotrophin
Hct	haematocrit
HCV	hepatitis C virus
HDL	high-density lipoprotein
HDR	high dose rate
HDU	High Dependency Unit
HELLP	haemolysis elevated liver enzymes & low platelets
HEV	hepatitis E virus
HFJV	high-frequency jet ventilation
HFOV	high-frequency oscillatory ventilation
Hib	*Haemophilus influenzae* bacterial infection
HIV	human immunodeficiency virus
HLA	histocompatibility antigen
HLA	human leucocyte antigen
HLC	Hospital Liaison Committees
HLHS	hypoplastic left heart syndrome
HNPU	has not passed urine
HOCM	hypertrophic obstructive cardiomyopathy
HPA	hypothalamic–pituitary–adrenal
HPV	human papilloma virus
HPV	hypoxic pulmonary vasoconstriction
HRT	hormone replacement therapy
HSDU	Hospital Sterilisation & Disinfecting Unit
HSV	Herpes simplex virus (types HSV1 & HSV2)
HSVI	Herpes simplex virus infection
HTIG	human tetanus immune globulin
HTLV	human T-cell lymphocytotrophic virus
HTST	higher temperature for a shorter time
HVS	high vaginal swab
IA	intra-articular
IABP	intra-aortic balloon pump
IAD	intraoperative autologous donation
IBD	inflammatory bowel disease
IBS	irritable bowel syndrome
ICD	implantable cardiac defibrillator
ICD	International Classification of Disease

ICE	in case of emergency
ICF	intracellular fluid
ICG	impedance cardiography
ICP	intracranial pressure
ICPM	intracranial pressure monitoring
ICPs	integrated care pathways
ICS	inhaled corticosteroids
ICS	intraoperative cell salvage
ICU	Intensive Care Unit
IDDM	insulin-dependent diabetes mellitus
IDS	intubation difficulty scale
IGS®	Implantable Gastric Stimulator
IHD	ischaemic heart disease
IHEB	inadvertent high epidural block
IJV	internal jugular vein
ILMA	intubating laryngeal mask airway
IM	intramuscular
IMG	international medical graduate
IMV	intermittent mandatory ventilation
INR	International Normalized Ratio
IO	intraocular
IOL	intraocular lens
IPF	idiopathic pulmonary fibrosis
IPPR	intermittent positive pressure respiration
IPPV	intermittent positive pressure ventilation
IR	infrared
IS	intra-synovial
ISTCs	Independent Sector Treatment Centres
IUCD	intrauterine contraceptive device
IUFB	intrauterine foreign body
IUGR	intrauterine growth retardation
IUI	intrauterine insemination
IV	intravenous
IVD	intra-vas device
IVF	in-vitro fertilisation
IVI	intravenous infusion
IVP	intravenous pyelogram
IVRA	intravenous regional anaesthesia
IVU	intravenous urography
IVUS	intravascular ultrasound
JVP	junctional venous pressure/pulse
KCl	potassium chloride

KOOS	knee injury & osteoarthritis outcome score
KUB	kidney, ureter and bladder
LA	local anaesthetic
LAB	lactic acid bacteria
LAFP	left atrial filling pressure
LARVH	laparoscopic-assisted radical vaginal hysterectomy
LASER	light amplification by stimulated emission of radiation
LASIK	laser-assisted in-situ keratomileusis
LASG	latex allergy support group
LAVH	laparoscopically assisted vaginal hysterectomy
LBBB	left bundle branch block
LBC	liquid-based cytology
LCD	liquid crystal display
LD	lethal dose
LDL	low-density lipoprotein
LDR	low dose rate
LED	light-emitting diode
LEEP	loop electrosurgical excision procedure
LFA	low friction arthroplasty
LH	laparoscopic hysterectomy
LIF	left ileac fossa
LIH	left inguinal hernia
LIP	lower inflection point
LLETZ	large loop excision of the transformation zone
LMA	laryngeal mask airway
LMP	last menstrual period
LMWH	low molecular weight heparin
LOR	loss of resistance
LOS	lower oesophageal sphincter
LREC	local research ethics committee
LSE	laser safety eyewear
LSH	laparoscopic supracervical hysterectomy
LSO	Laser Safety Officer
LT	laryngeal tube
LTH	laparoscopic total hysterectomy
LTSF	low temperature steam with formaldehyde
LUSCS	lower uterine segment Caesarean section
LVAD	left ventricular assist device
LVET	left ventricular ejection time
LVF	left ventricular failure
LVH	left ventricular hypertrophy
MAAS	motor activity assessment scale

MABP	mean arterial blood pressure
MAC	minimum alveolar concentration
MAOIs	monoamine oxidase inhibitors
MAP	mean arterial pressure
MAS	meconium aspiration syndrome
MAU	Medical Admissions Unit
MBF	myocardial blood flow
MBOS	maximum blood ordering schedules
MCI	mild cognitive impairment
MCP	metacarpophalangeal
MCS	minimally conscious state
MCSD	minimal clinically significant difference
MCV	mean cell volume
MD	muscular dystrophy
MDA	medical device alert
MDR	multi-drug resistant
ME	metabolic equivalents
ME	myalgic encephalomyelitis
MEA	microwave endometrial ablation
MEG	magnetoencephalography
MENS	microcurrent electrical neuromuscular stimulator
mEq	milliequivalent
MES	managed equipment service
MEWS	modified early warning scores
MFA	musculoskeletal function assessment
MH	malignant hyperthermia (hyperpyrexia)
MHA	Mental Health Act
MI	myocardial infarction
MIS	minimally invasive surgery
MISS	minimally invasive spinal surgery
MLAC	minimal local anaesthetic concentration
MMA	methylmethacrylate
MMC	Modernising Medical Careers
MMR	measles mumps & rubella
MMSE	Mini-Mental State Examination
MMV	mandatory minute volume
MND	motor neurone disease
MODS	multiple organ dysfunction syndrome
MOM	metal on metal
MPAP	mean pulmonary artery pressure
MPE	maximal permitted exposure
MPPS	most penetrating particulate size

MPWP	mean pulmonary wedge pressure
MRA	magnetic resonance angiography
MREC	multi-centre ethics committee
MRI	magnetic resonance imaging
MRS	magnetic resonance spectroscopy
MRSA	methicillin-resistant *Staphylococcus aureus*
MRT	magnetic resonance tomography
MS	multiple sclerosis
MSAFP	maternal serum alpha fetoprotein
MSbP	Munchausen's syndrome by proxy
MSG	monosodium glutamate
MSSA	methicillin-sensitive *Staphylococcus aureus*
MSSA	methicillin-susceptible *Staphylococcus aureus*
MSU	mid-stream urine
MTP	metarsophalangeal
MUA	manipulation under anaesthetic
MUGA	multiple-gated arteriography
MV	minute volume
MVC	motor vehicle collision
NAD	nicotinamide adenine dinucleotide
NAI	non-accidental injury
NASH	non-alcoholic steato hepatitis
NBM	nil by mouth
NCEPOD	National Confidential Enquiry into Peri-operative Deaths
ND	normal delivery
NDMR	non-depolarising neuromuscular relaxants
NET	neuroelectric therapy
NFR	not for resuscitation
NGT	nasogastric tube
NHBD	non heart beating donor
NHZ	nominal hazard zone
NIDDM	non-insulin-dependent diabetes mellitus
NIPPV	non-invasive positive pressure ventilation
NIV	non-invasive ventilation
NMA	non-medical anaesthetist
NMBA	neuromuscular blocking agent
NMJ	neuromuscular junction
NMP	neuromotor prosthesis
NMRI	nuclear magnetic resonance imaging
NOTES	natural orifice transluminal endoscopic surgery
NPDR	non-proliferative diabetic retinopathy
NPO	nil per os (nil by mouth)

Abbreviations

NPP	National Practitioner Programme
NPPV	non-invasive positive pressure ventilation
NRL	natural rubber latex
NRT	nicotine replacement therapy
NSAID	non-steroidal anti-inflammatory drug
NSCLC	non-small-cell lung cancer
NSS	neurological severity score
NTD	neural tube defect
OAB	overactive bladder
OCD	obsessive compulsive disorder
OCR	oculocardiac reflex
ODD	oesophageal detector device
ODR	organ donor register
OE	on examination
OELM	optimal external laryngeal manipulation
OGD	oesophago-gastro duodenoscopy
OHS	obesity hypoventilation syndrome
OHSS	ovarian hyperstimulation syndrome
OI	osteogenesis imperfecta
OLV	one-lung ventilation
OPD	outpatient(s) department
OPG	orthopantomogram
ORAC	oxygen radical absorbance capacity
ORIF	open reduction internal fixation
ORMIS	operating room management information system
ORSA	oxacillin-resistant *Staphylococcus aureus*
OSA	obstructive sleep apnoea
PA	pulmonary artery
PAC	pulmonary artery catheter
PACU	Post-Anaesthetic Care Unit
PAD	peripheral artery disease
PAD	pre-deposit autologous donation
PADSS	post-anaesthesia discharge scoring systems
PAF	platelet-activating factor
PAFC	pulmonary artery flotation catheter
PAH	pulmonary artery hypertension
PAL	powered assisted lipoplasty
PALS	Paediatric Advanced Life Support
PALS	Patient Liaison & Advice Service
PAOP	pulmonary artery occlusion pressure
PaP	papanicolaou (test) (cervix)
PARS	patient risk scores

PAS	physician-assisted suicide
PAWP	pulmonary artery wedge pressure
PBC	patient breathing circuit
PCA	patient-controlled analgesia
PCB	post-coital bleeding
PCD	programmed cell death
PCEA	patient-controlled epidural analgesia
PCOD	polycystic ovary disease
PCI	percutaneous coronary interventions
PCL	polycaprolactone
PCL	posterior cruciate ligament
PCPs	primary care providers
PCS	perioperative cell salvage
PCTs	Primary Care Trusts
PCV	packed cell volume
PCV	pressure control ventilation
PCWP	pulmonary capillary wedge pressure
PD	peritoneal dialysis
PDA	personal digital assistant
PDO	polydioxanone
PDP	paradichlorobenzene
PDPH	post-dural puncture headache
PDR	proliferative diabetic retinopathy
PE	pulmonary embolism
PEEP	positive end-expiratory pressure
PEG	percutaneous endoscopic gastrostomy
PEP	post-exposure prophylaxis
PERLA	pupils equal & reacting to light & accommodation
PET	polyethylene terephthalate
PET	positron emission tomography
PFCs	perfluorocarbons
PFCT	platelet function closure time
PFI	Private Finance Initiative
PFP	patient focused pricing
PFT	pulmonary function test
PG	prostaglandin
PGA	polyglycolide
PGD	pre-implantation genetic diagnosis
PH	pulmonary hypertension
PHN	post-herpetic neuralgia
PI	pressurised infusion
PIB	Pittsburgh compound-B

PICC	peripherally inserted central catheter
PID	pelvic inflammatory disease
PIH	pregnancy-induced hypertension
PIP	proximal interphalangeal (joint)
PLA	polylactic acid
PLV	partial liquid ventilation
PM	post-mortem
PMB	postmenopausal bleeding
PMCA	protein misfolding cyclic amplification
PMH	past medical history
PMHX	patient (past) medical history
PMMA	polymethylmethacrylate
PMR	percutaneous myocardial revascularisation
PMR	proportionate mortality rate
PN	postnatal
PNB	peripheral nerve block
PNS	peripheral nerve stimulator
PNS	post nasal space
POCU	Post Operative Care Unit
POD	Pouch of Douglas
POF	premature ovarian failure
POM	prescription only medicine
PONV	postoperative nausea & vomiting
POP	Plaster of Paris
POP	progesterone-only pill
PP	placenta praevia
PPD	para-phenylenediamine
PPE	personal protective equipment
PPG	photo-plethysmography
PPH	post-partum haemorrhage
PPH	primary pulmonary hypertension
PPI	proton pump inhibitor
PPM	parts per million
PPS	pentosan polysulphate
PR	per rectum
PR	prothrombin ratio
PRL	prolactin
PRN	pro-re nata (when required)
PrP	prion protein
PRVC	pressure-regulated volume control
PS	pressure support
PSA	prostate-specific antigen

PSA	puromycin-sensitive aminopeptidase
PSG	polysomnography
p.s.i.	pounds (per) square inch
PSI	patient state index
PSNS	parasympathetic nervous system
PSV	pressure support ventilation
PSVT	paroxysmal supraventricular tachycardia
PT	prothrombin time
Pt	patient
PTC	percutaneous transhepatic cholangiography
PTCA	percutaneous transluminal coronary angioplasty
PTH	parathyroid hormone
PTNS	percutaneous tibial nerve stimulation
PTRA	percutaneous transluminal renal angioplasty
PTT	partial thromboplastin time
PTT	pulse transit time
PTTK	partial thromboplastin time with kaolin
PTSD	post-traumatic stress disorder
PU	peptic ulcer
PV	per vagina
PVC	premature ventricular contraction
PVD	peripheral vascular disease
PVL	panton-valentine leukocidin
PVP	photo-selective prostate vaporisation
PVR	pulmonary vascular resistance
PVS	persistent vegetative state
PWV	pulse wave velocity
QA	quality assurance
QIPs	quality improvement programmes
RA	rheumatoid arthritis
RAO	right anterior oblique
RAOS	rheumatoid & arthritis outcome score
RAP	right atrial pressure
RASS	Richmond activity assessment scale
RBBB	right bundle branch block
RBC	red blood cell
RBS	random blood sugar
RCF	relative centrifugal force
RCT	randomised controlled (clinical) trial
RDA	recommended daily allowance
RDHB	rapid deployment haemostat bandage
RDI	recommended daily intake

REACH	registration, evaluation & authorisation of chemicals
REM	rapid eye movement
REMMS	reticulo-endothelial monocyte macrophage system
RF	rheumatoid factor
RFID	radiofrequency identification
RIDDOR	Reporting of Injuries, Diseases and Dangerous Occurrences Regulations
RIF	right iliac fossa
RIH	right inguinal hernia
RIV	respiratory-induced variations
RLS	restless leg syndrome
RPS	regional pain syndrome
RR	respiratory rate
RRT	renal replacement therapy
RSD	reflex sympathetic dystrophy
RSI	rapid sequence induction
RSI	repetitive strain injury
RTA	road traffic accident
RTC	road traffic collision
RV	residual volume
SAB	subarachnoid block
SABS	safety alert broadcast system
SACE	serum angiotensin-converting enzyme
SAD	supraglottic airway device
SAD(S)	seasonal affected disorder
SADS	sudden arrhythmic death syndrome
SAGM	saline-adenine glucose mannitol
SARS	severe acute respiratory syndrome
SAS	sedation assessment scale
SAT	syringe aspiration technique
SB	stillbirth
SBP	systolic blood pressure
SC	subcutaneous
SCBU	Special Care Baby Unit
SCN	suprachiasmatic nuclei
SCNT	somatic cell nuclear transfer
SCP	surgical care practitioner
SCS	spinal cord stimulator
SEDc	spondyloepiphyseal dysplasia congenital
SGOT	serum glutamic-oxaloacetic transaminase
SH	standard heparin
SHA	strategic health authority

SHOT	serious hazard of transmission
SI	système international d'units
SIADH	syndrome of inappropriate antidiuretic hormone secretion
SIB	self-inflating bulb
SICAT	siliconised catgut
SIDS	sudden infant death syndrome
SIMV	synchronised intermittent mandatory ventilation
SIRS	systematic inflammatory response syndrome
SLE	systemic lupus erythematosus
SLT	single lumen tube
SMR	submucous resection
SNPs	single nucleotide polymorphisms
SNS	sympathetic nervous system
SOD	superoxide dismutase
SOFA	sepsis-related organ failure assessment
SOP	standards of proficiency
SPD	serious personality disorder
SPF	skin protection factor
SPN	safer practice notice
SPOT	specialist practitioner of transfusion
SSI	sliding scale insulin
SSI	surgical site infection
SSRIs	selective serotonin re-uptake inhibitors
STD	sexually transmitted disease
STI	sexually transmitted infection
STM	symptom thermal method
SUI	stress urinary incontinence
SVP	saturated vapour pressure
SVR	systemic vascular resistance
SVT	supraventricular tachycardia
SWG	Standard Wire Gauge
T&As	tonsils & adenoids
TAH	total abdominal hysterectomy
TALS	Trauma Advanced Life Support
TB	tuberculosis
TBW	total body water
TCD	transcranial doppler
TCI	target controlled infusion
TCRE	transcervical resection of endometrium
TD	tetanus, diphtheria
TdP	Torsade de Pointes
TDT	Trieger Dot Test

TED	thromboembolism deterrent
TEF	theatre education facilitator
TENS	transcutaneous electrical nerve stimulation
TGI	tracheal gas insufflation
THA	total hip arthroplasty
THC	tetrahydrocannabinol
THR	total hip replacement
TIA	transient ischaemic attack
TIG	tetanus immunoglobulin
TIVA	total intravenous anaesthesia
TKP	total knee prosthesis
TKR	total knee replacement
TKVO	to keep vein open
TL	tubal ligation
TLC	trigger, limit, cycling
TMI	trans-mandibular implant
TMJ	temporomandibular joint
TMR	trans-myocardial revascularisation
TMS	transcranial magnetic stimulation
TMST	treadmill stress test
TNF	tumour necrosis factor
TNS	transcutaneous nerve stimulation
TNT	trinitrotoluene
ToF	train of four
TOE	trans-oesophageal echocardiogram
TOP	termination of pregnancy
TPA	tissue plasminogen activator.
TPN	total parenteral nutrition
TPR	temperature, pulse, respiration
TPR	thermo plastic rubber
TPR	total peripheral resistance
TQM	total quality management
T&S	type & screen
TSS	toxic shock syndrome
TSSU	Theatre Sterile Services Unit
TTJV	trans-tracheal jet ventilation
TTTS	twin-to-twin transfusion syndrome
TURBN	transurethral resection of bladder neck
TURP	transurethral resection of prostate (retrograde prostatectomy)
TURT	transurethral resection of tumour
TV	tidal volume

TVH	total vaginal hysterectomy
UA	urinalysis
UAL	ultrasonic-assisted lipoplasty
UARS	upper airway resistance syndrome
U&Es	urea and electrolytes
UHF	ultra high frequency
UHMW	ultra high molecular weight
UID	urinary incontinence device
URTI	upper respiratory tract infection
USS	ultrasound scan
UTI	urinary tract infection
UV	ultraviolet
VAD	ventricular assist device
VAE	venous air embolism
VAP	ventilation-associated pneumonia
Var	varicella (chicken pox)
VAS	visual analogue scale
VATS	video-assisted thoracic surgery
VC	vital capacity
VCD	volatile clotting time
VCH	vertebral canal haematoma
vCJD	variant Creutzfeldt–Jakob disease
VCUG	voiding cystourethrogram
VDA	vascular disrupting agents
VEGF	vascular endothelial growth factor
VF	ventricular fibrillation
VHF	very high frequency
VHP	vapour phase hydrogen peroxide
VI	virgo intacto
VIC	vaporiser inside circle
VIE	vacuum insulated evaporator
VILI	ventilator-induced lung injury
VLDL	very low density lipoprotein
VLE	virtual learning environment
VOC	volatile organic compound
VOC	vaporiser outside circle
VOC	vas-occlusive contraception
VP	vacuum pressure
VPAP	variable positive airway pressure
VRE	vancomycin-resistant *Enterococcus faecum*
VS	vegetative state
VSR	ventricular septal rupture

VSU	volatile substance abuse
VT	ventricular tachycardia
VTBI	volume to be infused
VTE	venous thromboembolism
VTOP	vacuum termination of pregnancy
VUR	vesicoureteral reflux
VVs	varicose veins
Vx	vertex
VZV	Varicella zoster virus
WAGs	waste anaesthetic gases
WBC	white blood cell
WPW	Wolff–Parkinson–White (syndrome)
Wt	weight
XDR-TB	extensive drug-resistant TB
YOB	year of birth

Medical terminology

a, an	without
ab	away from
acou(s)	hear
ad	towards
adeno	gland
adip	fat
aemia	blood
aesthesia	sensation
algia	pain
andro	man
angio	blood vessel
ankylo	crooked, curved
ante	before, in front
anti	against
arthro	joint
asis	state of
audio	hearing, sound
auto	self
bi, bis	two
bil	bile
bio	life
blepharo	eyelid
brach(i)o	arm
brachy	short
brady	slow
broncho	windpipe
bucco	cheek
calci	calcium
carcin	cancer
cardio	heart
carp	wrist
centi	a hundredth
cephal(o)	head
cerebro	brain
cervico	neck
chemo	chemical

chol	bile
choledocho	common bile duct
chondro	cartilage
cir(c)	around, about
co, col, com, con	together, with
colp	vagina
contra	against, counter
corpor	body
cost(o)	rib
costal	relating to the rib
crani(o)	skull
cryo	cold
cut(o)	skin
Cx	cervix
cyst(o)	bladder
cyt	cell
dacry	tear
dactyl	finger
de	removal or loss
deca	ten
deci	tenth
demi	half
dent	tooth
derm	skin
dextra	to the right
di, diplo	two, double
dia	through
dis	apart, away from
dors	back
dys	difficult, abnormal
ect	outside
ectomy	cutting out
em, en, end, ent	in, inside, within
embolo	plug
endo	within, into
entero	intestine
epi	upon, over
eu	good, normal
ex, exo	out of
extra	outside
ferro	iron
gastr(o)	stomach

gen	originate
genitor	genitals
genu	to bend, as at the knee
gingivo	gums
glosso	tongue
glycol	sugar
gram/graph	write/record
gravida	pregnancy
gyn(ae)	woman
haem	blood
hecta	one hundred
hemi	half
hepat	liver
hetero	unlike, dissimilar
hidro	sweat
hist	tissue
homeo	like
hydro	water
hygro	moisture
hyper	above
hypn(o)	sleep
hypo	below
hystero	uterus
idio	peculiar to, own
immuno	immunity, immune
infra	below
inter	between
intra	within
intro	inwards
isch	denotes suppression or deficiency
ischi	denotes the ischium
iso	equal
itis	inflammation
kilo	one thousand
lacto	milk
laevo	left
laparo	loins, abdomen
laryng(o)	larynx
later(o)	side
lept(o)	thin, slight, slender
leuc, leuk	white
lipo	fat

litho	stone
lordo	bent forward
lys(is)	dissolve
macro	large
mal	poor, abnormal
malac	soft
mammo	breast
mano	pressure
mast	breast
medi	middle
mega	big, enlarged
men/o	period
meso	middle
metron	measure
micr	small
micro	one-millionth
milli	one-thousandth
mono	single
morpho	form
mort	death
multi	many
myco	fungus
myelo	marrow
myo	muscle
narco	sleep, stupor
naso	nose
nato/natal	birth
neo	new
nephro	kidney
neuro	nerve
nil per os	nil by mouth
nocto	night
nulli	none
oct	eight
odont	tooth
odyno	pain
oesophago	oesophagus
oligo	difficult
oma	tumour
onco	tumour, cancer
oophoro	ovary
ophthalmo	eye

opia	vision
opsy	looking
orchid	testis
ortho	straight
os, oste	bone
osis	condition
ostomy	opening
otomy	cutting
paed	child
pan	all, entire
para	next to, adjacent
partum	given birth
patho	disease
penia	deficiency
penta	five
per	through
peri	around
pexy	fixing
phago	eat, destroy
phako (phaco)	lens of the eye
phlebo	vein
phobo	fear
phon	sound or voice
phoria	deviation
phyto	plants
pilo	hair
pimelo	fat
plega	paralysis
pneumo	lung
polio	grey
poly	many
post	after
pre	before, in front of
presbyo	old age
primi	first
proct(o)	anus
proto	first
proximo	near
pseudo	false
psycho	mind
pyo	pus, matter
pyr	heat, fever, fire

quadric	four
quinqu	five
re	again
retro	backwards
rhino	nose
rrhaphy	repair
sacro	sacrum
salping(o)	Fallopian tube
sclero	hard
scopy	looking
semi	half
serv	keep, maintain
servo	feedback
somato	body
son	sound
spiro	breath
spondylo	vertebrae
staphylo	cluster
steno	narrow
steth	chest
stom	mouth, opening
stoma	mouth
strepto	chain
sub	below
super	above
supra	above
syn	union/together
tachy	quick
tact	touching
terato	denotes a congenital abnormality
thermo	heat
thoraco	chest/thorax
thromb(o)	clot
tome	cutting instrument
toxico	poison
trans	through, across
tri	three
ultra	beyond
uni	one
uri	uric acid
vas, vaso	blood vessel
veno	vein

ventro	front
vesic(o)	vesicle
XX	female sex chromosome
XY	male sex chromosome
zym	enzyme, fermentation

A

Abdomen   **Quick Reference:** The area of the body between the chest and the pelvis.

Advanced Reference: The abdomen is separated from the chest by the diaphragm. The contents of the abdomen include stomach, small intestine, colon, rectum, liver spleen, pancreas, appendix, gall bladder.

Abdominal aortic aneurysm   **Quick Reference:** (an-your-ism) A ballooning or dilatation of the aorta within the abdominal cavity.

Advanced Reference: The aneurysm weakens the wall of the vessel and can result in rupture with potentially fatal consequences. As the diameter increases, the chances of rupture also increase. Men, usually over 60 years of age, are five times more likely than women to suffer this type of aneurysm. Also referred to as *triple-A*.

Abdominal hysterectomy   **Quick Reference:** Surgical removal of the uterus through a lower abdominal incision.

Advanced Reference: The procedure involves a number of approaches depending on the severity and/or spread, i.e. total, sub-total, pan and radical (*Wertheim's procedure*).

Abdominoperineal   **Quick Reference:** Pertaining to the *abdomen* and *perineum* regions of anatomy.

Advanced Reference: Includes the pelvic area, the female *vulva* and anus and the male anus and *scrotum*. The procedure synchronous combined abdominoperineal resection of the rectum involves excision of the lower colon, *rectum* and anus and is usually carried out by two surgeons working simultaneously.

Abduction   **Quick Reference:** The opposite *of adduction*. Away from the mid-line.

Advanced Reference: The movement of a limb away from the midline. Abduction of the legs is therefore to spread them outwards.

Aberrant   **Quick Reference:** A deviation or wandering from the normal or usual route.

Advanced Reference: Can be applied to the heart when the electrical system does not follow the expected conduction pathway.

Ablation   **Quick Reference:** Indicates removal or destruction.

Advanced Reference: Applies to body tissue, removal or destruction, usually by surgical means, the most common being ablation of the lining (endometrium) of the uterus which involves the application of heat (thermal balloon), electricity (roller-ball), *cautery*, *laser*, freezing, or radiofrequency. Similar methods are utilised for treatment of the *prostate*.

Abnormal lie   **Quick Reference:** Refers to when a baby is not in the normal head-down position in the uterus.

Advanced Reference: This may involve feet-first or *breech* position. Normal position is facing rearward towards the mother's back with the face and body turned to one side and is termed *cephalic* or vertex delivery.

Abortifacient   **Quick Reference:** Indicates causing abortion.

Advanced Reference: An agent, drug, or chemical that causes abortion. Also termed abortient.

Abortion   **Quick Reference:** The loss of a pregnancy. Removal of the fetus from the uterus.

Advanced Reference: The premature exit of products of conception (fetus, fetal membranes, placenta) from the uterus. Methods include: vacuum/suction, chemical, pharmaceutical and surgical (*hysterotomy*). A spontaneous abortion is commonly termed a *miscarriage*.

Abrasion   **Quick Reference:** The wearing away of an area.

Advanced Reference: Most commonly affects the skin, due to an abnormal mechanical process such as contact with a rough surface.

Abruption   **Quick Reference:** A sudden breaking off or tearing apart.

Advanced Reference: Placental abruption indicates the separation of the placenta from the normal positioning in the uterus leading to severe haemorrhage.

Abscess   **Quick Reference:** (ab-ses) A collection of *pus* as the result of (localised) infection.

Advanced Reference: An abscess forms as the result of infection. The area of infection becomes isolated from the healthy tissue and in time the dead white blood cells, bacteria and body fluids form pus.

Absolute zero   **Quick Reference:** (symbol – 0 K). Temperature at which nothing could be colder. A component of the Kelvin temperature scale.

Advanced Reference: At absolute zero no heat energy remains in a substance. It is the point at which molecules do not move (zero point energy).

ACE inhibitor   **Quick Reference:** Antihypertensive medication.

Advanced Reference: ACE inhibitors inhibit angiotensin-converting enzyme, which is important in the regulation of blood pressure.

Acetabulum   **Quick Reference:** A cup-shaped cavity on the outer side of the hip (innominate) bone.

Advanced Reference: Indicates the socket of the hip joint in which the head of femur moves (articulates).

Acetylcholine   **Quick Reference:** A neurotransmitter.

Advanced Reference: Involved in the transmission of nerve impulses between nerve endings and the muscles and within the parasympathetic nervous system. It is broken down normally by cholinesterase. Muscle relaxant drugs act by competing with acetylcholine at the neuromuscular junction.

Achalasia **Quick Reference:** (ak-al-aysea) Failure of a ring of muscle (*sphincter*) to relax.

Advanced Reference: Can affect the sphincter of the anus and oesophagus. Often treated through forced stretching (dilatation).

Achilles tendon **Quick Reference:** Tendon which runs from the calf muscle to the heel.

Advanced Reference: The achilles is responsible for drawing the foot downwards, hinging at the ankle joint. It is a weak point in certain activities and can rupture during activity and consequently requires surgical repair.

Achondroplasia **Quick Reference:** (ak-ondro-play-zea) Failure of the arms and legs to grow to normal size.

Advanced Reference: An inherited disorder that is mainly due to a defect in both bone and cartilage.

Acid–Base balance **Quick Reference:** Indicates a balance in the production and secretion of acids and bases.

Advanced Reference: A balance provides a stable concentration of hydrogen ions in the body.

Acidosis **Quick Reference:** Alteration of the acid–alkali balance towards acidity. Caused by an accumulation of acid or hydrogen ions or loss of bicarbonate.

Advanced Reference: In health, the slight alkalinity is held constant by the balance of dissolved carbon dioxide (acid) and sodium bicarbonate (alkali). Acidosis can be of either metabolic or respiratory nature. Also referred to as acidaemia. Someone who is suffering acidosis is said to be acidotic.

Acoustic shock **Quick Reference:** Temporary or permanent disturbance of the functioning ear or its related nervous system.

Advanced Reference: May be caused when a telephone user experiences sudden sharp rises in acoustic pressure, which can be a whistle, high-pitched bleep or unexpected noise. The condition is different from noise-induced hearing loss.

Acquired immunity **Quick Reference:** Form of immunity that is not innate (natural), i.e. has to be acquired.

Advanced Reference: Immunity may be acquired by infection, vaccination (active) or by transfer of antibodies from an immune person (passive).

Acromegaly **Quick Reference:** State produced by oversecretion of the *pituitary* growth hormone, commonly as the result of a tumour of the gland.

Advanced Reference: When it occurs in early life before the bones have stopped growing, the result is increased height or gigantism. After the bones have ceased to grow the patient develops a prominent forehead and cheekbones, a large jaw, hands and feet, a bent back combined with a hollow deep voice. Treatment is directed towards restoring hormone levels to normal.

Acrylic **Quick Reference:** (ac-rilic) Synthetic fibre, thermoplastic resin. Chemical compounds derived from acrylic acid.

Advanced Reference: An ethylene derivative combined with a vinyl. Used in the manufacture of dental prostheses and intraocular lenses. As they are resistant to weakened acids, alkalis and bleaches, they are useful in the production of containers, etc.

ACTH **Quick Reference:** Abbreviation for adrenocorticotrophic hormone.

Advanced Reference: A secretion of the pituitary gland which has the function of stimulating the cortex of the adrenal gland to secrete cortisol.

Action potential **Quick Reference:** Wave of electrical discharge that travels along the membrane of a cell. Created by a depolarising current.

Advanced Reference: Occurs when a neurone (nerve cell) sends information down an axon (nerve fibre) away from the cell body, carrying information within and between tissues.

Actrapid™ **Quick Reference:** Proprietary fast-acting preparation of insulin.

Advanced Reference: Used in the treatment of diabetes mellitus.

Acute **Quick Reference:** The opposite to *chronic*.

Advanced Reference: Any process which has a sudden onset and runs a relatively short course.

Acute abdomen **Quick Reference:** The sudden severe onset of abdominal pain.

Advanced Reference: Refers to a potential medical emergency, indicating a problem with one of the major abdominal organs, e.g. ruptured *appendix*, inflamed *gall bladder*, ruptured *spleen*.

Acute normovolaemic haemodilution **Quick Reference:** (ANH) Transfusion procedure/technique involving volume increase of *autologous* withdrawn blood.

Advanced Reference: The previously withdrawn blood is diluted and so increases the volume available for transfusion when required.

Adam's apple **Quick Reference:** Prominence at the front of the neck which is the underlying V-shape of the thyroid cartilage.

Advanced Reference: Positioned anteriorly to the larynx and visible as a protrusion externally. More prominent in men than women due to anatomical positioning.

Adduction **Quick Reference:** The opposite of *abduction*. To adduct is to move a limb, for example, towards the midline of the body.

Advanced Reference: The movement of a limb into (toward) the midline of the body. Adduction would thus bring the legs together.

Adenoids **Quick Reference:** Lymphatic glandular tissue present at the back of the nose.

Advanced Reference: May become enlarged as the result of *chronic* infection and obstruct the free passage of air, leading to mouth breathing and snoring.

In severe cases can lead to infection of the ***middle-ear*** or sinusitis and hearing loss. Infection and enlargement are associated with chronic tonsillitis.

Adenomyosis   **Quick Reference:** (aden-o-mio-sis) Uterine thickening.

Advanced Reference: Occurs when endometrial tissue, which normally lines the uterus, extends into the fibrous and muscular tissue of the uterus.

Adenosine   **Quick Reference:** Endogenous nucleoside. Drug used to treat supraventricular tachycardia (SVT).

Advanced Reference: Has a very short duration of action (half-life of 8–10 seconds). Also used as an aid to diagnosis by helping to identify the nature of other rapid rhythms.

ADH   **Quick Reference:** Antidiuretic hormone. Also known as vasopressin.

Advanced Reference: Released by the pituitary gland and promotes water reabsorption in the kidney tubules. Those suffering diabetes insipidus lack ADH. Is now used in the form of vasopressin as an alternative to adrenaline (epinephrine) during cardiopulmonary resuscitation (CPR).

Adhesion   **Quick Reference:** The joining or sticking together of two surfaces that are normally separate.

Advanced Reference: Adhesions can occur as a result of inflammation, which causes fibrous tissue to form. Peritonitis can cause adhesions, which may then lead to intestinal obstruction. Also often due to previous surgery.

Adipometer   **Quick Reference:** Instrument for measuring the thickness of skin folds.

Advanced Reference: Used in the assessment of weight gain and loss.

Adipose (tissue)   **Quick Reference:** The fatty tissue of the body.

Advanced Reference: Serves as an energy source and insulating layer. Adiposis (also termed liposis) is an abnormal accumulation of fatty tissue in the body. The protective layer of fat surrounding the kidney is referred to as the adipose capsule.

Adrenaline   **Quick Reference:** A hormone secreted by the medulla of the adrenal gland.

Advanced Reference: Also known by its pharmaceutical name, epinephrine. It has the actions of stimulating the heart, raising blood pressure, releasing glucose and increasing its metabolism, increasing muscular blood circulation, and relaxing air passages; hence its usefulness in shock and resuscitation settings.

Adrenergic   **Quick Reference:** Relates to nerve fibres that release ***noradrenaline***.

Advanced Reference: Noradrenaline is a chemical transmitter that stimulates muscles and glands, etc.

Adult-onset diabetes   **Quick Reference:** Also referred to as type 2 diabetes.

Advanced Reference: Usually manifests in middle and older age in conjunction with high blood glucose levels, high blood pressure, being overweight and lack of fitness, all leading to potential damage to the circulatory system.

Advocate   **Quick Reference:** One who acts on the behalf of another.

Advanced Reference: Anyone who acts in support of the patient, especially if they are unable to do so themselves because of age, understanding, status of consciousness, etc.

Adventitia   **Quick Reference:** (ad-ven-tisha) The outermost membranous covering of many anatomical structures.

Advanced Reference: Example, the outer coat of an artery.

Aeration   **Quick Reference:** The exchange of carbon dioxide for oxygen by the blood in the lungs.

Advanced Reference: The charging of a liquid with air or gas.

Aerobic   **Quick Reference:** Indicates the requirement of oxygen for life and growth.

Advanced Reference: An aerobe is any organism that requires oxygen in order to sustain life. The prefix aer(o) denotes air or gas.

Aerosol   **Quick Reference:** A fine mist or fog comprised of solid or liquid particles in a gas.

Advanced Reference: Commonly refers to a pressurised container containing a propellant and a spray mechanism for dispersing a fine mist of fluid droplets.

Afferent   **Quick Reference:** Towards the centre.

Advanced Reference: Afferent vessels and structures run throughout the body, i.e. the small arterioles entering the glomerulus of the kidney, the sensory nerve fibres that convey impulses from the periphery to the brain, and lymphatic vessels that lead from the tissues to a *lymph* gland.

Agar   **Quick Reference:** Culture medium.

Advanced Reference: Composed of seaweed with broth or blood added as a nutrient. It resists the action of bacteria and therefore is used as a medium on which cultures can be grown. Not all micro-organisms will grow in such a way outside of the body, viruses for example require living tissue to survive.

Agglutination   **Quick Reference:** The coming together of small particles in a solution to form clumps.

Advanced Reference: In blood, it is brought about by the action of antibodies on antigens carried by the red blood cells or bacteria and is therefore utilised to identify blood groups during cross-matching (X-matching). An agglutinin is an antibody that aggregates a particular antigen while an agglutinogen is any substance, when acting as an antigen, that stimulates production of an agglutinin.

Aggregate   **Quick Reference:** To gather together.

Advanced Reference: Indicates the total of a group of substances or components making up a mass or complex.

Agonal **Quick Reference:** Pertaining to death and dying.

Advanced Reference: An agonal ECG reading/trace indicates a rhythm displaying a dying heart.

Agonist **Quick Reference:** A contestant. Produces an action. Opposite of antagonist, which acts against and blocks an action.

Advanced Reference: An agonist muscle (prime mover) is one that is opposed/counteracted in action by another (antagonist). A drug that can combine with a receptor on a cell to produce a physiologic reaction.

Airway **Quick Reference:** Generic term for a wide range of oropharyngeal or nasopharyngeal adjuncts designed to maintain a clear airway.

Advanced Reference: *Guedel* is the most recognisable oral version, but there are numerous variations in design that include inflatable balloon cuffs at the distal tip, side-arms for supplemental oxygen, while the not-so-popular nasal version is available in a variety of sizes and materials. The *LMA* has undoubtedly reduced the use of oral and nasal airway usage in recent years.

Airway classification **Quick Reference:** Classification used to assess potential for airway ventilation and intubation and visualisation of the related structures.

Advanced Reference: There are a number of related classifications (i.e. ASA difficult airway algorithm, Mallampati's, Cormack and Lehane's) which all deal with the intubation and ventilation potential taking into consideration tongue size to pharyngeal size, landmark visualisation, anatomical obstructions, etc. Usually assessed with the patient sitting and with their head in the neutral position. The thyromental distance system bases intubation potential on the measurement from the *thyroid* notch to the tip of the jaw, while the sternomental distance uses a measurement from the *sternum* to the tip of the *mandible* (both with head extended). A measurement varying outside of an agreed norm is said to be an indication of *difficult intubation*.

Alberti **Quick Reference:** A protocol utilised in the treatment of *diabetes*.

Advanced Reference: The regime involves 10 units of insulin and 10 mmol of potassium chloride added to 500 ml of 10% dextrose and infused over 4 h. Said to be a fail-safe system that ensures that variations in infusion rate do not produce an imbalance of glucose and *insulin*, which could lead to *hypokalaemia*.

Albumin **Quick Reference:** A plasma protein.

Advanced Reference: Available as an intravenous preparation (plasma expander), *Human albumin solution (HAS)*.

Albuminuria **Quick Reference:** The presence of serum albumin, *globulin* and other proteins in the urine.

Advanced Reference: May be due to kidney disease, *nephritis* and inflammation of the lower urinary tract as well as heart disease, fevers, severe *anaemia* and the administration of certain drugs and poisons or even following strenuous exercise.

Alcohol   Quick Reference: Large class of organic compounds. Used mainly in the healthcare setting as cleaning, antiseptic and disinfecting agents.

Advanced Reference: Those relevant to medicine are methyl (wood alcohol – *methanol*) and ethyl alcohol (ethanol). Ethyl alcohol when free of water and impurities is called absolute alcohol (chemical formula C_2H_5OH).

Aldasorber™   Quick Reference: Passive scavenging system.

Advanced Reference: Prior to the standardisation of active scavenging systems in theatres, the Aldasorber passive system was used. It is comprised of a scavenging valve connected by tubing to a free-standing container of activated charcoal which absorbs halothane from expired gases. Disposal and exhaustion involved weighing the container and comparing this with the fresh weight stated on the packaging.

Aldehyde   Quick Reference: Colourless volatile fluid with a suffocating smell.

Advanced Reference: Obtained by oxidation of alcohol, during which the flammable liquid acetaldehyde is produced. Available in theatres as formaldehyde and as a sterilising agent, *glutaraldehyde*.

Aldosterone   Quick Reference: Hormone released by the renal cortex.

Advanced Reference: Responsible for the regulation of sodium levels, which it does by reabsorption in the kidney. In order to maintain an electrolyte balance, the hormone also plays a part in potassium excretion.

Alfentanil   Quick Reference: Narcotic analgesic, Rapifen™.

Advanced Reference: Suitable for use with short surgical procedures and outpatient/day-case surgery. Also used as an infusion during prolonged procedures.

Algorithm   Quick Reference: A set of rules, instructions or guidelines.

Advanced Reference: Allows for a solution or problem to be solved or achieved by breaking it down into simpler stages, without fully understanding the entire process. An example being cardiopulmonary resuscitation (CPR), an especially advanced technique which utilises a step-by-step approach.

Alimentary   Quick Reference: Refers to the alimentary canal or digestive tract.

Advanced Reference: Is composed of the mouth, pharynx, oesophagus, stomach and intestine.

Alkali   Quick Reference: Substance which neutralises acid to produce a salt.

Advanced Reference: Most common alkalis are oxides, hydroxides or carbonates and bicarbonates. Examples are sodium bicarbonate, calcium carbonate, magnesium carbonate, magnesium trisilicate and aluminium hydroxide. Alkalis turn litmus blue. *Alkalosis* is an increase in body alkali reserve, i.e. a rise in pH.

Alkalosis   Quick Reference: Condition in which the body's pH increases.

Advanced Reference: An acid–base imbalance in which there is a decrease in the hydrogen ion concentration and an increase/rise in the pH. Common causes are carbonic acid deficit or an excessive level of bicarbonate.

Allergy **Quick Reference:** Hypersensitivity to various substances (allergens), e.g. drugs, foods, insect bites.

Advanced Reference: It is due to an antigen–antibody reaction. Hay fever and asthma are examples of an allergic reaction. An allergen is a substance that causes the allergic reaction, and can be ingested, inhaled, injected or simply have skin contact.

Alloferin™ **Quick Reference:** Proprietary non-depolarising muscle relaxant.

Advanced Reference: Synthetic non-depolariser with a duration of 20–30 mins. Is a preparation of alcuronium chloride.

Allogeneic **Quick Reference:** Refers to transplanted tissue.

Advanced Reference: Allograft indicated tissue transplanted from one person to another.

Allograft **Quick Reference:** Type of graft or transplant.

Advanced Reference: Indicates between different species.

Alloimmunity **Quick Reference:** An immune response.

Advanced Reference: A condition in which the body gains **immunity** from another individual of the same species against its own cells. As occurs after: blood or plasma transfusion, *allograft*, and in the *fetus* after maternal *antibodies* have passed through the *placenta* into the fetus.

Alloy **Quick Reference:** Combination of metals.

Advanced Reference: A mixture of two or more metals or substances with metallic properties. Those with a medical application include amalgam (mercury and silver) used in tooth fillings, and many others used in the manufacture of implants.

Alpha-linolenic acid **Quick Reference:** A *fatty acid* found in fish and seeds. (Chemical formula – $C_{18}H_{30}O_2$.)

Advanced Reference: Used by the body in the formation of *prostaglandins*.

Alzheimer's disease **Quick Reference:** Degenerative brain disease.

Advanced Reference: Mainly affects those in middle and old age leading to *dementia*, resulting in progressive memory loss, impaired thinking and disorientation as well as character changes. Cause is unknown but there is found to be a deterioration in brain *neurones* and evidence of *amyloid plaque* deposits.

Amalgam **Quick Reference:** A group of *alloys* containing *mercury*.

Advanced Reference: Used in dentistry for tooth fillings. Made by mixing a silver–tin alloy with mercury.

Ambient **Quick Reference:** Surrounding, encompassing.

Advanced Reference: Relates to ambient temperature, ambient air pressure, the surrounding temperature and air pressure.

Ambu Bag® **Quick Reference:** Trade name of an airway device used primarily during CPR. A self-inflating bag.

Advanced Reference: Used as a general term to indicate an airway management device with a one-way valve, used mainly during CPR. The design is now more readily termed bag-valve-mask (BVM).

Ambulatory **Quick Reference:** Walking, able to walk.

Advanced Reference: Day-case surgical units are also referred to as ambulatory units. Indicates where patients do not require an overnight stay in hospital.

Amenorrhoea **Quick Reference:** Absence of menstruation.

Advanced Reference: Also referred to as menostasis.

Amides **Quick Reference:** Organic compound derived from *ammonia*.

Advanced Reference: Are formed when *amino acids* react to form *proteins*.

Amine **Quick Reference:** Organic compound containing *nitrogen*.

Advanced Reference: Formed by *ammonia* replacing *hydrogen* atoms.

Amino acids **Quick Reference:** Organic compound found in *proteins*.

Advanced Reference: There are 20 different amino acids which can formulate into numerous arrangements making a polypeptide chain, and are termed the building blocks.

Aminophylline **Quick Reference:** Bronchodilator.

Advanced Reference: Used to treat moderate forms of asthma and pulmonary oedema.

Amiodarone **Quick Reference:** Antiarrhythmic drug.

Advanced Reference: Used to treat *supraventricular* tachycardia (SVT). Now available as an alternative to *lignocaine*.

Ammonia **Quick Reference:** A gas with the chemical formula NH_3.

Advanced Reference: Is irritant to the lungs leading to *oedema* and bronchitis and can cause burns.

Amnesia **Quick Reference:** Loss of memory.

Advanced Reference: Caused usually by injury or emotional trauma. There is a specific form of memory loss that affects some individuals who have been artificially ventilated and sedated for a lengthy period.

Amniocentesis **Quick Reference:** Withdrawal of amniotic fluid from a pregnant uterus for diagnostic purposes.

Advanced Reference: Percutaneous transabdominal puncture of the uterus with a hollow needle in order to withdraw amniotic fluid from the sac surrounding the fetus.

Amniotic **Quick Reference:** Refers to amniotic fluid present in the pregnant uterus.

Advanced Reference: The amnion is a membranous bag containing the amniotic fluid, which is a watery liquid in which the baby floats until birth.

Amoxil™ **Quick Reference:** Proprietary antibiotic preparation.

Advanced Reference: Used in the treatment of systemic bacterial infections and those of the upper respiratory tract, ear, nose and throat, as well as the urogenital system. It is a preparation of the broad-spectrum penicillin, amoxicillin.

Amp **Quick Reference:** Ampere.

Advanced Reference: Unit used for the measurement of electrical current.

Amphetamine **Quick Reference:** (am-fet-amean) Agent that has a stimulant effect on both the central and peripheral nervous systems. (Chemical formula = $C_6H_5CH_2CH(NH_2)CH_3$).

Advanced Reference: Used in the treatment of **narcolepsy**, attention deficit hyperactivity disorder and at one time as an **anorexiant** in the treatment of obesity. Also a drug of abuse recognised with various names/terms, i.e. methamphetamine, P (pure), crystal-meth.

Ampicillin **Quick Reference:** Broad-spectrum **antibiotic**.

Advanced Reference: Similar in action to **tetracyclines**. Used in the treatment of urogenital tract, upper respiratory and ear infections. Many bacteria have now developed a resistance to this drug.

Amplitude **Quick Reference:** Width, breadth, range.

Advanced Reference: Maximum extent of vibration or oscillation from a position of equilibrium. The amplitude in relation to an ECG trace implies the height and strength of the signal.

Ampoule **Quick Reference:** Small glass or plastic container for drugs. Also called a vial.

Advanced Reference: Designed to contain a single dose of a drug or solution, as opposed to a multi-dose vial.

Amygdala **Quick Reference:** (am-ig-dela) The brain's emotion centre.

Advanced Reference: Anatomical term used to designate an almond-shaped structure. An almond-shaped mass of **grey matter** inside each **cerebral hemisphere**.

Amylase **Quick Reference:** An enzyme that breaks down starch and glycogen.

Advanced Reference: Present in the pancreatic juices and saliva, amylase acts as a catalyst in the hydrolysis of starch to sugar.

Amyl nitrite **Quick Reference:** A volatile flammable liquid with a pungent odour.

Advanced Reference: It is administered by inhalation in the treatment of cyanide poisoning where it produces **methaemoglobin** when it binds with the **cyanide**. Also used in cardiac diagnostic tests. Used as a drug of abuse to produce euphoria and sexual stimulation.

Anaemia **Quick Reference:** Condition in which there is an insufficient level of oxygen-carrying capacity in the blood.

Advanced Reference: There are various forms, e.g. iron-deficiency anaemia, haemolytic anaemia, pernicious anaemia, thalassaemia, sickle-cell anaemia.

Anaerobic   **Quick Reference:** Living/surviving without oxygen.

Advanced Reference: An aerobic micro-organism is one that can survive in the absence of oxygen, e.g. those that cause tetanus and gas gangrene or are found in wounds and body cavities which are either free of or low in oxygen, i.e. the bowel.

Anaesthesia   **Quick Reference:** Literally translates to 'without feeling'.

Advanced Reference: Term which is used to indicate both general and local anaesthesia and also used interchangeably with analgesia (without pain). Anaesthesia is commonly understood to indicate being put to sleep in order to undergo surgery.

Analgesia   **Quick Reference:** Indicates without pain.

Advanced Reference: Often used interchangeably with anaesthesia. Analgesia can be induced using drugs (analgesics), cold and electrical stimulation.

Anaphylaxis   **Quick Reference:** (anna-fil-axis) A category of shock caused by exposure to a foreign protein (allergen).

Advanced Reference: An acute systemic allergic reaction which occurs when a person has become sensitised to a substance or allergen and is again exposed to it. Symptoms include tachycardia, vasodilatation, hypotension, urticaria, sweating, bronchial swelling (oedema), dyspnoea. Anaphylactoid reactions, although similar, are not caused by an allergic reaction but instead by a non-immunological trigger. This can involve X-ray contrast media, certain IV fluids and even some morphine-based preparations.

Anastomosis   **Quick Reference:** The joining of two structures or ends.

Advanced Reference: In relation to surgery, anastomosis is the joining of two ends, usually following resection, i.e. between the two incised ends of the stomach following gastrectomy and likewise following bowel resection, and when joining blood vessel ends or one end to a vascular graft.

Anatomical snuff box   **Quick Reference:** Small hollow or depression on the lateral aspect of the wrist.

Advanced Reference: So-called as it is the place where snuff was traditionally placed prior to sniffing it into the nose. The area is formed by tendons reaching towards the thumb.

Androgen   **Quick Reference:** Hormone responsible for masculinisation.

Advanced Reference: Is in fact one of a group of steroid hormones that includes *testosterone* and androsterone that stimulate male sexual development, which involves the sex organs and male secondary sexual characteristics, i.e. deepening of the voice, beard growth, muscle development. The main source for these is the testis. Synthetic versions are used to treat a number of conditions including delayed puberty.

Aneroid   **Quick Reference:** Indicates the absence of fluid or not containing water.

Advanced Reference: Used to describe a device that is in contrast to one that utilises or contains fluid, e.g. an aneroid sphygmomanometer, which utilises mercury.

Aneurysm   **Quick Reference:** (an-your-ism) Localised dilatation of an artery, sometimes forming a sac.

Advanced Reference: May be congenital, due to inflammation, or caused by trauma. The pressure of blood causes the artery to distend as it weakens and becomes prone to rupture. Common sites are the abdominal aorta and carotid artery. There are a number of variations including dissecting aneurysm, in which a tear occurs in the lining and blood makes its way between the layers of the vessel, forcing them apart. Also, saccular aneurysm, which involves dilatation of only a part of the arterial circumference. Treatment for all usually involves surgery for repair, or grafting.

Angina pectoris   **Quick Reference:** Severe chest pain, felt behind the pectoral muscle.

Advanced Reference: Pectoris indicates the area of the chest around the pectoral muscles. The pain is due to narrowing or occlusion, usually by spasm, of the main arteries (coronary) supplying the heart. This leads to a lack of oxygen to the heart muscle itself, hence demand outstrips supply. It can be relieved by vasodilator drugs such as glyceryl trinitrate (nitroglycerine, GTN), which can be administered by injection, oral tablet or be absorbed from under the tongue (sublingual), as well as topically via a skin patch (dermally).

Angiogenesis   **Quick Reference:** The growth and formation of new blood vessels, revascularisation.

Advanced Reference: Used commonly in relation to the development of tumours. Also referred to as angiopoietic and vasculogenic.

Angiography   **Quick Reference:** X-ray of the cerebral vascular tree.

Advanced Reference: Involves imaging following the injection of a radio-opaque medium into a main neck artery. Often termed with arteriography, which is X-ray of an artery.

Angioplasty   **Quick Reference:** Actually indicates surgical reconstruction of a blood vessel but is most commonly referred to as a procedure to restore blood flow through an artery.

Advanced Reference: Balloon angioplasty involves dilatation of a constricted or blocked artery. The catheter is fed down the vessel and the distal balloon is inflated using gas or fluid to stretch/open the narrowing (usually due to *atherosclerosis*). In some procedures a stent is carried on the catheter and fixed in place to keep the vessel open following dilatation. There are a number of similar procedures, all carried out under X-ray control with the catheters being introduced via a cutaneous route and under local anaesthetic, i.e. percutaneous transluminal coronary angioplasty (PTCA), percutaneous coronary interventions (PCI), percutaneous transluminal renal angioplasty (PTRA), Percutaneous/peripheral transluminal angioplasty (PTA), the latter used for dilating more peripheral vessels such as femoral, iliac, popliteal arteries.

Angioscopy   **Quick Reference:** Use of an angioscope to visualise the lumen of blood vessels.

Advanced Reference: Also the visualisation of capillary blood vessels with a special (microscope) angioscope.

Angiospasm   **Quick Reference:** Spasm occurring in a blood vessel.

Advanced Reference: Mainly applies to arteries, with the spasm causing cramp in the muscles. Also a feature of Raynaud's disease, which effects the arteries supplying the fingers. Treatment can be with antispasmodic drugs or *sympathectomy* in unresponsive cases.

Anion   **Quick Reference:** A negatively charged ion.

Advanced Reference: An ion is an electrolysed solution that migrates to the anode. The anode is the positive pole; the cathode, the negative pole.

Ankylosing spondylitis   **Quick Reference:** (ankal-osing) Type of arthritis which causes deformity and stiffness in joints.

Advanced Reference: The resultant inflammation affects the joint capsule as well as the attached ligaments and tendons. If occurring in the area of the neck and spine, it can cause severe deformity (*kyphosis*) which may lead to airway management problems during anaesthesia.

Anode   **Quick Reference:** Positive node.

Advanced Reference: In an electrochemical cell, the electrode at which *oxidation* occurs, i.e. the positive electrode in an electrolytic cell or battery. The cathode is the negative node, i.e. the electrode at which reduction occurs.

Anodised   **Quick Reference:** Metal coated with a very thin layer of another metal.

Advanced Reference: Usually applied by *electrolysis*, common with surgical instruments to provide a non-glare finish.

Anorexia   **Quick Reference:** Dietary-related disease also known as slimmer's disease.

Advanced Reference: The correct term is anorexia nervosa. Symptoms include the sufferer refusing to eat or eating only under protest, often followed by them inducing vomiting to get rid of the food consumed. Leads to nutritional deficiency and hormonal imbalance. Occurs mainly in females between the ages of 14 and 17.

Anorexiant   **Quick Reference:** An appetite suppressant.

Advanced Reference: Also referred to as an anorectic. Amphetamines are foremost amongst this group and cause the release of noradrenaline.

Anosmia   **Quick Reference:** Impaired or complete loss of sense of smell.

Advanced Reference: Can be due to a simple cold, *hayfever*, medication as well as nasal *polyps* or even brain injury.

Antacid Quick Reference: Substance used to neutralise gastric acid.

Advanced Reference: In relation to the perioperative period, antacids are used for patients who are at risk of regurgitation, possibly due to hiatus hernia, and gastroesophageal reflux, they are given preoperatively. Sodium citrate is common for Caesarean section patients, while sodium bicarbonate, aluminium hydroxide and magnesium trisilicate are further examples of antacids.

Antagonist Quick Reference: An opposite or opposing action.

Advanced Reference: Examples would be the muscles, biceps and triceps: one relaxes as the other contracts. With reference to drugs, antagonist indicates one which blocks or reverses the action of another.

Antecubital fossa Quick Reference: Inside area of the elbow.

Advanced Reference: Area on the inside of the elbow where access for cannulation is regularly made via the *basilic* and *cephalic* veins. Ante = before, cubitus = forearm, fossa = depression or pit.

Anteflexion Quick Reference: Bending forward.

Advanced Reference: The uterus is a fine example of an organ that bends forward from its fixed point.

Antepartum Quick Reference: Before childbirth.

Advanced Reference: Actually indicates the three-month period prior to giving birth. An antepartum haemorrhage is bleeding from the uterus before delivery and is caused by the dislodged placenta lying below the baby/fetus.

Anterior Quick Reference: Indicates the front. Opposite of *posterior*.

Advanced Reference: Foremost, front surface of. *Ventral* is also used to indicate the front surface of the body.

Anteverted Quick Reference: Tilting forward.

Advanced Reference: Indicates the forward tilting of an organ, as with the uterus, which has a normal position of being tilted toward the front.

Anthropometry Quick Reference: Science which deals with measurements of the human body.

Advanced Reference: Includes weight, proportions and overall size.

Antiarrhythmic Quick Reference: (anti-a-rith-mik) Range of drugs used to regulate the heartbeat.

Advanced Reference: As there are a number of ways in which the heartbeat can become irregular, the range of drugs to treat this is broad. Irregularities include atrial and ventricular tachycardia, atrial flutter and fibrillation as well as the changes that may follow a heart attack. Common drugs in this category are digoxin, verapamil, lignocaine and amiodarone.

Antibacterials Quick Reference: Drugs and substances that destroy bacteria but may have less effect on other micro-organisms.

Advanced Reference: The major drug groups involved are antibiotics, although *sulphonamides* are sometimes categorised as such. They have specific uses or are administered in combination with antibiotics, especially when resistant strains or sensitivity is involved.

Antibiotic **Quick Reference:** A class of drugs used to treat infection (bacterial). Anti = against, biosis = life.

Advanced Reference: Collective name for a class of substances produced mainly from living organisms and are capable of destroying or hindering the growth of pathogenic organisms. The term is also used to cover similar synthetic compounds. Antibiosis is the action of one type of microbe opposing the growth of another (antagonism).

Antibody **Quick Reference:** Against (the body). Protein that is synthesised in response to a particular antigen.

Advanced Reference: Specific substances produced in the blood as a reaction to an *antigen* (foreign substance) and which circulate in the plasma ready to attack specific antigens.

Anticancer **Quick Reference:** Drugs and substances that act against cancer, i.e. mainly cytotoxics.

Advanced Reference: They work by interfering with cell replication and/or production and so prevent growth of new tissue. Inevitably, this means that normal cell production and proliferation are also affected and they are therefore prone to producing side-effects.

Anticholinergic **Quick Reference:** Drugs that inhibit the action, release or production of acetylcholine. They block the passage of impulses in the parasympathetic nervous system.

Advanced Reference: Acetylcholine plays an important role in the functioning of the nervous system, tending to relax smooth muscle. Anticholinergics inhibit the cholinergic enzyme from breaking down acetylcholine, so increasing its level and duration of action. Atropine is an example of an acetylcholine antagonist.

Anticholinesterases **Quick Reference:** (anti-coal-in-es-terase) Chemical that inhibits the cholinesterase enzyme from breaking down *acetylcholine*.

Advanced Reference: This action therefore increases both the level and duration of action of the neurotransmitter acetylcholine. They are used to increase neuromuscular transmission in such conditions as *myasthenia gravis*. Also referred to as acetylcholinesterase inhibitor.

Anticoagulant **Quick Reference:** Substance which prevents or reduces the formation of a clot in the blood.

Advanced Reference: The two most popular are the naturally occurring *heparin* and the synthetically produced *warfarin* (name taken from Wisconsin Alumni Research Foundation).

Antidote **Quick Reference:** Substance given to counteract or neutralise the effects of a poison, for example.

Advanced Reference: An example would be anti-venom (anti-serum) used to treat someone bitten/injected with snake venom.

Antiemetic **Quick Reference:** Drug administered to prevent nausea and vomiting.

Advanced Reference: These drugs work by either directly suppressing the vomiting centre in the brain or by stimulating stomach emptying.

Antigen **Quick Reference:** A substance treated as an alien or foreign substance within the body.

Advanced Reference: Any substance which invokes the action of an *antibody*. Something that has the properties of an antigen is said to be antigenic.

Antihaemorrhagic **Quick Reference:** An agent that prevents or stops haemorrhage.

Advanced Reference: May be a drug for injection, e.g. *aprotinin*, or a preparation applied directly to a bleeding point such as *Surgicel*™ or *bone-wax*.

Antihistamine **Quick Reference:** Drug which counteracts the effects of *histamine*.

Advanced Reference: Antihistamines work by blocking the receptors for histamine. Used in the treatment of drug allergies, allergic and itching rashes and *urticaria*.

Antimuscarinics **Quick Reference:** Group of drugs formerly termed *anticholinergics*.

Advanced Reference: They reduce intestinal motility and gastric secretion and are also used to treat some forms of *dyspepsia*.

Antioxidant **Quick Reference:** Any substance that delays or prevents oxidation.

Advanced Reference: Commonly used in relation to health to indicate any natural or synthetic substances that counteract the action of free radicals (reactive by-products of normal cell activity) in the body, such as vitamins C, E, A.

Antiplatelet **Quick Reference:** Refers to drugs that reduce *platelet aggregation*, e.g NSAIDs (non-steroidal anti-inflammatory drugs).

Advanced Reference: This group of drugs also inhibits *thrombus* formation, e.g. *aspirin*.

Antisepsis **Quick Reference:** The elimination of bacteria, fungus and viruses.

Advanced Reference: Includes all chemical and physical methods utilised to destroy micro-organisms that cause disease.

Antiseptic **Quick Reference:** Substance that destroys or arrests the development/multiplication of bacteria.

Advanced Reference: Used interchangeably but wrongly with disinfectant. One difference is that antiseptics can be safely applied to the body tissues, whereas disinfectants generally cannot or are not. Antiseptics are used primarily to prevent infection.

Antiserum **Quick Reference:** Serum containing antibodies (human or animal) that are specific to one or more antigens.

Advanced Reference: A method of passing on passive immunity; antiserum is obtained from an animal that has been immunised either by injection of an antigen or by infection with micro-organisms containing the antigen. Also referred to as antisera, antitoxin.

Antisialagogues **Quick Reference:** Used to dry salivary secretions.

Advanced Reference: Drugs in this group, atropine being the most common, have the action of drying both salivary and bronchial secretions. Useful as part of a premedication protocol.

Antispasmodic **Quick Reference:** Drug which counteracts the spasm in hollow organs.

Advanced Reference: They generally act on the smooth muscle of the gastrointestinal tract and ureters.

Antitoxin **Quick Reference:** Antibody formed in the blood in response to the presence of a toxin.

Advanced Reference: *Serum* containing antitoxin used to prevent or treat diseases such as *tetanus*. Toxins may originate from animals, plants or bacteria.

Antrum **Quick Reference:** A cavity or chamber.

Advanced Reference: One that is nearly closed and usually surrounded by bone.

Anuria **Quick Reference:** Condition in which no *urine* is produced.

Advanced Reference: Can be due to kidney failure, low pressure in the renal arteries or obstruction/blockage within the urinary system. Ischuria indicates retention or suppression of the urine.

Anus **Quick Reference:** End of the *alimentary* tract.

Advanced Reference: The position where the *rectum* opens to the exterior. It is surrounded by two *sphincters*.

Anxiolytic **Quick Reference:** Anti-anxiety. Drugs used in the treatment of anxiety.

Advanced Reference: Drugs which produce *sedation*. *Tranquillisers* are commonly included in this category. *Benzodiazepines* are an example.

AO system **Quick Reference:** Range of systems and instruments associated mainly with orthopaedic surgery.

Advanced Reference: Arbeitsgemeinschaft Osteosynthesefragen – Association for the Study of Internal Fixation (AO/ASIF). Founded (1958) and developed by a group of Swiss orthopaedic and general surgeons with the aim of improving methods of fracture treatment.

Aorta **Quick Reference:** Main artery of the body.

Advanced Reference: Beginning in the chest at the left ventricle, curves up, over and then down to pass through the *diaphragm* into the abdominal cavity then eventually dividing into the left and right common iliac arteries. During its course it gives off many branches, e.g. renal arteries.

Aortic regurgitation   **Quick Reference:** Involves the retrograde flow of blood from the aorta to the left ventricle (LV) during *diastole*.

Advanced Reference: Eventually leads to LV dilatation and hypertrophy and a low cardiac output. Causes include ischaemic heart disease (IHD), *endocarditis* and rheumatic fever, or may be congenital.

Aortic valve   **Quick Reference:** Heart valve.

Advanced Reference: Positioned between the left ventricle and entrance to the *aorta*. Also termed the semilunar valve, it consists of three flaps which help to maintain unidirectional blood flow.

Aortocaval compression   **Quick Reference:** Indicates obstruction to flow through the vessels due to compression by other organs, the fetus in pregnancy or a tumour. Also referred to as aortocaval occlusion.

Advanced Reference: Most commonly associated with late pregnancy when the *vena cava* and sometimes the *aorta* are compressed between the pregnant uterus and vertebral column, leading to reduced venous return and impaired cardiac output. Hence the reason for tipping the patient to the left or positioning in full left *lateral* when attending for *Caesarean section*.

Apache   **Quick Reference:** Acute Physiology and Chronic Health Evaluation.

Advanced Reference: A scoring system of severity of illness in ITU patients.

Aperient   **Quick Reference:** A mild oral laxative. Purgative.

Advanced Reference: May be a medicine or food. An alternative to *enema* and *suppository*.

Aperture   **Quick Reference:** An opening or hole.

Advanced Reference: May be present in an object or anatomical structure.

Apex   **Quick Reference:** The summit, top or peak of anything cone shaped.

Advanced Reference: Used with reference to the apex beat of the heart, located or felt at the level of the fifth intercostal space in the midclavicular line.

Apgar scale   **Quick Reference:** A scoring system used to assess the newborn.

Advanced Reference: Involves assessment of pulse/heart rate, respiratory effort, muscle tone, grimace/irritability and colour. Each is awarded a value of (0, 1, 2) and the total score indicates condition, with the maximum being 10 and below 9 suggesting that the baby requires attention; a score of less than 6 indicates that resuscitation is needed. Taken at 1- and 5-min intervals after birth.

Aphakia   **Quick Reference:** Absence of the lens of the eye.

Advanced Reference: Is the state of the eye after a *cataract* has been removed.

Aphasia   **Quick Reference:** Loss of power of speech, reading and writing.

Advanced Reference: Caused by damage to the parts of the brain concerned with these functions.

Aplasia **Quick Reference:** Lack of development of an organ or tissues.

Advanced Reference: A congenital absence of an organ or tissues. Can also indicate the cessation of normal regenerative processes in organs and tissues.

Apnoea **Quick Reference:** Cessation of breathing.

Advanced Reference: Caused by a number of factors including reduced central respiratory drive due to drugs, peripheral nerve lesious and respiratory muscle weakness.

Apoptosis **Quick Reference:** Pertaining to a pattern of cell death. Disintegration of cells.

Advanced Reference: A natural process of self-destruction in certain cells. Also called programmed cell death (PCD). The body's method of controlling cell numbers and eliminating cells that may threaten survival.

Appendicectomy **Quick Reference:** Surgical removal of the appendix.

Advanced Reference: Identification of the appendix is at the ileo-caecal junction, i.e. the distal aspects of the ileum and the proximal aspects of the ascending colon. *McBurney's* point marks the incision site. A *Grid-Iron* is the term used to indicate the lie of the muscles that have to be divided and a *purse-string* suture technique is used to close the location from where the appendix is removed.

Apposition **Quick Reference:** Two bodily structures being in close contact.

Advanced Reference: Making a fist brings the fingers together. Appose is to bring two structures together, as with tissue edges being brought together for suturing/stapling, etc.

Approximate **Quick Reference:** To bring together; into *apposition*.

Advanced Reference: Used commonly in relation to wound edges being brought together for suturing, etc.

Apronectomy **Quick Reference:** A plastic surgery procedure carried out to remove abdominal tissue. Also termed abdominoplasty.

Advanced Reference: Involves removal of an apron of skin and underlying tissue/fat from the abdominal-pelvic region, mainly for cosmetic reasons.

Aprotinin **Quick Reference:** An antifibrinolytic drug.

Advanced Reference: An *antihaemorrhagic* used to reduce perioperative blood loss during such procedures as cardiopulmonary bypass.

Arachnoid **Quick Reference:** One of the *membranes* covering the *brain*.

Advanced Reference: Named because of its resemblance to a spider's web.

Aramine™ **Quick Reference:** Vasoconstrictor drug.

Advanced Reference: Proprietary form of metaraminol. Used to raise blood pressure or in conditions of severe shock. Used during anaesthesia/surgery as an infusion.

ARDS **Quick Reference:** Adult respiratory distress syndrome.

Advanced Reference: Serious condition involving the lungs. It has a high mortality rate, and is a form of respiratory failure due to a number of causes.

Predisposing factors include aspiration of gastric contents, sepsis, fluid overload and lung contusion.

Arm board   **Quick Reference:** Piece of equipment used to support and position the patient's arm(s) during surgical procedures.

Advanced Reference: Positioned and usually fixed to the side of the operating table at shoulder level as a support when the arm is at an angle to the table. Intended to provide access to the arm/hand for IV use and BP readings, etc., as well as keeping the arm clear of the surgical site. There are a number of inherent hazards involved in the utilisation of arm boards:

1. The angle of the board must not exceed 90° as this could cause **brachial plexus** injury.
2. The board can drop below the table level causing a drag on the shoulder joint and associated nerves.

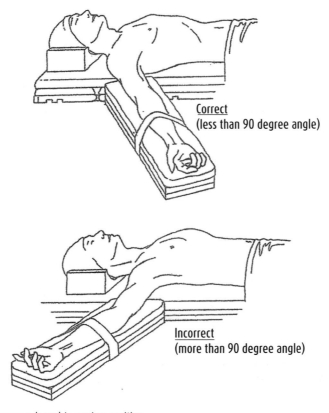

Fig. 1. Arms on arm board in supine position

3. As some are made of metal, earthing of the patient's skin is possible if unprotected.
4. There are opposing views over whether the arm/hand should lie palm up or palm down.

Also, are there any benefits of the patient's head being turned to face the arm that is out on a board, as it may reduce anatomical stress? Having both arms out on boards simultaneously also creates the potential for injury if necessary precautions are not identified. There are designs of board available for both attaching to the table and sliding under the table mattress.

Arm support   **Quick Reference:** Device for securing the patient's arms while positioned on the operating table.

Advanced Reference: Numerous designs are available but all are a variation on an L-shape. Intended to fit under the mattress with the upper section holding the arms, whether positioned at the side or folded across the chest. If wrongly applied, can cause damage to the arm itself and/or the ulnar nerve at the elbow as well as skin injury if placed directly under the patient rather than the mattress.

Aromatase inhibitors   **Quick Reference:** A group of drugs used to stop the natural production of *oestrogen*.

Advanced Reference: They are used in the treatment of breast cancer, sometimes in conjunction with alternative medications. Examples are anastrozole, exemestane, letrozole.

Arrhythmia   **Quick Reference:** (a-rith-me-a) Any irregularity in the rhythm of the heartbeat.

Advanced Reference: Actually indicates no rhythm, the more accurate term is *dysrhythmia*. Drugs used to treat arrhythmias are referred to as antiarrhythmics. Lignocaine and amiodarone are commonly used in the treatment of tachyarrhythmias.

Artefact   **Quick Reference:** Artificially made, produced.

Advanced Reference: A false signal on an ECG trace caused by interference.

Arteriosclerosis   **Quick Reference:** Hardening of the arteries.

Advanced Reference: Loss of elasticity of the arterial walls due to thickening and calcification. Leads to a raised blood pressure.

Artery forceps   **Quick Reference:** An instrument for holding bleeding vessels securely during surgery.

Advanced Reference: All artery forceps have serrate jaws designed to hold bleeding vessels securely. Some have sharp teeth at the ends of the jaws which provide a stronger grip on tougher tissues. They come in many sizes and shapes, with some of the most common being Mosquito, Halstead, Spencer Wells, Kelly, Kocher. Also referred to as a clamp.

Arthritis   **Quick Reference:** Inflammation of a joint.

Advanced Reference: Term applied to many types of joint disease, although not always accurately. A degenerative condition in which the restriction of movement is a prominent symptom. The three common types are rheumatoid, osteoarthritis and gout.

Arthropathy   **Quick Reference:** Indicates any disorder or disease affecting a joint.

Advanced Reference: Arthro = joint, path(o) = disease.

Arthroplasty   **Quick Reference:** Replacement of a joint with an artificial implant.

Advanced Reference: The joint is replaced by a prosthesis; arthro meaning joint and plasty indicating a false moulding, i.e. total knee arthroplasty, where the distal end of the femur and the head of the tibia are both replaced with a prosthesis.

Articular   **Quick Reference:** Pertaining to a joint.

Advanced Reference: Indicates a joint or the movement of a joint.

Arytenoid   **Quick Reference:** (aret-noid) Two cartilages of the larynx.

Advanced Reference: Their function is to adjust the tension of the vocal cords to which they are attached.

ASA   **Quick Reference:** American Society of Anesthesiologists.

Advanced Reference: Refers to the criteria laid down by the ASA which involve a patient's preoperative assessment and classification which utilises a scale of 1–5 ranging from healthy to moribund, and also includes status in emergency situations.

Asbestos   **Quick Reference:** Combination of minerals including magnesium silicate. At one time used as insulating medium in the building trade.

Advanced Reference: Inhalation of the dust can lead to pulmonary fibrosis and cancer. Asbestosis indicates accumulation of the fibres in the bronchioles. One particular type is responsible for mesothelioma. Now closely controlled under the Health and Safety laws.

Ascending   **Quick Reference:** (a-sending) Indicating to rise.

Advanced Reference: Ascending infection is one that rises through organs or structures such as infections from the bladder via the ureters to kidneys.

Ascites   **Quick Reference:** (a-site-ease) Accumulation of fluid in the peritoneum.

Advanced Reference: Leads to abdominal swelling. There are many causes including infections (such as tuberculosis), portal hypertension, liver-related conditions (cirrhosis), heart failure. Paracentesis is the drawing off of fluid, usually via needle aspiration.

Asepsis   **Quick Reference:** Absence of any living organisms.

Advanced Reference: Term often used wrongly to indicate sterility. In relation to theatres it indicates an area intended to be free of micro-organisms by the use of antiseptics, barriers, washing techniques, etc.

Asphyxia **Quick Reference:** Suffocation, due to lack of oxygen.

Advanced Reference: Brought about by obstruction of the air passages, by lack of, or reduced, oxygen in the air or by gases interfering with the utilisation of oxygen within the body.

Aspiration **Quick Reference:** To withdraw fluids, usually with suction. The release of fluid and/or contents from a body cavity.

Advanced Reference: In relation to theatre practice and anaesthesia, refers to the inhalation of gastric contents into the lungs.

Aspiration pneumonitis **Quick Reference:** Lung infection that develops when oral or gastric contents enter the bronchial tree. Also termed aspiration *pneumonia* or chemical pneumonitis.

Advanced Reference: This includes food, saliva or nasal secretions. Dependent on the acidity of the aspirate, a chemical pneumonitis can develop. Anaerobic bacteria from the gut can add to the inflammation. There is much debate over whether the condition is a bacterial infection or a chemical inflammation process. Prominent amongst the causes are regurgitation and aspiration during general anaesthesia.

Aspirin **Quick Reference:** Proprietary name for acetylsalicylic acid.

Advanced Reference: An effective analgesic and anti-inflammatory, used for lowering body temperature during fever; it has *antiplatelet* properties.

Asthma **Quick Reference:** Condition which produces attacks that cause breathing difficulties.

Advanced Reference: Asthma attacks produce obstruction to expiration because of narrowing of the bronchi caused by hypersensitivity to certain substances. Usually treated initially with a bronchodilator to ease breathing difficulties and/or adrenaline.

Astringent **Quick Reference:** Agent that causes contraction of tissues upon topical application.

Advanced Reference: Used locally on skin and mucous membranes to stem blood flow from capillary bleeding. Examples are aluminium acetate and potassium permanganate.

Astrocytoma **Quick Reference:** Malignant tumour of nerve tissue.

Advanced Reference: Tumour of the brain and found throughout the *central nervous system*.

Asymmetrical **Quick Reference:** Unequal in size and/or shape.

Advanced Reference: Different in placement and arrangement. Not forming a conventional pattern.

Asystole **Quick Reference:** (a-sist-o-lee) Absence of a heartbeat or output.

Advanced Reference: Confirmed when there is no functional ventricular activity. As seen on the ECG trace, it is not a flat line but the absence of organised electrical activity.

Ataxia   **Quick Reference:** Impaired ability to coordinate movement.

Advanced Reference: Involves posture imbalance, causing someone to stagger.

Atelectasis   **Quick Reference:** Incomplete expansion of the lung.

Advanced Reference: A term that can cover a number of causes and effects in both adults and infants. Affects premature babies and those who have inhaled damaging substances. Failure to produce the lubricating agent **surfactant** is also grouped under this condition. Also described as collapse of the lung.

Atenolol   **Quick Reference:** A beta-blocker drug.

Advanced Reference: Used to reduce heart rate and the force of contraction.

Atherectomy   **Quick Reference:** Surgical procedure for removing arterial *plaque*.

Advanced Reference: The procedure utilises a rotating shaver on the end of a catheter which is introduced through an arm or leg vein and then advanced through the blocked coronary artery. The shaver then grinds down the plaque. The procedure is often followed by balloon angioplasty.

Atheroma   **Quick Reference:** Fatty deposit.

Advanced Reference: Composed of fatty substances such as cholesterol, it can lead to arterial obstruction and reduced blood supply to an area.

Atherosclerosis   **Quick Reference:** Disease affecting the walls of the arteries.

Advanced Reference: The arterial walls become thickened, stiff and sometimes swollen following the laying down of atheromatous deposits.

Atomic   **Quick Reference:** Pertaining to or consisting of atoms.

Advanced Reference: Extremely minute. Atomic energy is the energy derived from nuclear fission. Atomic weight indicates the average mass of an atom of an element usually expressed in relation to the atomic mass of carbon 12.

Atopy   **Quick Reference:** Having a *genetic* predisposition to hypersensitivity reactions.

Advanced Reference: Involves *hereditary* allergies characterised by such symptoms as hayfever and *asthma*; produced upon exposure to specific *antigens*.

ATP   **Quick Reference:** (adenosine triphosphate.) Involved in the storage of energy by the cells of the body.

Advanced Reference: Supplies large amounts of energy to cells for various biochemical processes, including muscle contraction and sugar metabolism.

Atracurium   **Quick Reference:** Non-depolarising muscle relaxant.

Advanced Reference: *Tracrium*™. Undergoes spontaneous breakdown within the body due to a process known as Hoffman elimination.

Atresia   **Quick Reference:** Congenital absence of a normal body orifice or tubular organ. Also referred to as clausura.

Advanced Reference: Incomplete development resulting in the obliteration of a passage such as the anus, oesophagus or vagina. Biliary atresia causes obstructive jaundice in infancy and ***tricuspid*** atresia obstructs the blood flow within the heart from the right atrium to the right ventricle.

Atria   **Quick Reference:** The two smaller chambers of the heart (right and left). Also referred to as the auricles.

Advanced Reference: The atria receive blood from the veins and pump it on into the ***ventricles***.

Atrophy   **Quick Reference:** Wasting away of tissue or an organ.

Advanced Reference: Usually due to degeneration of cells through disuse, aging or malnourishment.

Atropine   **Quick Reference:** An anticholinergic.

Advanced Reference: Its source is the deadly nightshade plant (belladonna). Used to counteract bradycardia and as part of a premedication regime to dry secretions. Most commonly seen being used in combination with neostigmine as a reversal for non-depolarising muscle relaxants. Also as a topical pupil dilator in ophthalmic procedures.

Atypical   **Quick Reference:** (a-tip-ical) Not typical, irregular.

Advanced Reference: Not like the usual, does not conform to the normal. When a disease does not follow the normal or expected course or does not display expected signs and symptoms.

Auditory   **Quick Reference:** Pertaining to the sense of hearing.

Advanced Reference: Audiology is the science of dealing with hearing and audiometry is the measurement of the power of hearing.

Augmentation   **Quick Reference:** To add on, enlarge, increase in size.

Advanced Reference: Breast augmentation is a commonly used term to indicate enlargement with implants.

Augmentin™   **Quick Reference:** Commonly used antibiotic.

Advanced Reference: Proprietary preparation of the penicillin-like antibiotic amoxicillin combined with an extending agent (clavulanic acid).

Augustine guide   **Quick Reference:** Device enabling blind oral intubation.

Advanced Reference: Considered when cervical spine injury is an issue, it consists of an anatomically shaped channel guide and special stylet. The endotracheal tube is loaded over the guide and the stylet is used to detect the trachea. It combines features of the pharyngeal airway, standard stylet, bougie and oesophageal detector. Its use is associated with a high degree of laryngopharyngeal trauma.

Aura   **Quick Reference:** The forewarning of various cerebral-related attacks.

Advanced Reference: Experienced before ***epileptic*** and ***migraine*** attacks. Characterised in epileptics by a peaceful coolness passing over the body and in migraine by the presence of flickering lights and blurring of vision.

Auscultation   **Quick Reference:** Method of examining the body by use of hearing.

Advanced Reference: Mostly applies to areas such as the chest and heart when they are examined with a stethoscope.

Autoclave **Quick Reference:** A machine for sterilising theatre products and equipment.

Advanced Reference: A machine that utilises steam and pressure to sterilise. It will destroy most micro-organisms, such as human immunodeficiency virus (HIV) but not the agent of *Creutzfeldt–Jakob disease (CJD)*.

Autograft **Quick Reference:** Grafting from one part of the same body to another.

Advanced Reference: Auto indicates self. A graft where the donor is also the recipient, e.g. skin graft.

Autoimmune disease **Quick Reference:** An immune reaction to one's own tissues.

Advanced Reference: It is not fully understood why in some instances individuals produce an immune reaction to one of their own tissues and the autoantibodies set up an inflammatory response which damages the organ or tissue involved. Examples of disease states that occur in this way are: pernicious and haemolytic *anaemia, myasthenia gravis, nephritis, ulcerative colitis* and rheumatoid arthritis and some *thyroid* conditions.

Autologous **Quick Reference:** Indicates self.

Advanced Reference: An autologous graft involves the donor also being the recipient, i.e. blood collected, stored and then infused when required into the same patient. Usually withdrawn and stored over a six-week period prior to surgery.

Autonomic nervous system **Quick Reference:** Responsible for regulating body functions other than voluntary movement and conscious sensation.

Advanced Reference: Composed of the *sympathetic* and *parasympathetic* nervous systems whose actions are generally opposed, e.g. the sympathetic accelerates the heart rate and the parasympathetic slows it down. In the intestine they function in the opposite manner.

Autoregulation **Quick Reference:** The process that occurs when some action or mechanism within a biological system detects changes and makes adjustments.

Advanced Reference: An example is the body trying to maintain a constant blood flow despite changes in arterial pressure or the adjustment of blood flow through an organ in order to provide for its metabolic needs.

Autosomal **Quick Reference:** The non-sex chromosomes. Auto = self, somal = body.

Advanced Reference: There are 22 pairs of autosomal chromosomes in each cell together with the 2 sex chromosomes, XY in the male and XX in the female.

AV fistula **Quick Reference:** Fistula indicates a false or abnormal passage connecting one structure with another.

Advanced Reference: Atrioventricular (AV) fistula is the anastomosis of an artery to a vein for the purpose of haemodialysis in patients with renal failure. It provides access for the artificial kidney machine.

Avian influenza   **Quick Reference:** Bird flu. Has its origins in Asia and the East. Is of concern because of its potential to cross over into humans. Avian means of or pertaining to birds.

Advanced Reference: There are three main types of flu virus: A, B and C. C displays mild problems in humans, B may cause more serious illness and seasonal epidemics, but bird flu involves type A which has the ability to change and adapt more readily. The birds shed the virus in their faeces, saliva and nasal secretions.

AV node   **Quick Reference:** Atrioventricular node of the heart.

Advanced Reference: Conductive node situated between the atria and ventricles which transmits impulses and forms a pathway in the cardiac conduction system.

Avulsion   **Quick Reference:** (avul-shon) To tear away.

Advanced Reference: To forcibly wrench away, as in avulsion of the toenail when just the nail is removed but not including the nail bed. Also, avulsion of varicose veins.

AxiaLIF®   **Quick Reference:** Axial lumbar interbody fusion. A minimally invasive technique used for lumbar spine fusion.

Advanced Reference: A treatment for L5/S1 degenerative disc disease, spinal stenosis and spondylolisthesis (slipping forward of the vertebral body), which avoids major invasive surgery by entering through a small incision adjacent to the sacral bone (tailbone) and inserting and feeding a probe up toward the affected area under X-ray control. The instrumentation is used to fill the vacated space with bone graft and/or to stabilise the fused structures with a screw-like titanium implant.

Ayer's T-piece   **Quick Reference:** (airs) Paediatric anaesthetic circuit.

Advanced Reference: Corresponds to the *Mapleson* E system. Suitable for children up to 20 kg. The *Jackson-Rees* modification added an open-ended bag which enabled artificial ventilation.

Asphyxia   **Quick Reference:** (as-fix-ea) A reduction in oxygen.

Advanced Reference: Suffocation. Caused by a lack of or reduced levels of oxygen in the lungs and tissues. Causes include choking, drowning and smoke inhalation.

B

Babcock **Quick Reference:** A tissue-holding forceps used during bowel surgery.

Advanced Reference: This design of forceps has a hollow end for picking up bowel without causing damage to the delicate tissue involved.

Bacillus **Quick Reference:** Term used originally to mean a rod-shaped microorganism.

Advanced Reference: The many diseases caused by this group include anthrax, diphtheria, gasgangrene, tetanus, tuberculosis and typhoid.

Bacillus cereus **Quick Reference:** Bacterium that causes food poisoning.

Advanced Reference: Food-borne illness, significantly diarrhoea and vomiting, that occurs due to the survival of the bacterial spores when food is improperly cooked.

Back **Quick Reference:** Pertaining to the posterior surface.

Advanced Reference: Refers to the rear surface of the patient's trunk. The dorsum of an anatomical surface. The dorsum of the hand as used for intravenous cannulation.

Back-bar **Quick Reference:** Connecting block that seats the anaesthetic *vaporiser*.

Advanced Reference: The back-bar is situated between the *flowmeters* and the connecting fresh gas flow pipeline within the anaesthetic machine. Commonly the back-bar contains the *Selectatec*™ seating pins for the vaporiser to be positioned in line. More modern back-bars allow for multiple vaporisers to be fitted with interlocking mechanisms designed to prevent simultaneous delivery from the vaporisers.

Back blows **Quick Reference:** Airway clearing method used to relieve choking.

Advanced Reference: A manoeuvre used as a first step in relieving foreign body airway obstruction where blows with the flat of the hand are delivered to the upper-middle of the back.

Back support **Quick Reference:** A half-moon-shaped support offering stabilisation and protection for the patient in the *lateral* position.

Advanced Reference: A back support, often termed lumbar support, is used to stabilise the patient on the operating table. A patient in the lateral position can be precarious and this requires them to be protected from falls. A table clamp holds the support in place and it has an adjustable arm with antistatic/protective padding covering the metal areas.

Bacteria   **Quick Reference:** Single-cell microbes that have the capacity to multiply.

Advanced Reference: Bacteria can become harmful to humans through the increase in number of bacterial cells. Bacterial spread requires a nutritional substance, warm temperature and, for certain types (aerobic), the presence of oxygen. Common forms of bacteria are cocci, bacilli and spirochaetes. Through these bacterial forms poisonous toxins are spread via exotoxins (which freely diffuse outward from the bacterial cell and spread throughout the body) and endotoxins (which are released once the bacteria itself has become dysfunctional).

Bacterial filter   **Quick Reference:** A filter attached to the patient-end of a breathing circuit, intended to prevent the spread of infection.

Advanced Reference: Bacterial filters are used more routinely to prevent expired bacteria from being transmitted into a breathing system that will later be attached to other patients. The filter contains a 22-mm male–female connector allowing secure fitment between the circuit and patient airway device. Similar inline devices are used within ventilator circuits.

Bacterial translocation   **Quick Reference:** Indicates the movement of resident bacteria from their normal site to another body area.

Advanced Reference: Most commonly the passage of bacteria from the gastrointestinal tract to other extra-intestinal sites, such as the mesenteric lymph nodes, liver, spleen, kidneys and blood. Causes include excess growth of gastroenteric bacilli, impaired immune defence, injury to the intestinal mucosa (*mucous membrane*).

Bain breathing system   **Quick Reference:** A breathing system used in conjunction with an anaesthetic machine.

Advanced Reference: The Bain circuit attaches to the fresh-gas outlet and comprises a reservoir bag at the machine end along with the expiratory valve. The system has two channels (coaxial): the narrower inner tubing carries the fresh gas to the patient and the broader outer channel conveys expired gases away and out via the valve. As a safety measure involving disconnection the inner tubing is usually of a distinctive colour (red, black) so that it can be seen and examined through the outer transparent tubing. The Bain equates to the *Mapleson* D classification.

Bair Hugger™   **Quick Reference:** (bare) A warm-air overblanket system, unlike previous water and electric-element underblankets.

Advanced Reference: Designed primarily for intraoperative use but has a place during other treatment phases and locations.

Baker's cyst   **Quick Reference:** A cyst found in the *popliteal* space.

Advanced Reference: Formed from synovial fluid that has escaped from the *bursa*, usually secondary to some other condition.

Balanced anaesthesia **Quick Reference:** Indicates the traditional or a preferred general anaesthetic technique, as opposed to other options such as *TIVA* and *regional*.

Advanced Reference: More precisely refers to a combination of premedication, intravenous opioid, muscle relaxants, volatiles and the possible addition of a regional technique.

Balfour retractor **Quick Reference:** A self-retaining retractor used regularly during abdominal surgery.

Advanced Reference: Is of a frame design with fixed blades and a removable centre blade with a curved shape and a distal lip which is screwed and fixed into position.

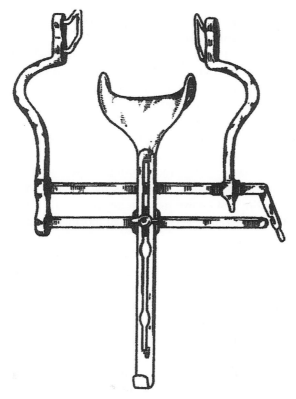

Fig. 2. Balfour self-retaining retractors

Balkan frame   **Quick Reference:** Also referred to as Balkan beam. A traction device used in orthopaedics.

Advanced Reference: A frame that fixes to the bed and is used for attaching splints for continuous traction using weights and pulleys and also useful when an immobilised patient wants/needs to change position.

Balloon pump   **Quick Reference:** Also termed intraaortic balloon pump, it is a device inserted into the descending *aorta* in the management of left ventricular failure (LVF).

Advanced Reference: The balloon is positioned within the descending aorta at the beginning of *diastole* and deflated immediately before *systole*. Introduced via the *femoral* artery and inflated with helium or carbon dioxide. Its function is synchronised with the ECG and arterial trace and increases coronary blood flow and improves oxygen supply to the myocardium. It is a temporary measure in left ventricular failure, cardiogenic shock, after myocardial infarction (MI) and before or after cardiac surgery.

Banding   **Quick Reference:** Rubber-band ligation.

Advanced Reference: The application of a small *Silastic*® band, commonly used in haemorrhoidectomy, placed around the *pedicle* of each *haemorrhoid*.

Bar   **Quick Reference:** Unit of pressure.

Advanced Reference: $100\,kPa = 1\,bar \approx 1$ atmosphere ≈ 15 psi $= 750\,mmHg$.

Barbiturate   **Quick Reference:** Group of drugs used mainly as sedatives and anaesthetics.

Advanced Reference: Derived from barbituric acid, with a wide range of essentially depressant actions. They work by direct actions on the brain. *Thiopentone* is the best known barbiturate anaesthetic induction agent.

Barbotage   **Quick Reference:** Technique used mostly during spinal anaesthesia to disperse drugs.

Advanced Reference: Involves injection, aspiration and re-injection in order to cause turbulence within the cerebrospinal fluid (CSF) and so disperse distribution of drugs; however, the technique has limited effect with the current use of small-bore needles.

Bard Parker   **Quick Reference:** Name of a surgical blade (scalpel) holder.

Advanced Reference: Often referred to as the Bard Parker handle and comes in different lengths and holds different sizes of blade.

Bariatric   **Quick Reference:** The branch of medicine that specialises in treating being overweight and obesity.

Advanced Reference: Involves the study and treatment of the cause and prevention of obesity.

Barium   **Quick Reference:** A flexible soft silvery metallic element.

Advanced Reference: The properties of barium allow it to be detected by X-rays and it is used for barium meal diagnostic procedures when the patient ingests the compound prior to having films taken of their digestive tract. Barium enema is also used for visualisation of the colon. Many invasive devices are impregnated or coated with barium so as to make them detectable by X-ray, i.e. intravenous cannulae, endotracheal tubes.

Barium lime   Quick Reference: Carbon dioxide absorbent used in anaesthetic *closed circuits* (re-breathing).

Advanced Reference: Consists of 80% calcium hydroxide and 20% barium hydroxide.

Barometric   Quick Reference: Relates to atmospheric pressure.

Advanced Reference: A barometer is an instrument used to measure the pressure that the atmosphere exerts on the Earth. Barotrauma is an injury caused by pressure (i.e. the differential between ambient pressure and that in the cavity) especially in enclosed cavities such as the *Eustachian tube*, *middle ear* and lungs.

Baroreceptor   Quick Reference: Type of receptor that is stimulated by changes in pressure. The body contains a collection of sensory nerve endings sensitive to changes in blood pressure. Also termed baroceptor and pressoreceptor.

Advanced Reference: They are present in the carotid sinuses, aortic arch, the heart and the walls of some major arteries and veins; they are sensitive to stretching of vessel walls due to pressure changes. They communicate changes to the *medulla*, which acts in turn to normalise pressure via adjustment of blood vessel resistance and cardiac output.

Barotrauma   Quick Reference: Tissue injury caused by a change in pressure.

Advanced Reference: A change which compresses or expands gas contained in various body structures. Examples are the middle ear or paranasal sinuses due to an imbalance between the *ambient* pressure and pressure within the cavity.

Barré-Guillain syndrome   Quick Reference: A condition that causes paralysis of the nervous system.

Advanced Reference: The disorder encourages the body's immune system to attack the peripheral nervous system, leading to a varying degree of tingling sensations usually commencing in the arms and legs then spreading throughout the body. Can be life threatening and may result in complete paralysis leaving the patient hospitalised and needing life-support measures.

Barrett's oesophagus   Quick Reference: Chronic peptic ulcer of the lower oesophagus. Also known as Barrett's syndrome.

Advanced Reference: Involves abnormal changes in cells of the lower end of the oesophagus caused by damage from chronic acid exposure or *reflux* oesophagitis. Considered to be a premalignant condition.

Bartholin's gland   Quick Reference: Pair of glands, one on either side of the opening of the vagina, that secrete a lubricant.

Advanced Reference: Situated in the labia majora, with their ducts opening outside of the vulva. These glands can become infected and cause a painful abscess.

Baseline **Quick Reference:** The normal value of a reading.

Advanced Reference: Baseline readings can apply to the initial physiological parameters of a patient before surgical, medical and anaesthetic interventions.

Basic metabolic rate **Quick Reference:** Minimum amount of energy (calories) expended while at rest.

Advanced Reference: Considered as the amount of energy measured in calories expended by the body in order to sustain life.

Basilic **Quick Reference:** A prominent vein that runs along the back of the forearm.

Advanced Reference: A vein on the inner side of the arm at the bend of the elbow; it is sometimes chosen for venipuncture.

Bassinis operation **Quick Reference:** Reconstruction of the inguinal canal.

Advanced Reference: Carried out during an inguinal *hernia* repair.

BAWO **Quick Reference:** Bilateral antrum washout.

Advanced Reference: Involves the insertion of a cannula under the inferior turbinate in order to flush out pus, etc. from the maxillary sinus using saline.

BCC **Quick Reference:** Basal cell carcinoma.

Advanced Reference: May appear as a nodule or as a small, unstable ulcerating area with persisting crusting. Depending on size, it may be removed under local anaesthetic but larger examples need a general anaesthetic due to the more radical surgery involved.

Beating heart transplant **Quick Reference:** Heart transplant technique.

Advanced Reference: The technique involves keeping the heart beating following *harvesting* rather than being stopped and cooled prior to transplantation. Potassium solution is used to bring about cessation of function and storage temperature is around 4 °C with no longer than four hours being recommended between removal and transplantation.

Bed sore **Quick Reference:** Pressure sore; also known as *decubitus ulcer*. Also termed pressure sore.

Advanced Reference: Ulcerated area of the skin caused by continuous pressure and irritation from lying in the one position in bed.

Beer's knife **Quick Reference:** A triangular-shaped knife used in eye surgery.

Advanced Reference: The Beer's knife has similarities to a diamond knife. Essentially the knife is used to make an incision into the cornea. The curve-shaped incision allows access for removal and replacement of the lens of the eye. It is named after a German ophthalmologist, G. J. Beer (eighteenth century).

Belfast roller **Quick Reference:** A patient transfer device.

Advanced Reference: A board-like device comprised of rollers, approximately 8 ft or 2.5 m long, covered with rubber which turns on the rollers. The entire device is inserted under the patient and the draw sheet under the patient is used to pull them across it and onto the receiving surface. Its use was discontinued when it was found that the rollers could cause damage to bony prominences.

Belladonna **Quick Reference:** Name of a plant and of the alkaloids produced from it.

Advanced Reference: Atropine and hyoscine are two of the most well-known drugs to come from this source.

Bellows **Quick Reference:** A concertina and cylindrical-shaped rubber component contained within a mechanical ventilator.

Advanced Reference: Bellows are the extendable rubber aspect of mechanical ventilators that indicate gas volume delivered to the patient.

Bell's palsy **Quick Reference:** Paralysis that occurs down the side of the face.

Advanced Reference: Often due to oedema being present around the facial nerve, injury during surgery, accidental pressure by the face-mask during anaesthesia or pressure sustained during wrongful positioning of the head when in the *prone* position.

Benign **Quick Reference:** (ben-ine) A non-life-threatening tumour that is in most cases treatable.

Advanced Reference: A tumour or stricture that is present and treatable. Usually localised and has not spread to other parts of the body. Benign tumours in the oesophagus on X-ray show a distinct tapering shape compared to malignant tumours, which display a significant shape.

Bennett's fracture **Quick Reference:** Fracture of the thumb.

Advanced Reference: Associated with falling on to the outstretched hand with the thumb taking the force. Bennett's describes the initial dislocation of the metacarpal from its location and a triangular section of the base becomes detached. Treatment involves reduction of the thumb and direct pressure on the base to realign the bone fragments, followed by application of a Plaster of Paris cast (or scotch cast), which is usually removed after 4–6 weeks.

Benzocaine **Quick Reference:** Local anaesthetic agent.

Advanced Reference: Available as a spray, cream, ointment, aerosol or even lozenges and utilised for topical use in endoscopy as well as intubation.

Benzodiazepines **Quick Reference:** A group of drugs with sedative properties that also act upon the central nervous system.

Advanced Reference: Primarily used as sedatives or hypnotics, e.g. diazepam, nitrazepam, lorazepam.

Beta-blocker **Quick Reference:** Medications whose effect is to reduce the rate and force of the heartbeat.

Advanced Reference: They oppose certain actions of the sympathetic nervous system, in particular stimulation of the heart. Principally used to treat hypertension.

Betadine™ **Quick Reference:** A skin preparation and surgical scrub solution.

Advanced Reference: Betadine™ is a trade name for an iodine-based solution. Iodine is used to minimise the spread of bacteria on the skin's surface and can be clearly identified by its unique dark-brown appearance which stains yellow on the skin.

Biceps **Quick Reference:** Muscle of the upper section of the arm.

Advanced Reference: Biceps are connected to the shoulder joint and are held to the radius by tendons. They participate in the mechanics of lifting of the forearm by counteracting the action of the triceps.

Biconcave **Quick Reference:** A structure that has inwardly curved depressions on both sides.

Advanced Reference: The inwardly facing structures often present themselves in various pieces of equipment as transmitters of light from one focal point to another.

Biconvex **Quick Reference:** A structure that has outward curvatures.

Advanced Reference: Can be found, as with biconcave structures, in devices that transmit light.

Bicuspid **Quick Reference:** Indicates having two projections or cusps.

Advanced Reference: The mitral valve of the heart positioned between the left atrium and left ventricle is also known as a bicuspid valve due to its significant shape.

Bier's block **Quick Reference:** (beers) Regional anaesthesia technique used on limbs.

Advanced Reference: Bier's block is a regional anaesthetic technique used primarily for upper limbs and, to a lesser extent, the legs. It involves the use of a double tourniquet cuff, where the *proximal* cuff is inflated followed by local anaesthetic solution injection into a vein. With onset of the local anaesthetic, the distal cuff is inflated and when fully inflated the proximal cuff is deflated. The *distal* cuff would thus be over an area that is affected by the local anaesthetic solution. Following the procedure, the cuff should be deflated slowly or in stages to minimise the volume of local anaesthetic entering the circulation.

Bifid **Quick Reference:** Forked or split into two parts.

Advanced Reference: To form a cleft or two branches. Abnormality that can occur in many parts of the body, e.g. the uterus, ribs.

Bifidobacteria **Quick Reference:** A group of *anaerobic* bacteria and form of *probiotic*.

Advanced Reference: A major strain of resident gut *flora* that have health benefits, one being that they assist in producing a lower incidence of *allergy*.

Bifurcate **Quick Reference:** The division of a structure into two branches.

Advanced Reference: Blood vessels continually bifurcate throughout the body, dividing into the right and left structures of the same name; and the trachea bifurcates into the two main bronchi. The bifurcation point of the trachea is the *carina*.

Bigeminy **Quick Reference:** Refers to a cardiac *dysrhythmia*.

Advanced Reference: Term that relates to *ectopic* beats appearing in pairs on an *ECG* trace. Bi = two.

Bigorexia **Quick Reference:** Term applied to body builders. Also termed muscle dysmorphia.

Advanced Reference: A psychological condition affecting mainly male body builders who, as with *anorexics* and bulimics, view themselves differently than what may be the reality, but with this condition the perception is of being smaller than they actually are. A degree of depression, anxiety and obsessive compulsive disorder is involved. Those affected are referred to as bigorexics.

Bilateral **Quick Reference:** Indicates both sides. Bi = two, lateral = side.

Advanced Reference: Regularly used in surgical terminology to indicate both sides, i.e. bilateral inguinal hernia repair.

Bile **Quick Reference:** A liquefied enzyme that is secreted by the liver and stored in the gall bladder.

Advanced Reference: A yellow-green coloured liquid that becomes concentrated in the storage pouch (bile duct) of the biliary tree. Travels from the gall bladder, along the cystic duct, down through the common bile duct and into the duodenum. The main function of bile is to assist in the breakdown of emulsifying fats.

Bilharzia **Quick Reference:** (bel-hart-sia) Chronic illness caused by parasitic worms. Also referred to as schistosomiasis.

Advanced Reference: Mostly found in the tropics due to infestation by *flukes* picked up in infected water, gaining entry through bathing or drinking and via the skin. Affects the *liver*, *lungs*, spleen, *intestines* and urinary system. Symptoms include fever, headache, cough and *diarrhoea*, and later the *liver* and *spleen* may become enlarged.

Biliary tree **Quick Reference:** Refers to the components associated with the production and passage of bile.

Advanced Reference: The main components are: liver, gall bladder, cystic duct, common bile duct, ampulla of Vater, head of pancreas and associated blood vessels.

Bilirubin **Quick Reference:** Orange-coloured substance produced by the destruction of *haem*.

Advanced Reference: Bilirubin is conveyed to the liver within the plasma, later to be filtered by the liver and eventually excreted in the bile. The accumulation of bilirubin in the blood and tissues results in the yellowish pigmentation of the patient's skin and eyes. This discoloration is associated with *jaundice*.

Billroth **Quick Reference:** A type of gastrectomy.

Advanced Reference: Named after an Austrian surgeon who developed the technique of removing the majority of the lesser curvature of the stomach and the pyloric segment. The remaining section of the fundus and antrum of the stomach are then anastomosed to the duodenum.

Bimetallic strip **Quick Reference:** A temperature-compensating device found within modern vaporisers.

Advanced Reference: A bimetallic strip containing two dissimilar metals that are fused together and expand at different rates when heated. If one metal is heated and starts to expand, the other counteracts and prevents full expansion of the other. This process is utilised in vaporisers to maintain the regulated percentage of volatile agent being delivered, irrespective of surrounding temperature changes.

Bioabsorbable polymers **Quick Reference:** Refers to substances such as modified plastics that the body can break down and absorb.

Advanced Reference: Many devices are manufactured from bioabsorbable materials, i.e. sutures, staples, drug capsules, stents, meshes as well as orthopaedic screws and bone plates. They are broken down and absorbed harmlessly by the body, in some cases the end-product being carbon dioxide or lactic acid which are then excreted in the normal manner. They negate the need for later removal and problems with adverse reactions.

Bioavailability **Quick Reference:** The degree to which a drug becomes available to the target tissue after administration.

Advanced Reference: It is the ratio of the amount of drug reaching the circulation to the amount present if the drug had been given intravenously. A drug can have oral and intramuscular bioavailability. It is expressed as a percentage, such that a drug given intravenously has a bioavailability of 100%.

Biocide **Quick Reference:** A chemical substance capable of killing differing forms of organisms.

Advanced Reference: Can be an antimicrobial, germicide, antibacterial and antiviral agent as well as antibiotics.

Biocompatible **Quick Reference:** Being harmonious with life.

Advanced Reference: Not having toxic or injurious effects upon biological function.

Biodegradable **Quick Reference:** Readily decomposed by bacterial action.

Advanced Reference: There are many biomedical materials that are biodegradable, absorbable sutures being one group.

Biodiversity **Quick Reference:** The number and variety of organisms found within a specified geographical area.

Advanced Reference: The variability among living organisms on Earth, including the variability between species and ecosystems.

Bioequivalent **Quick Reference:** A value indicating the rate at which a substance enters the bloodstream and becomes available to the body.

Advanced Reference: Having the same strength and similar *bioavailability* in the same dosage form as another specimen of a given drug.

Biohazard **Quick Reference:** Any biological process that presents a hazard or risk.

Advanced Reference: Examples are needle-stick injury, chemical spillage, body fluids and diathermy plume.

Biological death **Quick Reference:** Refers to permanent brain death.

Advanced Reference: This death is final as opposed to *clinical death*.

Biomechanics **Quick Reference:** The science concerned with the mechanics of living organisms.

Advanced Reference: Involves the internal and external forces acting on the human body and the effects produced.

Biometrics **Quick Reference:** Bio = life, metron = measure.

Advanced Reference: The study of automated methods for uniquely recognising humans based on one or more physical traits.

Biopsy **Quick Reference:** Process by which a small sample of tissue for examination is obtained.

Advanced Reference: Biopsy samples are usually taken for study under a microscope and can assist with the diagnosis of a patient's condition or underlying disease. There are different types of biopsy procedures, e.g. needle biopsy, frozen section.

BiPAP **Quick Reference:** Bilevel Positive Airway Pressure. Patient ventilation mode. Also referred to as Variable Positive Airway Pressure (VPAP).

Advanced Reference: Used primarily in the treatment of sleep apnoea and other lung-related conditions such as emphysema. Unlike CPAP (Continuous Positive Airway Pressure) it provides two different pressures, i.e. a higher one during inspiration (Inspired Positive Airway Pressure; IPAP) and a lower one during expiration (Expiratory Positive Airway Pressure; EPAP). EPAP guarantees alveolar ventilation and a higher IPAP gives increased volume for diffusion.

Bipolar **Quick Reference:** Device or structure with two poles.

Advanced Reference: Refers to bipolar *diathermy* in which the current flows down one arm of the forceps and back up the other. Also used in psychiatry to describe certain conditions.

Birkett **Quick Reference:** Long, curved artery forceps.

Advanced Reference: Fine curved-tip artery forceps that are used during abdominal surgery, the fine tips being useful for clamping vessels and structures when dissecting the mesentery from the intestinal system.

Birmingham hip   **Quick Reference:** Also referred to as hip resurfacing.

Advanced Reference: With this procedure the ball of the hip is resurfaced with a metal shell rather than being removed and replaced. The socket is replaced as in traditional hip replacement but without cement.

Birth canal   **Quick Reference:** Relating to the passage through the uterine cervix.

Advanced Reference: The birth canal is the channel formed by the cervix, vagina and vulva through which the fetus is expelled during normal birth.

Bispectral index   **Quick Reference:** (BSI) Technique for assessing intraoperative awareness and depth of anaesthesia.

Advanced Reference: Involves the measurement of brain activity on a scale, with 100 signifying awake and 0 relating to electrical silence. A measurement of 40–65 is considered as suitable for absence of awareness during general anaesthesia.

Bisphosphonates   **Quick Reference:** Class of drugs that inhibit the resorption of bone.

Advanced Reference: A calcium-regulating agent used in the treatment of *osteoporosis*, bone cancers and *Paget's* disease. May be taken intravenously or orally, but when taken via the latter route they can cause stomach upset and erosion of the oesophagus.

Bite guard   **Quick Reference:** Also referred to as a bite-block, it is a device used to shield and protect the patient's teeth.

Advanced Reference: Usually made of silicone or rubber, bite guards are used primarily during intubation as well as during such procedures as electroconvulsive therapy (ECT). In all instances the intention of their use is to prevent injury to teeth, tongue and lips. Also, it is not uncommon for an oropharyngeal airway to be inserted during general anaesthesia with an intubated patient so as to act as a bite guard while additionally preventing the patient from biting-down and occluding the endotracheal tube.

Bi-valve   **Quick Reference:** Consisting of two similar separate parts.

Advanced Reference: Slang/colloquial term for splitting of a Plaster of Paris cast. Separating into two halves when either removing or leaving in place for continuing immobilisation/support then securing it in place with bandaging.

Bladder   **Quick Reference:** A sac or container able to hold a volume of fluid.

Advanced Reference: Involves mainly two anatomical structures, i.e. the urinary bladder and gall bladder. The former collects urine from the kidney; ureters then expel it to the exterior via the urethra. The latter is a component of the biliary system acting as a storage chamber for bile until it is expelled into the duodenum.

Bladder sand   **Quick Reference:** Term applied to small kidney stones.

Advanced Reference: The stones are formed primarily of calcium oxalate.

Blade Quick Reference: Refers to a scalpel blade.

Advanced Reference: Scalpel blades come in different sizes and shapes and are attached to a compatible handle such as a Bard Parker. Also refers to disposable scalpels.

Bleach Quick Reference: A generic term regularly used interchangeably with disinfectant.

Advanced Reference: Bleach can indicate a number of chemical forms and compounds. *Sodium hypochlorite* (NaOCl) is referred to as chlorine bleach while *hydrogen peroxide* (H_2O_2) is termed oxygen bleach, and sodium percarbonate is a peroxide-releasing compound also used in hair dyes.

Bleeding time Quick Reference: Test done to assess platelet function.

Advanced Reference: Normal values are between 2 and 9 min. This is dependent on a number of factors involving related conditions and current medication.

Blepharoplasty Quick Reference: Correction of excessive tissue of the eyelids.

Advanced Reference: Performed to reduce any excess/loose tissue from the upper and lower eyelids. Considered as a cosmetic procedure.

Blink Quick Reference: Rapid, reflex opening and closing of the eyelid.

Advanced Reference: We blink approximately 10–15 times every minute with each blink having a duration of 100–150 ms. The intention of blinking is to moisten and oxygenate the *cornea*.

Blood Quick Reference: Red fluid contained within the blood vessels.

Advanced Reference: Blood circulates via the heart and blood vessels, supplying oxygen and nutrients to all parts of the body. Consists of approximately 55% fluid and 45% solids (cells). Adult volume is about 5 litres. Blood plasma is the fluid part of the blood in which the cells are suspended and the fluid left after blood has clotted is called serum. Blood flow is defined as perfusion pressure divided by resistance ($P \div R$).

Blood–brain barrier Quick Reference: The membranes between the blood and brain.

Advanced Reference: A permeable membrane that supports movement of water, oxygen, carbon dioxide and other substances such as alcohol and drugs. Essentially, the blood–brain barrier maintains a distinctive separation of the blood from direct contact with the brain itself but supports the passage of essential substances.

Blood clotting Quick Reference: Indicates the solidifying of blood. *Coagulation*.

Advanced Reference: It is a natural mechanism in response to injury but, as well as happening externally in such cases, it can be brought about within the vessels, i.e. intravascular clotting (IVC) and *disseminated intravascular coagulation (DIC)*.

Blood gas analysis   **Quick Reference:** Blood gas measurement involves the analysis of heparinised fresh arterial blood.

Advanced Reference: The parameters measured are arterial blood oxygen and carbon dioxide partial pressure and the pH of arterial blood. From these, other parameters can be ascertained, for example bicarbonate, base excess.

Blood patch   **Quick Reference:** Carried out in an attempt to alleviate post-spinal headache following dural puncture. Also referred to as epidural blood patch (EBP).

Advanced Reference: Involves the injection of 10–20 ml of autologous venous blood injected into the extradural space immediately after removal from a peripheral vein with the intention of plugging the hole made by the dural puncture and so stopping the flow of cerebrospinal fluid and easing the potential for headache. Meticulous attention to sepsis is observed during blood collection and injection.

Blood poisoning   **Quick Reference:** A term used to signify the presence in the blood of bacteria, their *toxins* or infected matter.

Advanced Reference: Bacteraemia is the result of an infection with organisms virulent enough to invade the bloodstream and multiply there; *septicaemia* is the presence of their toxins and pyaemia is the release of fragments of an infected *clot* or *pus*.

Blood pressure   **Quick Reference:** Pressure exerted by the blood on the walls of the arteries.

Advanced Reference: Blood is driven through the arteries by the pressure and force of the heartbeat. The pressure is at its greatest when the heart contracts (systole) and lowest when it relaxes (*diastole*). Although standards and norms are quoted for adults and children, these can alter with factors such as age, disease state, fitness and emotion.

Blood products   **Quick Reference:** Refers to the products present in or obtained from donated blood.

Advanced Reference: Plasma-reduced blood or packed cells have had a portion of plasma removed in order to use it to provide fresh frozen plasma (FFP), platelets and factor VIII.

Blood sugar   **Quick Reference:** Amount of glucose in the circulating blood.

Advanced Reference: Expressed in millimoles per litre, the normal range is said to be 3.5–5.5 mmol/l.

Blood transfusion   **Quick Reference:** Indicates the transfer of blood or administration of donated blood.

Advanced Reference: May be donated from another person of the same blood group or by oneself (autotransfusion). Involves the administration of stored (or removed) blood into the circulatory system via a blood-giving set. Transfusion is carried out for a number of both medical and surgical reasons, e.g. blood loss, anaemia.

Blood warmer   **Quick Reference:** Device for warming transfused blood.

Advanced Reference: A number of designs are available (e.g. coil through warmed water, electric element), all intended to prevent the adverse effects of transfused blood taken straight from the fridge.

Blue baby   **Quick Reference:** Refers to a neonate born with *cyanosis*, which may be the result of a *congenital* cardiac or pulmonary defect that causes inadequate oxygenation of the blood.

Advanced Reference: May be due to either a large portion of the venous blood bypassing the lungs because of narrowing of the pulmonary artery, or profound anaemia following incompatibility between fetal and maternal blood when the infant's red cells are destroyed by *antibodies* in the mother's blood.

Blunt dissection   **Quick Reference:** The separation of tissues with an instrument that has no cutting ability.

Advanced Reference: Required around delicate structures such as nerves and blood vessels, and usually done with fingers or blunt forceps and scissors.

BMI   **Quick Reference:** Body mass index (BMI) of an individual can be used to calculate desirable weight and the obesity risk to health.

Advanced Reference: $BMI = \frac{weight\ (kg)}{height\ (m^2)}$

BNF   **Quick Reference:** *British National Formulary.*

Advanced Reference: Drugs and medicines catalogue. Includes descriptions, preparation, dosages/strengths, etc. of all medicines in current use in the UK.

Bobbin   **Quick Reference:** Constituent part of a gas flowmeter/rotameter on an anaesthetic machine or gas delivery system.

Advanced Reference: The bobbin is the measuring indicator within a flowmeter and alters as the needle valve is adjusted to provide more or less gas. The reading of gas flow is taken at the top of the bobbin.

Bodok seal   **Quick Reference:** A rubber washer with an outer metal circumference which acts as a seal where medical gas cylinders connect to anaesthetic machines.

Advanced Reference: They were first developed by the British Oxygen Company (BOC) and were designed primarily as a seal between the two metal surfaces of the cylinder head and yoke of the connection block but also assisted in reducing friction.

Bohr effect   **Quick Reference:** An effect by which there is an increase of carbon dioxide in the blood.

Advanced Reference: The outcome is a decrease in pH, which results in a decrease of the affinity of haemoglobin for oxygen.

Boiling point   **Quick Reference:** The temperature at which a substance changes from the liquid to the gaseous state.

Advanced Reference: Boiling point occurs when the vapour pressure of a liquid is equal to atmospheric pressure. This explains why water boils at a lower temperature at altitude, where air pressure is decreased. Is of relevance to the use of volatile anaesthetic agents and temperature-compensated vaporisers.

Boiling water   Quick Reference: Not considered now as a reliable sterilising method.

Advanced Reference: Is only a method of disinfection or pasteurisation as it cannot be guaranteed to kill spores and a host of other pathogenic organisms.

Bolsters   Quick Reference: Rubber or plastic lengths of tubing used with retention sutures.

Advanced Reference: The suture is fed through the bolster, bridging the wound in order to prevent cutting into the patient's skin.

Bolus   Quick Reference: A single, one-off dose.

Advanced Reference: Bolus can be referred to in two different contexts: (1) a bolus of food is soft after mastication and swallowed, (2) a bolus of drug for injection describes a single amount of medication given as one dose.

Bone marrow   Quick Reference: The internal substance of bones.

Advanced Reference: Red marrow is found in the skull, ribs, pelvis, sternum, vertebrae and the ends of long bones. It is actively involved in the production of red cells. Yellow marrow is full of fat and is the main constituent of long bones in adult life.

Bone nibblers   Quick Reference: A surgical instrument of heavy or fine design depending on need.

Advanced Reference: Used during orthopaedic or neurosurgery to remove (nibble) small pieces of bone.

Bone wax   Quick Reference: A haemostatic material.

Advanced Reference: Used mostly in neuro and spinal surgery on bleeding cancellous bone surfaces.

Botox®   Quick Reference: Trademark name for a preparation of Botulinum toxin type A.

Advanced Reference: Used to smooth facial wrinkles in cosmetic procedures as well as for muscle dystonia (abnormal tonicity of tissue), *strabismus* and blepharospasm.

Bougie   Quick Reference: (boo-gee) An intubation aid.

Advanced Reference: Name given to an adjunct originally made of *malleable* gum-elastic used as an intubation aid during *difficult intubation*. In the event of poor visualisation during laryngoscopy, the catheter Bougie is fed via the *vocal cords* into the *trachea* and the *endotracheal tube* (ETT) is introduced over it.

Bourdon   Quick Reference: A pressure gauge usually fitted to high-pressure cylinders, e.g. oxygen.

Advanced Reference: The gauge works on the Bourdon tube principle, namely that when pressure is exerted into a curved tube the end begins to straighten, thus manipulating the rack and the pivotal point of the needle to show the reading on calibrated markings.

Bovie cleaner   **Quick Reference:** Surgical instrument scraper. Also termed a scratch-pad.

Advanced Reference: A rough-surfaced pad used to clean the diathermy point during surgical procedures.

Bowel   **Quick Reference:** Refers to the intestines.

Advanced Reference: The bowel is commonly referred to as either the small or large intestines. The small bowel comprises the duodenum, jejunum, ileum and terminates at the ileo-caecal valve, where the large bowel begins and becomes the ascending colon, transverse colon, descending colon, sigmoid, rectum and anus.

Bowel clamp   **Quick Reference:** A surgical instrument used to occlude the bowel.

Advanced Reference: Bowel clamps are either crushing or non-crushing and are used in pairs during surgery. Some of the most common are Doyen and Payr's.

Bowie-Dick   **Quick Reference:** A test used to measure the efficiency of steam autoclaves.

Advanced Reference: Prior to the daily use of an autoclave the test is carried out and consists of placing a small section of paper, to which is adhered a cross of autoclave tape, between a pile of folded surgical drapes and putting it through a sterilising cycle. The tape should change colour, confirming penetration but not necessarily sterilisation.

Bowman's capsule   **Quick Reference:** Structure within the kidney nephron, proximal to the tubules.

Advanced Reference: Opening area of the nephron, a cup-shaped structure which surrounds the glomerulus.

Boyle-Davis gag   **Quick Reference:** Mouth gag used in throat surgery.

Advanced Reference: Used specifically in tonsillectomy and fitted between the teeth to keep the mouth open. Comes with both split and fixed tongue plates.

Boyle's   **Quick Reference:** Indicates a number of anaesthetic-related adjuncts and named after Henry Boyle, an English anaesthetist.

Advanced Reference: The standard anaesthetic machine is named after him and his early design and even though they have undergone much change, modern machines are still referred to as Boyle's. The Boyle's bottle is an early design of vaporiser that was designed for ether and has been superseded today by calibrated temperature-compensated vaporisers.

Brachial plexus   **Quick Reference:** A network of nerves at the root of the neck supplying the upper limbs.

Advanced Reference: The complex is formed chiefly by the lower four cervical nerves and the first thoracic nerve. Lies partly within the axilla and supplies nerves to the chest, shoulder and arm. It is one of the areas of injury risk related to poor patient positioning, especially when using a board for the outstretched arm, when placing the board at 90° or more to the table can lead to stretching of the plexus.

Brachytherapy   **Quick Reference:** Form of *radiotherapy*.

Advanced Reference: Involves the placement of a radioactive source within or close to the area requiring treatment, i.e. prostate, head and neck tumours.

Bradycardia   **Quick Reference:** Patient (adult) with a slow pulse rate below the level of 60 beats per minute (bpm).

Advanced Reference: Brady refers to slow and cardia the heart. A bradycardia can occur at any time but must not be confused in a patient who normally at rest has a relatively slow pulse, i.e. athletes or those on medication. Monitor the patient rather than the reading.

Bradykinin   **Quick Reference:** A *polypeptide* that forms from blood plasma *globulin*.

Advanced Reference: Is a potent vasodilator, which stimulates pain receptors and the contraction of smooth muscle, and is involved in the inflammatory process.

Brain   **Quick Reference:** Control centre of the central nervous system, contained within the skull.

Advanced Reference: The brain is a multifunction organ that has two hemispheres, with one for logical thinking and the other for abstract thinking. The brain receives and sends messages to all other systems. Areas of the brain include, the cerebrum, midbrain, cerebellum, medulla oblongata and pons Varolii.

Brain attack   **Quick Reference:** Increasingly used term for a stroke (cerebro-vascular accident or CVA).

Advanced Reference: The thinking is that the approach to transient ischaemic attacks (TIAs) and stroke should be similar to that of cardiac resuscitation, i.e. early intervention in an attempt to improve outcomes, much as cardiopulmonary resuscitation or CPR has done.

Brain death criteria   **Quick Reference:** Protocol designed to confirm irreversible brain death. Also referred to as brain death test.

Advanced Reference: Usually performed for patients on life support by two physicians over a set period.

Involves testing of vital reflexes, i.e. pupillary response (reaction to light and irritating the cornea to instigate a blink), gag/cough reflex (e.g. stimulation of the pharynx with a suction catheter), level of consciousness (by pressure and pinching/painful stimulus of sensitive areas such as the nose) and cold water injected into the ears to assess eye movement. Respiration viability is assessed lastly by switching off mechanical ventilation. As organs for donation may be involved, the criteria dictate that transplant surgeons should not be involved in the assessment.

Brainstem   **Quick Reference:** The enlarged extension of the spinal cord within the skull.

Advanced Reference: Consists of the *medulla oblongata, pons* and *midbrain*.

Brainstem death   **Quick Reference:** Permanent irreversible cessation of brain function.

Advanced Reference: Often confused with coma or vegetative state but, unlike these, brainstem death is a permanent state.

Breathing systems   **Quick Reference:** A term that describes the apparatus needed for gas flow to and from the patient.

Advanced Reference: These involve anaesthetic circuits of many designs as well as those used with ventilators and the non-rebreathing types used in resuscitation, i.e. Ambu and Bag-Valve-Mask (BVM).

Breech   **Quick Reference:** Indicates buttocks first.

Advanced Reference: Applies to the lie/position of the fetus in the uterus when it presents buttocks first rather than the normal head first.

Bretylium   **Quick Reference:** (bret-eel-e-um) An antihypertensive and antiarrhythmic drug. Bretylate.

Advanced Reference: Used primarily to treat cardiac dysrhythmias and tachycardia.

Brietal   **Quick Reference:** Anaesthetic induction agent. Alternative name is methohexitone.

Advanced Reference: A short-acting induction agent available as a powder for reconstitution with water into a 1% solution. Causes hiccoughing and contraindicated in epilepsy. Mostly now been replaced by the use of *Diprivan® (propofol)*.

British Horse Power   **Quick Reference:** BHP. Unit of power in British engineering.

Advanced Reference: 1 BHP = 550 foot pounds-force per second or 745.7 watts. Brake Horse Power is a measure of an engine's horse power without the loss in power caused by the likes of the gearbox and generator.

Brittle bone disease   **Quick Reference:** Osteogenesis imperfecta, also referred to as OI.

Advanced Reference: Disease which runs in families signified by higher than normal bone fracture incidence. An absence or reduced level of collagen is thought to be part of the cause.

Broad ligaments   **Quick Reference:** Ligaments related to attachment of the female uterus.

Advanced Reference: The broad ligaments support the blood vessels to the uterus and uterine tubes and consist of folds of peritoneum which extend from the uterus to the sides of the pelvis.

Bronchial blocker   **Quick Reference:** Design of tracheal tube used in thoracic surgery to isolate one lung or a portion thereof.

Advanced Reference: Term also used broadly to indicate endobronchial and double-lumen tubes such as Robert-Shaw, Gordon-Greene and Carlins.

Bronchitis   **Quick Reference:** Inflammation of the bronchi.

Advanced Reference: May be *acute* or *chronic* and the infection may be caused by bacteria or a virus.

Bronchodilator   **Quick Reference:** Any agent that relaxes the smooth muscles of the bronchial passages.

Advanced Reference: There are many causes of spasm and closure of the bronchial muscles, most common are asthma and bronchitis. Best known bronchodilators are salbutamol and aminophylline.

Bronchomalacia   **Quick Reference:** (bronco-mal-ace-ea) Deficiency in the cartilaginous wall of the bronchus.

Advanced Reference: Often accompanied by a degree of tracheomalacia (softness of the tracheal cartilage) which may lead to *atelectasis* or obstructive *emphysema*.

Bronchopleural fistula   **Quick Reference:** Abnormal connection between the tracheobronchial tree and the pleura.

Advanced Reference: Occurs after surgery (pneumonectomy), following trauma, infection or damage due to tumour.

Bronchoscopy   **Quick Reference:** Procedure for visually examining the trachea, main bronchus and lung.

Advanced Reference: Carried out using either fibre-optic or rigid broncho-scope. Usually under general anaesthesia when ventilation is maintained using a Venturi injector.

Bronchospasm   **Quick Reference:** (bronco-spasm) Narrowing of the bronchi.

Advanced Reference: Narrowing is due to muscular contraction because of a stimulus such as happens in *asthma* and *bronchitis*. May be relieved by the administration of *bronchodilator* drugs.

Bronchus   **Quick Reference:** Windpipe or bronchial tube.

Advanced Reference: The bronchi refer to the two primary divisions of the trachea that lead, respectively, into the right and left lung.

Brooks airway   **Quick Reference:** Type of oropharyngeal airway.

Advanced Reference: An airway designed for use in mouth-to-mouth resuscitation but allows for non-contact between rescuer and victim. It has a mouth guard/cover which is designed to form an airtight seal. Has been replaced by a number of designs including the Laerdal Pocket mask™.

Brown fat   **Quick Reference:** Specialised adipose tissue involved in the generation of heat.

Advanced Reference: Of special importance in neonates. Distributed throughout the body (mainly upper back and shoulder area) of the newborn, it allows for an increase in the metabolism and thus heat production, while simultaneously using up the fat itself.

Bruit   Quick Reference: Alternatively referred to as a ***murmur***.

Advanced Reference: Is a noise heard via a stethoscope and is due to turbulent blood flow within the heart and larger blood vessels.

Buccal   Quick Reference: Pertaining to the mouth or cheek.

Advanced Reference: The buccal cavity is the mouth and consists of two parts, the outer or vestibule, which is the space outside of the teeth and within the lips and cheeks, and the inner part which communicates with the oropharynx.

Bucket-Handle movement   Quick Reference: Relates to the chest and rib-cage movement during breathing.

Advanced Reference: Specifically relates to the upward and outward movement of the rib cage in the manner of a bucket handle being lifted for carrying. In children the anterior/posterior expansion of the chest is limited due to the rib shape, therefore they may lack this movement.

Buffer   Quick Reference: A solution in which the concentration of hydrogen ions remains constant despite the addition of an alkali or acid.

Advanced Reference: Sodium bicarbonate is the body's chief buffering system.

Bulimia   Quick Reference: (bul-eem-ea) Eating disorder associated with a fear of becoming fat.

Advanced Reference: Depressive illness linked to ***anorexia nervosa***, characterised by bouts of over-eating and a craving for food followed by intervals of starvation and involving self-induced vomiting and excessive purging.

Bullard laryngoscope   Quick Reference: Rigid *fibre-optic* scope.

Advanced Reference: An aid in ***difficult intubation*** situations, the design helps with visualisation of the glottic opening when there is an inability to align the oral, pharyngeal and laryngeal axis. Compared to conventional direct laryngoscopes this design requires minimal head and neck movement so is of value in situations involving cervical spine injury as well as for patients with minimal mouth-opening ability. The design also allows for oxygen ***insufflation*** via the suction port. Inserted in the neutral head position, the blade tip retracts the ***epiglottis*** and allows for the endotracheal tube to be fed over the integral ***stylette***.

Bulldog   Quick Reference: A surgical clamp used primarily in vascular surgery.

Advanced Reference: A small vascular clamp designed to hold the vessel securely but without causing trauma.

Bundle branch block   Quick Reference: An irregularity in the cardiac conduction system.

Advanced Reference: Involves a delay in conduction along either side (right or left) of the atrioventricular (AV) bundle and related to heart block; detected on an ECG trace.

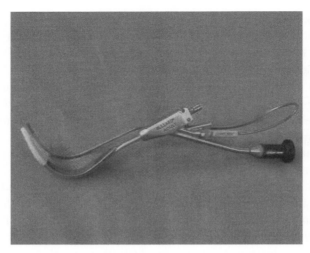

Fig. 3. Bullard laryngoscope used with permission. http://vam.anest.ufl.edu

Bundle of His **Quick Reference:** Large collection of neuromuscular fibres that pass through the middle of the heart (septum).

Advanced Reference: The Bundle of His starts with the atrioventricular node that collects the electrical activity generated by the sinoatrial node. The electrical charge is transmitted down and through the fibres and then brings about contraction within the ventricles.

Bung **Quick Reference:** A rubber end or plastic cap that is used to close off the end of an intravenous cannula.

Advanced Reference: Bungs can also be found as caps on blood bottles. Leur-lock caps can be referred to as bungs.

Bunion **Quick Reference:**. A deformity of the joint at the base of the big toe.

Advanced Reference: Caused by friction and pressure from shoes, forming a bursa. Severe forms require surgery, with the operation being termed hallux valgus. A bursa is a fibrous sac lined with synovial membrane and contains a small quantity of synovial fluid.

Bupivacaine **Quick Reference:** A local anaesthetic agent that has a longer action than *lignocaine*.

Advanced Reference: Bupivacaine has a slow onset of action but has the distinct advantage of lasting longer than most alternative local agents. Often used for skin infiltration around a wound site to give a degree of pain relief following surgery. Heavy marcain is a form of bupivacaine with glucose added to use for spinal anaesthetic.

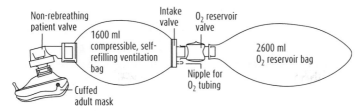

Child (Intended for patients between 7 and 30 kg)
Flow rate of 10 l/min required to deliver an O_2 concentration of 90%–95%.

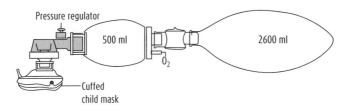

Infant (Intended for patients weighing less than 7 kg)
Low rate of 5 l/min required to deliver an O_2 concentration of 90%–95%.

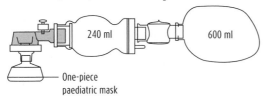

Benefits
• Creates an artificial barrier between the arrest victim & the rescuer, thus reducing the risk of contact with potentially infectious vomitus, saliva & blood.

• When connected to an oxygen supply, allows delivery of high concentrations of oxygen (90%–95% O_2) with an appropriate flow rate

Adult (Intended for patients over 30 kg)
Flow rate of 15 l/min required to deliver an O_2 concentration of 90%–95%.

Fig. 4. (cont.)

Burette **Quick Reference:** Piece of infusion equipment.
  Advanced Reference: A measuring chamber which attaches to the IV fluid bag or giving set allowing monitored infusion volumes. Used when volume and dose are critical, i.e. paediatrics and drug administration.

Burr **Quick Reference:** Surgical drill bit.
  Advanced Reference: Used for drilling or cutting bone and teeth. A burr hole is drilled into the skull to relieve pressure inside the cranium.

Bursa **Quick Reference:** Small fibrous sac containing *synovial* fluid.

Advanced Reference: Intended to reduce friction where structures move over one another, i.e. around joints, between a tendon and a bone, although they can also be formed in some locations by friction and pressure.

Buscopan®   **Quick Reference:** Antispasmodic drug used to relax the intestinal wall.

Advanced Reference: Buscopan® is the trade name of hyoscine butylbromide. The drug is usually given 20–30 min prior to a patient's having a gastroscopy or a sigmoidoscopy. Relaxing the intestines allows greater flexibility for the scope to be advanced through the intestinal system, avoiding trauma. Provides for a lighter relief of pain during the diagnostic procedure.

Butterfly needle   **Quick Reference:** A type of intravenous access needle.

Advanced Reference: Has plastic side wings which act as a grip for insertion and an anchor on the skin when laid flat. Available in a range of sizes and gauges.

Butyrophenones   **Quick Reference:** Class of antipsychotic agent.

Advanced Reference: They are potent *neuroleptics*. The prototype of the group was haloperidol.

BVM   **Quick Reference:** Bag-valve-mask. A self-inflating breathing circuit.

Advanced Reference: Used mainly for resuscitation purposes, and has more or less replaced the Ambu-bag. Can be used remotely when it delivers 21% oxygen (atmosphere); attached to an oxygen supply, where it can deliver up to 60%; or with an additional reservoir, which allows for approximately 95% being delivered.

Bypass   **Quick Reference:** Indicates diversion of flow from the normal route.

Advanced Reference: Can refer to *cardiopulmonary* bypass as used in open cardiac surgery, aorta-bifemoral bypass in vascular surgery and when using a shunt in carotid artery bypass.

C

CABG **Quick Reference:** Coronary artery bypass graft. Referred to as cabbage.

Advanced Reference: A surgical procedure to bypass diseased and blocked coronary arteries using the patient's own veins, usually the saphenous from the leg.

Cachexia **Quick Reference:** A profound state of general ill-health and malnutrition.

Advanced Reference: Characterised by loss of appetite, weight loss, muscle wasting. Commonly occurs during chronic illness.

Cadaver **Quick Reference:** A corpse.

Advanced Reference: Refers to a dead body used for dissection or harvesting of organs.

Caecostomy **Quick Reference:** Surgical creation of an artificial opening between the caecum and abdominal wall.

Advanced Reference: A constructed connection between the first part of the large intestine and the exterior via an opening or *stoma* in the abdominal wall. Also referred to as typhoplasty.

Caecum **Quick Reference:** (see-cum) First part of the large intestine.

Advanced Reference: Lies in the lower right side of the abdominal cavity. The appendix opens off the caecum.

Caesarean section **Quick Reference:** Delivery of a baby through an abdominal incision.

Advanced Reference: Performed for a variety of reasons and conditions, e.g. fetal distress and placenta praevia. There is continuing debate about the origins of the name. One view is that Julius Caesar was born via this method, whereas another states that it stems from a dictate issued by Caesar proclaiming that all women dying during childbirth should be cut open in order to save the life of the baby.

Caffeine **Quick Reference:** An *alkaloid* found in tea, coffee and plants.

Advanced Reference: A weak stimulant to the nervous system which also has *diuretic* properties.

Calcium **Quick Reference:** Metallic element.

Advanced Reference: Calcium levels in the blood are approximately 0.01%. A deficiency or excess can seriously disturb the function of nerve cells and muscle fibres. Calcium is also necessary in the blood clotting process. The correct concentration is maintained by the action of hormones of the *parathyroid* gland.

Calcium antagonist **Quick Reference:** Group of drugs used as antihypertensives. More correctly termed calcium channel blockers.

Advanced Reference: Used in the treatment of hypertension, they act by reducing calcium entry into heart cells, which then reduces the force of the heartbeat and therefore lowers blood pressure (BP).

Calcium oxalate **Quick Reference:** (CaC_2O_4) A salt of oxalic acid.

Advanced Reference: High levels in the urine lead to *calculus* formation.

Calculus **Quick Reference:** Stone. A hard insoluble mass. The term calculi indicates an accumulation of stones.

Advanced Reference: Calculi (stones) are formed from substances normally soluble in body fluids but which accumulate and form a mass that can go on to cause obstruction to function. Common sites are kidneys, bladder, gall bladder and salivary glands.

Caldwell-Luc **Quick Reference:** Surgical procedure to drain the maxillary sinus.

Advanced Reference: Also referred to as antrostomy. Involves the creation of an opening through the upper jaw opposite to the second molar tooth.

Calibrate **Quick Reference:** To calculate or correlate readings with a set standard.

Advanced Reference: Can refer to calibration of manometers (mechanical, electronic, digital), a transducer used for measuring such parameters as central venous pressure. Invasive arterial reading is calibrated to atmosphere before connecting to a patient as this sets a constant standard.

Calliper **Quick Reference:** A two-pronged device used to exert traction.

Advanced Reference: Used as part of a traction apparatus when treating bone fractures, especially those of the lower limb. A calliper can also be a measuring instrument used in engineering.

Callus **Quick Reference:** Hard substance formed at the site of a broken bone.

Advanced Reference: Callus collects around and between the bone ends. When a bone is fractured, *osteoblasts* multiply and form irregular bone, which knits the ends together as new bone develops.

Calorie **Quick Reference:** Unit of energy.

Advanced Reference: By definition, it is the amount of heat required to warm 1 kg of water by 1°C. The calorie (calorific) value of food is the number of calories it would yield if it were completely burnt.

Calorimetry **Quick Reference:** Measurement of the amount of heat absorbed or given out.

Advanced Reference: A calorimeter is the apparatus used to measure heat flow.

Canal **Quick Reference:** Passageway.

Advanced Reference: Examples are the anal canal and auditory canal.

Cancellous **Quick Reference:** Indicates a lattice-like bone structure.

Advanced Reference: During bone development and in the consolidation phase of fracture repair, cancellous bone is laid down by osteoblasts.

Cancer   **Quick Reference:** A disorder of cell growth.

Advanced Reference: A carcinogen is any substance liable or able to cause cancer. The term carcinoma is used generally but actually indicates cancers arising in or covering membranes.

Candela   **Quick Reference:** SI unit of luminosity.

Advanced Reference: A measure of the intensity of luminosity.

Canine   **Quick Reference:** Third tooth from the midline of each jaw. Also termed the eye tooth.

Advanced Reference: There are therefore four canines, two in each jaw, in both the *deciduous* and *permanent* teeth.

Cannulation   **Quick Reference:** To make access to a vessel, with a cannula.

Advanced Reference: Term most commonly used in relation to the insertion of an intravenous cannula. Can also indicate entry to an artery and several other invasive techniques. Often used interchangeably with catheterisation but this tends to involve a longer device, i.e. CVP line or as in bladder catheterisation via the urethra.

Canthoplasty   **Quick Reference:** Surgery of the eyelid where the canthal tendon is either reconstructed or strengthened (canthopexy).

Advanced Reference: The procedure is designed to strengthen the tissues at the outer corner of the eyelid and so give improved support.

Capacitance   **Quick Reference:** To store. Stored electrical charge.

Advanced Reference: Something with capacitance has the ability (capacity) to retain an electrical charge. A capacitor consists of a conductor separated by an insulator and so prevents (stores) flow of (direct-DC) current and maintains it ready for discharge. A defibrillator is charged to the required energy (joules) ready to deliver the shock and the capacitor stores the energy which is then delivered as and when required.

Capillary   **Quick Reference:** Smallest blood vessel.

Advanced Reference: A minute vessel which is the pathway between an arteriole and venule. It is in the capillary that the blood and the tissue fluids exchange gases, food and waste products.

Capnograph   **Quick Reference:** A device which displays carbon dioxide (CO_2) concentration.

Advanced Reference: Capnography utilises *infrared* light absorption to measure carbon dioxide, usually end-tidal CO_2, when it is displayed in both numerical and wave form. End-tidal CO_2 approximates to alveolar partial pressure of CO_2 (PCO_2), which in turn indicates arterial CO_2 tension. Capnometry indicates measurement only or the reading of carbon dioxide.

Capsule   **Quick Reference:** Fibrous *sheath* enclosing an organ.

Advanced Reference: The tough flexible casing of a joint strengthened with ligaments and lined with synovial membrane.

Caput medusa Quick Reference: Term used to describe a bluish-purple discoloration of the skin around a *stoma*.

Advanced Reference: Caused by dilation of the *cutaneous* veins.

Carbohydrate Quick Reference: Substance which includes *carbon, oxygen* and *hydrogen*. [Chemical formula – $C_X(H_2O)$.]

Advanced Reference: There are many carbohydrates and they form the sugar and starchy components of food. They are broken down to provide energy, being metabolised to water and *carbon dioxide*.

Carbolic acid Quick Reference: Phenol.

Advanced Reference: One of the first antiseptics. Still used as a standard to measure newer germicides.

Carbon Quick Reference: Non-metallic element.

Advanced Reference: Numerous pieces of theatre-related equipment are impregnated with carbon intended as a conductor for static electricity, i.e. anaesthetic tubing and trolley wheels.

Carbon dioxide Quick Reference: Colourless gas which is found at 0.038% in atmospheric air. A product of body metabolism. Chemical formula CO_2.

Advanced Reference: Formed following the metabolism of oxygen in the body and carried via the blood and plasma in the veins to the lungs where it forms approximately 3%–4% of expired air. When dissolved in water, forms carbonic acid.

Carbon monoxide Quick Reference: Chemical formula CO. Colourless, odourless gas formed by the incomplete burning of fuels. Most common example is car exhaust.

Advanced Reference: When inhaled, it combines with the *haemoglobin* much more readily than oxygen and thus leads to carbon monoxide poisoning, which is a type of *asphyxia*. However, it produces a bright pink complexion (cherry-red) rather than the blue appearance (*cyanosis*) associated with lack of oxygen in the tissues.

Carboxyhaemoglobin Quick Reference: *Haemoglobin* combined with *carbon monoxide*.

Advanced Reference: Most significant during use of a pulse oximeter when readings can be misleading as a higher oxygen saturation reading is displayed.

Carcinoma Quick Reference: From the Greek, Karkinoma and Karkinos (crab). Used as a term to denote *cancer*.

Advanced Reference: A malignant growth made up of *epithelial* cells tending to infiltrate the surrounding tissues. A carcinogen is any substance that may instigate cancer. Carcinogenesis indicates the growth and progress of a cancer cell from a normal cell.

Cardex Quick Reference: Equipment/procedure preference cards for individual doctors.

Advanced Reference: System for recording both surgeon and anaesthetist requirements for individual procedures.

Cardiac arrest   **Quick Reference:** Cessation of the heartbeat/output.

Advanced Reference: Indicates sudden cardiac/circulatory stoppage. Signs include cyanosis, apnoea, absent pulse. Treatment is immediate institution of *CPR*.

Cardiac catheterisation   **Quick Reference:** Passage of a catheter under X-ray guidance through a vein until it reaches the heart. Access is via the cutaneous route with the femoral being a common vessel for this purpose.

Advanced Reference: Used in the diagnosis and treatment of heart disease and related conditions, i.e. coronary angioplasty.

Cardiac cycle   **Quick Reference:** The period between one heartbeat and the next.

Advanced Reference: In adults this period lasts approximately less than a second (0.8 s) and takes in contraction of the atria ($\times 2$) and ventricles ($\times 2$) and expulsion of the circulation into the aorta.

Cardiac massage   **Quick Reference:** Manual compression of the heart. Can be internal as well as external.

Advanced Reference: Rhythmic compression of the heart performed in order to re-establish or sustain sufficient circulation. External cardiac massage involves compression of the heart between the sternum and spinal column; internal is direct handling and squeezing of the organ.

Cardiac output   **Quick Reference:** Volume of blood expelled from the heart (each minute).

Advanced Reference: Is dependent on stroke volume (litres) and heart rate, i.e. = stroke volume $\times$ heart rate (bpm), where bpm = beats per minute.

Cardiology   **Quick Reference:** Speciality dealing with cardiac conditions and care.

Advanced Reference: A cardiologist is a physician who specialises in disease of the cardiac system. As many related procedures are now non-invasive or performed under X-ray control these are carried out by the cardiologist, e.g. cardiac catheterisation.

Cardiomyopathy   **Quick Reference:** A chronic disorder of the heart muscle.

Advanced Reference: A general diagnostic term indicating a primary disease of the heart often of obscure or unknown origin, hence why the term is used in such a broad manner.

Cardiomyoplasty   **Quick Reference:** Surgical procedure where the patient's own body muscle is wrapped around the heart to provide support for a weakened, damaged and failing heart.

Advanced Reference: Usually the back muscle (latissimus dorsil) is used and for some time is connected to a pulse generator which is triggered to copy the heart muscle contraction.

Cardiopulmonary   Quick Reference: Relating to the heart and lungs.

Advanced Reference: Term applied to many activities related to heart and lung conditions, i.e. cardiopulmonary resuscitation (CPR), cardiopulmonary bypass.

Cardiopulmonary bypass   Quick Reference: A form of *extracorporeal* circulation used in cardiac surgery.

Advanced Reference: Diversion of the flow of blood from the heart directly to the *aorta* via a pump oxygenator (*Heart–lung machine*) therefore bypassing the heart and *lungs.*

Cardiovascular   Quick Reference: Terminology relating to the heart and blood vessels.

Advanced Reference: Takes in the systemic and pulmonary circulations and the entire network of veins and arteries throughout the body.

Cardioversion   Quick Reference: Application of synchronised DC electric current to restore normal cardiac sinus rhythm.

Advanced Reference: Use of the defibrillator at varying energy levels to treat atrial flutter/fibrillation, ventricular tachycardia and supraventricular tachycardia. The defibrillator is synchronised to deliver the shock to coincide with the R-wave of the ECG trace, as delivering it during the repolarisation phase can induce ventricular fibrillation.

Care pathway   Quick Reference: A hospital-wide multi-professional approach to patient care. Standardised holistic care.

Advanced Reference: Theoretically should involve all necessary professional disciplines playing their part in the patient's hospital stay, the objective being to deliver standardised quality care.

Care plan   Quick Reference: A tool for planning patient care during the perioperative phase of their treatment. Individualised care.

Advanced Reference: A care plan will help staff assess, plan, implement and evaluate the operative needs of each patient.

Caries   Quick Reference: Decay and death of a bone.

Advanced Reference: Most commonly applied to teeth.

Carotene   Quick Reference: Natural red-yellow pigment found in many dark-green, yellow and leafy vegetables.

Advanced Reference: Is fat soluble and converted to *vitamin A* by enzyme action in the intestinal wall and liver.

Carotenoid   Quick Reference: Any of a group of pigments that are tallow to deep red in colour.

Advanced Reference: Examples are *carotene* and *lycopene.*

Carotid   Quick Reference: Usually refers to the main artery of the neck/head.

Advanced Reference: The carotid artery supplies the head and brain with blood. It has two branches, i.e. the external and internal carotid arteries.

Carpal tunnel syndrome **Quick Reference:** Syndrome related to the wrist. Chronic wrist pain.

Advanced Reference: Compression of the median nerve at the wrist which causes pain, paraesthesia, tingling and numbness in the fingers and muscle weakness in the forearm and hand. Carpal tunnel release or decompression is the surgical procedure used to correct the disorder and involves dividing the transverse carpal ligament, whether performed via an open or endoscopic technique.

Carter-Braine **Quick Reference:** Patient arm support used during surgery.

Advanced Reference: Type of support used for the upper arm when the patient is placed in the lateral position for such procedures as hip replacement and kidney surgery. Precautions should be taken to minimise the risk of the patient's touching the metal section of the support.

Cartilage **Quick Reference:** Gristle, a tough supporting bodily tissue.

Advanced Reference: The majority of bones are originally formed from cartilage and when the bone is fully developed, the cartilage remains at the bone ends only, forming an articulating surface.

Cast **Quick Reference:** Piece of material moulded into a required shape.

Advanced Reference: Usually refers to a Plaster of Paris (POP) cast.

CAT or CT **Quick Reference:** Computerised axial tomography; a CAT scan.

Advanced Reference: An image taken to show structures lying in a selected plane of the body. Along with X-rays and magnetic resonance imaging (MRI), one of three main imaging systems used as diagnostic tools. Originally used to examine the brain but is now utilised for the entire body. As X-rays are limited, especially in being able to pick up minor changes, the CT scan, by feeding images into a computer and creating a reconstructed image, is able to identify minor changes not possible with X-ray.

Catabolism **Quick Reference:** A chemical breakdown of substances in the body.

Advanced Reference: A chemical process by which complex substances are broken down to form simpler substances, and with it the release of energy.

Catalyst **Quick Reference:** Substance which brings about a chemical change.

Advanced Reference: More precisely, brings about a change without undergoing a change itself. Enzymes are an example of a catalyst.

Cataract **Quick Reference:** Opacity of the lens of the eye.

Advanced Reference: Causes dimness in vision and if not treated may lead to complete loss of vision. Correction involves removal of the lens, and with it the ability to focus. Often an artificial lens is implanted in place of the natural one.

Catecholamines **Quick Reference:** Group of agents having *sympathomimetic action*.

Advanced Reference: Examples are *dopamine*, norepinephrine (*noradrenaline*) and epinephrine (*adrenaline*).

Catgut   **Quick Reference:** A suture material made from the intestines of sheep. However, no longer used due to the potentially related problems of bovine spongiform encephalopathy (BSE).

Advanced Reference: Suture or ligature material, woven into different strengths. Available as a plain catgut or as one treated with chromic acid (chromic catgut) which extended its absorption time.

Catheter mount   **Quick Reference:** Anaesthetic adjunct that connects the endotracheal tube to circuit tubing.

Advanced Reference: Use much less now, following introduction of the laryngeal mask airway, and not part of the circuit where uncut endotracheal tubes are the norm.

Cation   **Quick Reference:** Ion with a positive charge.

Advanced Reference: Due to the positive charge, a cation moves towards a cathode in the presence of an electric field (electrolysis).

Cauda equina   **Quick Reference:** Terminal end of the spinal cord.

Advanced Reference: Tail-like appendage which contains the bundle of sacral and lumbar nerves.

Caudal   **Quick Reference:** Towards the back or tail.

Advanced Reference: A regional anaesthetic technique produced by injection of local anaesthetic into the caudal or sacral canal.

Cautery   **Quick Reference:** An instrument used to seal a bleeding point during surgery.

Advanced Reference: A surgical instrument which applies heat to tissues in order to arrest bleeding. A function of the diathermy machine along with a separate or combined cutting facility.

Cavity   **Quick Reference:** A walled/enclosed area within the body.

Advanced Reference: A well-defined space within the body, e.g. chest cavity, abdominal cavity and pelvic cavity.

c.c.   **Quick Reference:** Cubic centimetre.

Advanced Reference: As a measurement, millilitre (ml) is the more exact term.

CCF   **Quick Reference:** Congestive cardiac failure.

Advanced Reference: Describes the state in which there is both right and left ventricular failure combined with systemic and pulmonary symptoms.

CDH   **Quick Reference:** Congenital dislocation of hip.

Advanced Reference: Deformity resulting from developmental abnormality. Involves failure in development and thus the fit/seating of the head of the femur and acetabulum.

Cefotaxime   **Quick Reference:** Broad-spectrum antibiotic. Proprietary preparation is called Claforan®.

Advanced Reference: One of the cephalosporins used to treat a wide range of bacterial infections. Cefuroxime is another of this group with similar actions and is used in the treatment of upper respiratory tract and urinary tract infections.

Cell   **Quick Reference:** A single-cell unit from which the body is constructed.

Advanced Reference: A microscopic single-celled mass made up of protoplasm, a nucleus and cytoplasm, which is able to reproduce itself by *mitosis*.

Cell salvage   **Quick Reference:** Perioperative use of patient's own blood. An *autologous* blood transfusion.

Advanced Reference: Intra-surgical blood loss is collected and reused after passing through a process that involves centrifugal cell separation.

Cellulite   **Quick Reference:** (sel-u-lite) Deposits of fat.

Advanced Reference: Occurs usually in pockets just under the skin with the hips, thighs and buttocks being most commonly affected.

Cellulitis   **Quick Reference:** Inflammation of cellular tissue.

Advanced Reference: Commonly due to infection by streptococci, usually from infected/contaminated wounds. Treated with antibiotics and/or sulphonamides.

Cellulose   **Quick Reference:** (cell-u-lows) A type of carbohydrate.

Advanced Reference: Composed of glucose chains and makes up the cell walls of many plants. Not easily or readily digested by humans but is an important source of dietary fibre.

Celsius   **Quick Reference:** Temperature-measuring scale. Formerly referred to as centigrade. Named after Andreas Celsius.

Advanced Reference: Scale originally based on the melting point of ice which is 0 °C and the boiling point of water, taken as 100 °C. Now in universal use and referred to as the Celsius scale.

Cement   **Quick Reference:** Refers to bone cement used in orthopaedic surgery.

Advanced Reference: Bone cement is not an adhesive but functions by filling up a space and so forming a better mechanical fit. Most common cements are acrylic. Prepared at the time of need (during surgery) by mixing a liquid, which contains a monomer and stabiliser, with a powder that includes a catalyst to initiate polymerisation. Also included is a radio-opaque material and an antibiotic. Known to cause a reaction (anaphylactoid) which can lead to severe hypotension upon application.

Centesis   **Quick Reference:** (sen-tee-sis) Denotes to puncture or perforate.

Advanced Reference: Amniocentesis is puncture and biopsy of *amniotic* fluid from the *uterus*.

Centilitre   **Quick Reference:** (symbol cl) Metric unit of volume.

Advanced Reference: Equal to one-hundredth of a litre.

Central nervous system   **Quick Reference:** (CNS) The *brain* and spinal cord.

Advanced Reference: It is responsible for the integration of all nervous activities. Does not indicate the *peripheral* and *autonomic nervous systems*.

Central veins **Quick Reference:** Term used to indicate the larger and accessible veins as compared to the smaller peripheral vessels.

Advanced Reference: Namely the vena cava (inferior and superior), internal and external jugular, subclavian and femoral. Used mainly for CVP insertion, whereas the more peripheral *basilic*, cephalic and median veins are used for intravenous cannulation.

Centrifuge **Quick Reference:** A machine used for separating materials of different densities and particles suspended in a liquid.

Advanced Reference: When the centrifuge spins at high speed (approx. 50 000 rpm+), particles are forced outwards and downwards. Used commonly in haematology laboratories for separating blood and blood products.

Cephalic **Quick Reference:** (cef-alic) Pertaining to the head.

Advanced Reference: Cephalagia = headache. The cephalic index is the relation of the length of the head to its breadth.

Cerclage **Quick Reference:** Encircling of a part with a ring or loop.

Advanced Reference: A common example would be suturing of the non-competent uterus.

Cerebellum **Quick Reference:** The hindbrain.

Advanced Reference: Situated behind the brainstem, it is involved with balance, muscle tone and coordination of movement.

Cerebral **Quick Reference:** Of or relating to the *cerebrum*.

Advanced Reference: The cerebral *hemispheres* are the two lateral halves of the cerebrum. Cerebral *palsy* is a disability caused by brain damage before, during or immediately after birth resulting in poor muscle coordination.

Cerebrovascular accident **Quick Reference:** CVA. Referred to as a stroke.

Advanced Reference: Caused by a haemorrhage, thrombus or embolus, often leaving the sufferer paralysed down one side.

Cerebrum **Quick Reference:** The largest part of the brain.

Advanced Reference: Includes the two cerebral hemispheres but sometimes used to indicate the brain as a whole.

Cervarix™ **Quick Reference:** *Cervical* cancer vaccine.

Advanced Reference: Prevents the virus that leads to most cases of cervical cancer.

Cervical **Quick Reference:** Of the neck.

Advanced Reference: Pertaining to the region, e.g. cervical spine.

Cervical smear **Quick Reference:** A diagnostic test for cervical cancer.

Advanced Reference: Involves the sampling of cells from the neck of the womb which are then stained and examined under a microscope in order to form a diagnosis of malignancy or pre-malignancy.

Cervix **Quick Reference:** The adjoining neck-like structure between the *vagina* and cavity of the uterus.

Advanced Reference: Measures approximately 2 cm in length and is capable of variations in dilatation to accommodate childbirth.

CETP inhibitors **Quick Reference:** Class of drug being used in the fight against heart disease caused by high *cholesterol* levels.

Advanced Reference: CETP (cholesterol ester transfer protein). They are thought to encourage good cholesterol (high-density lipoproteins or HDLs) and regulate the size of cholesterol particles, which influences the formation of *plaque* in the arteries.

Cetrimide **Quick Reference:** A detergent with antiseptic properties.

Advanced Reference: Cetrimide is often combined with chlorhexidine and used as a skin preparation.

CFCs **Quick Reference:** Chlorofluorocarbons.

Advanced Reference: Class of chemicals containing carbon, hydrogen, chlorine and fluorine. Originally used as propellants and solvents as well as cooling agents in fridges. Mostly banned or discontinued now due to their detrimental effect on the ozone layer and contribution to global warming.

Chelate (Chelator) **Quick Reference:** Chemical compound containing a metal *ion*. Substance that combines particular ions, removing them from a solution.

Advanced Reference: Chelating agents are used in metal poisoning. The metal binds to the chelating agent and is excreted safely from the body.

Chemo-Brain **Quick Reference:** Slang term related to *chemotherapy*.

Advanced Reference: Refers to the suspected effects of chemotherapy drugs which include seizures and memory loss.

Chemotherapy **Quick Reference:** A chemical agent used to arrest the progress of, or to eradicate, a disease. Most commonly associated with cancer treatment.

Advanced Reference: This group of agents can be administered orally, intramuscularly or intravenously. They are intended to have a detrimental effect on the diseased area without causing irreversible injury to healthy tissue. Involves mainly the cytotoxic and sulphonamide groups.

Cheyne–Stokes respiration **Quick Reference:** A pattern of breathing found in patients in a deep coma or close to dying.

Advanced Reference: Instead of a normal breathing rhythm, there is a cycle wherein breaths become slower until they stop, then speed up before decreasing again.

Chin support **Quick Reference:** Device used to support the chin during general anaesthesia (GA).

Advanced Reference: Involves a spatula or similar implement used in conjunction with a head-harness (*Clausen*), which then supports the jaw and maintains the open airway during spontaneous breathing mask anaesthesia. Mostly obsolete now due to the use of the *laryngeal mask airway (LMA)*.

Chlamydia Quick Reference: (clam-id-ea) Type of micro-organism.

Advanced Reference: Classified as a bacteria but has virus-like behaviour in that it can only multiply within cells. Responsible for a number of diseases, e.g. trachoma and urethritis in men, but it is predominantly associated with cervicitis and salpingitis in women, which can lead to infertility. The organism is sensitive to tetracyclines and erythromycin.

Chloral hydrate Quick Reference: Sedative and hypnotic agent used to induce sleep.

Advanced Reference: Usually given by mouth and absorbed rapidly in the alimentary tract and used primarily with children and the elderly.

Chloramphenicol Quick Reference: A broad-spectrum antibiotic popular in ophthalmology.

Advanced Reference: It is administered topically in the form of eye drops, ear drops, cream or in tablet form.

Chlorhexidine Quick Reference: An antimicrobial solution used to prevent bacterial multiplication.

Advanced Reference: Chlorhexidine forms the basis of many antiseptics (skin preps, hand-washing agents) used within theatre. Often seen as a pink-coloured solution that is used as a skin prep. Once an alcohol version has been applied to the skin, it should be left long enough for the alcohol to work before being dried-off so as to avoid diathermy ignition.

Chlorine Quick Reference: Chemical element with symbol Cl.

Advanced Reference: A pale-green gas with a suffocating odour and powerful oxidant used in bleaches and disinfectants.

Chlorine dioxide Quick Reference: (ClO_2) An oxidising agent, commonly used as a bleach.

Advanced Reference: Useful as a bactericide, fungicide and also used for disinfecting drinking water.

Chloroacne Quick Reference: A form of acne. Also referred to as chlorine acne.

Advanced Reference: Caused by exposure to chlorine-containing compounds.

Chloroform Quick Reference: A colourless volatile liquid once used as an anaesthetic.

Advanced Reference: Administered as an anaesthetic inhalation agent but no longer in use as it was discovered to cause cardiac problems, liver damage and pollution.

Choanal atresia Quick Reference: Congenital anomaly of the anterior skull base which causes narrowing or blocking of the nasal airway by membranous or bony tissue.

Advanced Reference: Characterised by closure of one or both posterior nasal cavities. As a congenital condition it can cause respiratory distress at birth.

Cholangiogram **Quick Reference:** X-ray image of the biliary tract.

Advanced Reference: The introduction of radio-opaque dye to define the biliary tree and related structures.

Cholangitis **Quick Reference:** (col-an-gitis) Inflammation of the *bile* ducts.

Advanced Reference: Commonly due to obstruction by *gall stones* often leading to *jaundice*. Any associated infection is treated with *antibiotics* and often requires surgical intervention.

Cholecystectomy **Quick Reference:** Surgical removal of the gall bladder.

Advanced Reference: Usually performed for the removal of symptomatic gall stones and most commonly through a right subcostal (Kocher's) incision or increasingly via a laparoscopic technique.

Cholecystitis **Quick Reference:** Inflammation of the gall bladder.

Advanced Reference: Has symptoms of acute pain radiating through the back causing nausea and vomiting. Usually due to stone formation lodged in the cystic duct.

Choledochal **Quick Reference:** (col-e-doke-al) Pertaining to the common bile duct (CBD).

Advanced Reference: A choledochotomy is a surgical procedure to open the CBD to remove stones. Choledochoplasty is plastic surgery repair of the CBD.

Cholera **Quick Reference:** Acute infection of the small intestine.

Advanced Reference: Caused by the bacterium *Vibrio cholerae*. Involves severe vomiting and *diarrhoea* which can lead to *dehydration*. Contracted from food or contaminated drinking water. Treatment involves antibiotics and fluid/IV salt solutions.

Cholestasis **Quick Reference:** Stagnation of bile in the liver.

Advanced Reference: Usually due to obstruction of the bile passage and is a common cause of jaundice.

Cholesterol **Quick Reference:** Fat-like substance found in most tissues as well as cell membranes.

Advanced Reference: Blood contains about 0.2% cholesterol (in health). It is the main component of deposits in the lining of arteries and so is associated with *arteriosclerosis*.

Choline **Quick Reference:** An amine found in the body and present in egg yolk and fat. Also a vitamin of the B complex.

Advanced Reference: Plays an important part in the metabolism of fats and the functioning of the nervous system in the form of acetylcholine.

Cholinesterase **Quick Reference:** Enzyme involved in the destruction of acetylcholine.

Advanced Reference: Cholinesterase hydrolyses acetylcholine at the neuro-muscular junction; the depolarising muscle relaxant suxamethonium is also rapidly hydrolysed by cholinesterase.

Chronic **Quick Reference:** A disease or condition of long duration.

Advanced Reference: Chronic conditions often have a gradual onset. Opposite of acute, which often has a rapid onset but is of short duration. Examples would be chronic renal failure and acute renal failure.

Chronic cough   **Quick Reference:** Also referred to as persistent cough. Defined as a cough that lasts for more than eight weeks.

Advanced Reference: Suspected causes include *asthma*, drugs, heartburn and environmental triggers. Most common in obese adults.

Chronic fatigue syndrome   **Quick Reference:** (CFS) Prolonged fatigue. Also known as myalgic encephalomyelitis (ME).

Advanced Reference: Of unknown origin but suspected causes include stress, toxins or viruses. Characterised by headaches, sore throat, muscle aches and sometimes depression.

Chyle   **Quick Reference:** A milky fluid found in the lymphatic system.

Advanced Reference: It is the end-product of digested fats, which are absorbed through the lymph vessels in the intestinal wall.

Chyme   **Quick Reference:** Partly digested stomach contents.

Advanced Reference: A semi-liquid acid mass of undigested food that passes into the small intestine.

Ciclosporin   **Quick Reference:** Powerful immunosuppressant.

Advanced Reference: Particularly used to limit tissue rejection with transplantation. A patient taking ciclosporin is particularly vulnerable to infection because of the overall suppressive effect on the immune system.

Cide   **Quick Reference:** Suffix indicating to kill.

Advanced Reference: Examples are bactericide and Cidex trade name for a glutaraldehyde preparation. Homicide indicates the killing of a person by another.

Cilia   **Quick Reference:** Fine hair-like structures.

Advanced Reference: Present on the surface of certain cells, they have an undulating action which sweeps matter along body passages, e.g. those in the air passages.

Circadian rhythms   **Quick Reference:** Refers to the body clock and the daily rhythmic activity cycle.

Advanced Reference: Based on 24-hour intervals. A routine or activities that are carried out or happen at the same time each day.

Circulation   **Quick Reference:** The flow of blood through the arteries and veins.

Advanced Reference: Indicates fluid movement in a circular motion or around a circuit. The circulatory (blood) system refers generally to the systemic circulation but should include more accurately the pulmonary, portal, coronary and collateral circulations. The pulmonary involves the passage of blood from the right ventricle through the pulmonary artery, lungs and back to the heart via the pulmonary veins. The portal circulation is the route of the blood from the alimentary tract, pancreas and spleen via the portal vein through the liver and into the hepatic veins. The coronary circulation is the system of vessels which supply the heart muscle itself, while the collateral indicates the vessels which have the action of establishing blood flow to an area when the main system fails.

Circulator Quick Reference: Refers to the member of the theatre team who provides for the scrub practitioner and surgical team during surgery.

Advanced Reference: Also called a runner or a scout in the USA. The name refers to the comparison with the scrub practitioner who by nature is relatively static at the operating site.

Circumcision Quick Reference: Removal of the foreskin of the penis.

Advanced Reference: Removal of a portion of the foreskin (prepuce) is a better description. Carried out for either medical and religious/cultural reasons. Medical reasons involve *phimosis* and *paraphimosis*.

Cirrhosis Quick Reference: (sir-o-sis) Disorder of the liver.

Advanced Reference: Leads to the development of fibrous tissue in the organ with consequent scarring, hardening and loss of function. There are a number of causes, e.g. chronic alcoholism, chronic *hepatitis* (types B and C).

Cisatracurium (besylate) Quick Reference: Non-depolarising neuromuscular blocking agent.

Advanced Reference: Provides an intermediate onset and duration of action and is cardio-stable. An *isomer* of *tracrium* available as Nimbex®.

Citanest® Quick Reference: Proprietary local anaesthetic.

Advanced Reference: It is a preparation of prilocaine hydrochloride. Used regularly as a local anaesthetic in dental practice. Also available containing a vasoconstrictor (octapressin).

CJD Quick Reference: Creutzfeldt–Jakob disease. A new-variant form of mad-cow disease. Also known as bovine spongiform encephalopathy (BSE).

Advanced Reference: CJD destroys brain cells leading to confusion, disability and eventual death. It cannot be destroyed by normal sterilisation methods, i.e. autoclaving. Wherever possible, disposable instruments are to be used on a known or potential case. There are national policies and guidelines for the use of instruments used in such cases.

Clamps Quick Reference: Surgical instrument used for gripping, closing or holding tissues.

Advanced Reference: There are numerous for specialist procedures, e.g. bowel clamp, arterial clamp. Their design and shape generally allow them to grip tissue or occlude vessels without causing too much trauma. Common versions are Bulldog, Cooley, DeBakey and Glover.

Claudication Quick Reference: Limping. Name derived from Emperor Claudius who was disabled.

Advanced Reference: Cramp-like pain in the legs which comes on during mild exercise due to inadequate blood supply to the muscles usually because of diseased arteries.

Clausen head harness   **Quick Reference:** A head harness used to hold the anaesthetic face mask in place on the patient's face.

Advanced Reference: A three-tailed rubber antistatic harness that helps secure the face mask in position, leaving the anaesthetist's hands free. Although still available, the increasing use of the *laryngeal mask airway (LMA)* has made it almost redundant.

Clavicle   **Quick Reference:** The collarbone.

Advanced Reference: Bone joined at its inner end to the breastbone and at its outer end to the shoulder blade.

Clear airway   **Quick Reference:** Term with a specific meaning but broad in application in relation to creating or maintaining a patent airway for functional breathing.

Advanced Reference: In anaesthesia the term *sniffing* position is utilised, while in recovery and *CPR* settings the head-tilt/chin-lift method is popular, and in a situation where neither of these may be suitable, such as cervical spine injury, the jaw-thrust manoeuvre is recommended.

Cleft palate   **Quick Reference:** Defect in the roof of the mouth.

Advanced Reference: Cleft indicates a fissure or opening. A congenital condition due to failure of the medial plates of the palate to meet and consequently has an effect on speech. Often found in conjunction with *harelip*.

Clindamycin   **Quick Reference:** Semi-synthetic version of the natural *antibiotic* lincomycin from which it is produced.

Advanced Reference: Both are primarily effective against *Gram-positive* bacteria.

Clinical   **Quick Reference:** Associated with a clinic or indicates, in medical terminology, to the bedside.

Advanced Reference: Refers to actual observation and treatment of patients, as distinguished from theoretical treatment. In hospitals and health-care settings, staff can be referred to as clinical or non-clinical (management, administration, etc.).

Clinical death   **Quick Reference:** Indicates that the heartbeat and breathing have stopped. May be averted or reversed.

Advanced Reference: Best thought of as 'near' death as opposed to *biological death*. Situation where the heart is stopped intentionally, i.e. as for cardiac or neurological surgery when the patient is cooled. Also referred to as suspended animation.

Clinical trials   **Quick Reference:** Trials carried out in the clinical setting. Can involve drugs, equipment, or new procedures.

Advanced Reference: Carried out to determine if a treatment is viable, safe and suitable and to make comparisons with current practice.

Clitoris   **Quick Reference:** The female counterpart of the male *penis*.

Advanced Reference: From the Greek meaning 'little hill', it contains erectile tissue which is activated during sexual stimulation.

Clone   **Quick Reference:** A living organism which is an exact copy of another individual.

Advanced Reference: Cloning is an artificial process engineered by humans, originally used in the breeding of plants and then animals; now various techniques involving human cloning are being explored.

Clonidine   **Quick Reference:** Originally an antihypertensive. Also used in the treatment of migraine.

Advanced Reference: Is also used for its sedative/antianxiety effects. May be administered orally or by injection.

Closed circuit   **Quick Reference:** Alternative name used for the circle anaesthetic breathing system. Also referred to as the bottom circuit.

Advanced Reference: So-called due to the patients re-breathing their own gases which are recycled via the closed system. Consequently there is a build-up of carbon dioxide, hence the use of soda-lime within the circuit as an absorber. Use of this circuit has a number of advantages; for example, use of low flows, therefore it is cost-saving and creates less pollution, and it maintains humidification from the patient's own exhaled breaths.

Clostridium   **Quick Reference:** A genus of anaerobic spore-forming bacteria which are rod-shaped and Gram-positive.

Advanced Reference: Includes those bacteria responsible for tetanus and gas gangrene. They thrive in the absence of oxygen with most strains of *Clostridium* being found in soils, and infection through this route is common. The main types include *C. botulinum, C. tetani, C. perfringens, C. novyi, C. welchii* and *C. difficile*.

Clostridium difficile   **Quick Reference:** Bacterium naturally present in the intestine.

Advanced Reference: Most commonly a hospital-acquired infection following *antibiotic* therapy. Can cause enterocolitis (entero-, the intestine + *colitis*, inflammation of the colon) affecting both small intestine and colon.

Clot   **Quick Reference:** Usually a semi-solid mass.

Advanced Reference: Formed from liquids such as blood, lymph, etc.

Clubbing   **Quick Reference:** Indicates clubbing of the fingers due to poor circulation.

Advanced Reference: Involves both toes and fingers, due to chronic heart and respiratory conditions.

CNS   Quick Reference: Central nervous system.

Advanced Reference: Incorporates the spinal cord and brain but not the peripheral nervous system.

Coagulation   Quick Reference: Refers to the clotting of blood.

Advanced Reference: Circulating fibrinogen is converted into insoluble fibrin, which forms the framework for a clot. The change from fibrinogen to fibrin is brought about by an enzyme, thrombin, not normally present in the blood but is produced from prothrombin by the action of thromboplastin, which is produced when tissue cells are injured. Platelets (thrombocytes) and calcium are also involved in the clotting process.

Coagulopathy   Quick Reference: Bleeding disorder or irregularities.

Advanced Reference: Any disorder adversely affecting the blood clotting or coagulation factors. Dilutional coagulopathy occurs during or after a large intravenous infusion.

Coarctation   Quick Reference: Abnormal narrowing of a vessel.

Advanced Reference: The aorta is a common site for this. Often a congenital cause and involves constriction which reduces blood flow and supply to those parts downstream of the stricture. Compensatory mechanisms involve the establishment of a collateral circulation. Surgical intervention is usually required to restore adequate circulation.

Coaxial   Quick Reference: More than one component or channel. Refers primarily to patient breathing circuits that have separate channels for inspiration and expiration.

Advanced Reference: The most common designs are the Lack and *Bain*. The former allows fresh gas to come in via the outer channel and the expired gases to exit through the inner channel, whereas the Bain has the opposite arrangement. The design corresponds to the Mapleson D arrangement.

Cobalt   Quick Reference: (symbol Co) Metallic element used chiefly for magnetic and high-temperature alloys. Atomic number 27.

Advanced Reference: Inhalation of cobalt dust can lead to *pneumoconiosis* and exposure to the powder can cause dermatitis.

Cobalt–chrome   Quick Reference: Term used in reference to chrome–cobalt *molybdenum alloy*.

Advanced Reference: Used in the manufacture of surgical instruments and prosthetic implants, in this form, usually in conjunction with *polyethylene* as the opposite half of a joint, such as with total hip replacements (THR).

Cocaine   Quick Reference: CNS stimulant.

Advanced Reference: Used mainly as an anaesthetic for topical application in ear, nose and throat (ENT) surgery and in eye drops. Once used as a constituent in elixirs prescribed to treat pain in terminal care.

Coccus   Quick Reference: Spherical-shaped bacteria.

Advanced Reference: Cocci are arranged in various groups, i.e. the staphylococcus in bunches like grapes, streptococcus in chains and the diplococcus in pairs.

Coccyx **Quick Reference:** The lower end of the back bone.

Advanced Reference: A small triangular bone projecting beyond the sacrum and consists of four tiny vertebrae fused together. It is a remnant of a human tail.

Cochlea **Quick Reference:** Part of the inner ear.

Advanced Reference: Shaped like a spiral shell, the cochlea contains the hearing apparatus. A cochlea implant is an electronic device inserted under general anaesthesia and whose function it is to stimulate the auditory nerve in an attempt to restore partial hearing in profound sensory deafness.

Cockpit drill **Quick Reference:** Alternative term used to describe anaesthetic machine checking.

Advanced Reference: As the induction and reversal/reawakening processes are often likened to the take-off and landing of an aeroplane, the term was adopted for checking and preparing anaesthetic equipment akin to the cockpit safety checks carried out by pilots.

Codeine **Quick Reference:** Alkaloid drug derived from opium.

Advanced Reference: Closely related to morphine but less potent and less habit forming. Used for pain relief alone and in combination with other drugs such as aspirin.

Coeliac disease **Quick Reference:** (seal-e-ac) Disorder of the small intestine.

Advanced Reference: Involves malabsorption due to the lining of the intestine not tolerating a component of *gluten*, which is a protein found in wheat, barley and rye.

Cognition **Quick Reference:** The mental act or process of perceiving knowledge. Cognitive. From the Latin meaning 'to know'.

Advanced Reference: Also includes perception, judgement and intuition. Cognitive behavioural therapy is based on the belief that psychological problems are due to faulty ways of thinking about one's surroundings and environment.

Colic **Quick Reference:** Intermittent pain, often severe, arising from internal organs.

Advanced Reference: Due to contraction of involuntary muscles which in turn stretch sensory nerve endings. Can be due to inflammation, obstruction of a bile duct or obstruction within a kidney (renal colic).

Colitis **Quick Reference:** Inflammation of the colon.

Advanced Reference: Usually refers to and affects the large bowel. Causes include bacterial food poisoning and various types of *dysentery*.

Collagen **Quick Reference:** An insoluble protein.

Advanced Reference: A group of proteins whose fibres form long bundles. The principal fibrous component of connective tissue. Many body tissues are regularly broken down and re-synthesised but when collagen is degraded there is little regeneration. This is why age is said to be a condition of connective tissue.

Collateral   **Quick Reference:** Alternative route for blood flow.

Advanced Reference: Refers to blood supply which develops as an alternative route when the main arterial supply is interrupted. It involves the enlargement and activation of smaller networks.

Colles' fracture   **Quick Reference:** Fracture of the wrist.

Advanced Reference: Usually due to a fall onto the palm of the hand, consequently the radius breaks off and is displaced backwards. Due to the connection between the radius and ulna, injury to adjoining ligaments is also involved. Treatment is reduction and immobilisation.

Colloid   **Quick Reference:** A suspension of particles rather than an actual solution.

Advanced Reference: The term is used to indicate a group of solutions used as intravenous plasma expanders. Composed of large molecules which causes them to remain in the circulation once infused as they cannot pass through the blood vessel walls and so exert osmotic pressure that draws fluid from the surrounding tissues.

Colon   **Quick Reference:** The majority portion of the large intestine.

Advanced Reference: The colon begins in the right iliac fossa, where the small intestine joins the caecum at the ileo-caecal junction. It continues with the ascending colon, transverse colon, descending colon, which becomes the sigmoid colon, and terminates with the rectum.

Colorectal   **Quick Reference:** Pertaining to the **colon** and *rectum*.

Advanced Reference: Both are parts of the large intestine (bowel). The term is regularly used with reference to anatomical sites and disease states.

Colostomy   **Quick Reference:** A surgical procedure to form a temporary or permanent opening onto the surface of the abdomen.

Advanced Reference: A colostomy takes over the natural function of the rectum. It is performed when there is an obstruction in the large intestine. The intestinal (faeces) contents are collected into a colostomy bag.

Colporrhaphy   **Quick Reference:** (col-pora-fee) Surgical repair of the vagina.

Advanced Reference: There are two related procedures, namely anterior and posterior colporrhaphy. Anterior repair is required when the bladder has prolapsed into the vagina (cystocele) often following childbirth. The posterior version involves prolapse of the rectum into the vagina (rectocele).

Colposcopy   **Quick Reference:** Performed for patients with an abnormal *pap smear* suggestive of *dysplasia*.

Advanced Reference: A diagnostic examination to identify abnormal cells in the cervix such as dysplasia and carcinoma.

Coma   **Quick Reference:** A state of deep unconsciousness.

Advanced Reference: A depth of consciousness from which the sufferer cannot be roused, with reflexes such as coughing and blinking being totally absent; nor do they respond to painful stimuli.

Combined spinal/epidural   **Quick Reference:** (CSE) Regional analgesia which involves gaining access to both the subarachnoid and epidural spaces in one technique.

Advanced Reference: Can be achieved by inserting the epidural and spinal needles through separate lumbar interspaces or the same space by using the 'needle-through-needle' technique, where the epidural is inserted into the epidural space, followed by a finer gauge spinal needle of longer length introduced into the subarachnoid space, the epidural needle then acting as a guide or introducer. Advantages include rapid onset of the spinal combined with the facility for top-up of analgesia via an indwelling epidural catheter.

Combitube   **Quick Reference:** Emergency airway device.

Advanced Reference: Is a double-lumen tube, one with a blunt end which functions as an *oesophageal obturator* and the other as an endotracheal tube. Intended to be introduced blindly. Besides its intended use in emergency and trauma scenarios, it has been considered for use in *difficult intubation* situations.

Commensal   **Quick Reference:** An organism that lives in or on another species.

Advanced Reference: This organism can live in harmony within or on the body without causing ill effects.

Comminution   **Quick Reference:** (com-yin-u-shon) Bone breakage.

Advanced Reference: A comminuted fracture is when the bone is broken into small fragments.

Common bile duct   **Quick Reference:** The duct that conveys bile from the gall bladder to the duodenum.

Advanced Reference: Can become blocked with stones requiring cholecystectomy (open surgery), laparoscopic removal or shock-wave therapy.

Compartment syndrome   **Quick Reference:** Involves the compression of blood vessels and nerves within an enclosed space. Swelling of the muscles within a compartment.

Advanced Reference: The term usually relates to limbs and involves the swelling of the muscle within a compartment and leads to raised pressure so that blood supply to the muscle is cut off causing *ischaemia* and further swelling. The compression obstructs the microvascular system and accompanying *oedema* further elevates intra-compartmental pressure. Other areas of the body can be affected, i.e. abdominal compartment syndrome.

Compliance   **Quick Reference:** Indicates the degree of stiffness of the lungs.

Advanced Reference: Also involves the elasticity and distensibility of the chest wall and a number of related factors, e.g. respiratory disease and anatomical anomalies. A decrease in compliance results in the need for a greater effort during respiration. If the lungs inflate easily they are said to have a high compliance; therefore, a low compliance indicates difficult inflation.

Compos mentis   **Quick Reference:** Sane, sound of mind.

Advanced Reference: Responsible for own behaviour and decisions. To be non-compos mentis renders a person not legally responsible.

Compound   **Quick Reference:** A mixture. Substance or thing made up of a number of parts or ingredients.

Advanced Reference: When two or more elements (a pure substance that is composed of atoms of the same kind and which cannot be broken down into simpler substances in ordinary chemical reactions) combine chemically in definite proportions in a substance to produce molecules held together by chemical bonds.

Concentric   **Quick Reference:** Having a common centre.

Advanced Reference: Extending out equally in all directions from a common centre. Concentric objects share the same centre, e.g. circles, tubes, cylinders, discs.

Concussion   **Quick Reference:** Shaking of the brain, caused by a blow to the head causing temporary loss of consciousness.

Advanced Reference: Any damage to the head can cause the brain to shake violently within the skull. This then causes damage to the brain and the tissues become bruised, often followed by loss of consciousness.

Condensation   **Quick Reference:** The act or process of reducing a gas or vapour to a liquid or solid form.

Advanced Reference: The process by which a substance changes from the gaseous state to the liquid state and in the process loses energy and cools.

Conduction   **Quick Reference:** May involve temperature, as with patient heat loss, electrical conduction of the cardiac or nervous system, or be used in relation to local analgesia.

Advanced Reference: In relation to heat loss, it is the process by which heat is transferred from one substance to another due to differences in temperature.

Conduction anaesthesia   **Quick Reference:** Alternative name indicating regional anaesthesia.

Advanced Reference: Indicates drugs that act locally to block nerve impulses before they reach the *CNS*.

Conduit   **Quick Reference:** Channel or pipe for conveying fluids.

Advanced Reference: An ileal conduit is a procedure that uses a segment of ileum to convey urine to the exterior, implanted into a piece of isolated bowel fixed to the interior abdominal wall following the removal of the urinary bladder.

Cone biopsy **Quick Reference:** Gynaecological procedure where an inverted cone of tissue is excised from the cervix.

Advanced Reference: Although considered a diagnostic procedure, a large enough sample of tissue is excised in the hope of removing suspect cells. Usually carried out following *Pap* smear and *colposcopy* when precancerous cells have been detected. Alternative methods to cone biopsy are loop diathermy (LEEP or loop electrosurgical excision procedure) and laser ablation. Cryotherapy is also often used.

Confidentiality **Quick Reference:** Relates to disclosure of information.

Advanced Reference: In medical ethics involves the limits on how and when health-care providers have permission to disclose information provided by a patient to a third party.

Congenital **Quick Reference:** Present at birth.

Advanced Reference: A condition that is recognised at birth or believed to have been present since birth.

Congestion **Quick Reference:** To overload or clog.

Advanced Reference: An overloading which leads to congestion and an accumulation, as with blood and fluid in *congestive heart failure*.

Congestive heart failure **Quick Reference:** Condition in which the heart weakens and fails to keep the blood flowing adequately. Also referred to as left ventricular failure (LVF).

Advanced Reference: The reduced function and capability leads to fluid accumulation and further kidney failure leading to a build up of water and *sodium*. The resultant increase in volume creates more work for the already weakened heart causing vascular congestion which goes on to cause pulmonary *oedema*.

Conjoined **Quick reference:** Indicates a joining together.

Advanced Reference: Used with reference to 'Siamese' twins, physically joined together at some bodily part at birth.

Conjunctiva **Quick Reference:** The transparent covering of the eye.

Advanced Reference: The delicate membrane covering the inside of the eyelid and the front of the eye.

Conjunctivitis **Quick Reference:** Inflammation of the *conjunctiva* of the eye.

Advanced Reference: Characterised by redness, swelling and pain. Can be due to many causes including *allergic* reactions, infection and exposure to *ultraviolet* light.

Connective tissue **Quick Reference:** The body's packing tissue, which supports and binds more specialised tissue. Forms a matrix.

Advanced Reference: Classified as loose or dense according to the concentration of fibres.

Consent   Quick Reference: To give permission.

Advanced Reference: Patient consent, an essential part of the preoperative process involving the patient giving their permission for treatment to take place. Consent can be expressed in writing, verbally or given on behalf of another, i.e. legal guardian or appointed person in the case of a minor or unconscious patient.

Constipation   Quick Reference: Infrequent or absent movement of the *bowel*.

Advanced Reference: May be due to a variety of causes including blockage of the intestine or dietary imbalance involving lack of *fibre* and insufficient fluid. Many analgesics such as *morphine* also have a constipating effect and in old age it can be due to decreased muscle tone.

Continuous positive airway pressure   Quick Reference: (CPAP) A breathing mode employed on most intensive care unit ventilators.

Advanced Reference: This technique produces a similar effect to *positive end-expiratory pressure* (*PEEP*) but may be utilised during either spontaneous or mechanical ventilation and has the effect of elevating lung pressure throughout the whole respiratory cycle, having the effect of improving *functional reserve capacity (FRC)* and oxygenation.

Continuous spinal anaesthesia   Quick Reference: Involves the introduction of an indwelling catheter via the spinal needle into the subarachnoid space for continuous injection.

Advanced Reference: Due to the small size of the needles (approx. 26 g) and catheters (approx. 30 g) involved, and the subsequent difficulty of insertion and injection, it has proved to be unpopular.

Continuous suture   Quick Reference: Wound closure suturing technique.

Advanced Reference: Consists of tying off only the first and final stitch as opposed to an interrupted technique, when each throw is knotted. Not widely popular because a break at any point may mean disruption to the entire suture line.

Contraception   Quick Reference: Birth control. To prevent pregnancy.

Advanced Reference: Artificial prevention of a pregnancy by using various methods, i.e. contraceptive pill, condom, cap and the symptom-thermal (STM) method, which observes body temperature and cervical secretions.

Contrast medium   Quick Reference: Substance used in radiography to visualise body structures and activity.

Advanced Reference: Because of the difference in absorption of X-rays by contrast medium and surrounding tissues, this allows radiographic visualisation of structures.

Controlled drugs   Quick Reference: Term used in relation to medications whose use and handling are controlled under law.

Advanced Reference: A number of evolving laws (Dangerous Drugs Act, Controlled Drugs, Misuse of Drugs Act) have overseen the control, security, recording, handling and use of certain classified drugs.

Contusion   **Quick Reference:** A bruise.

Advanced Reference: Injury to deep tissue through intact skin.

Convection   **Quick Reference:** As with *conduction*, involves the process of heat moving through a material, i.e. liquid, gas.

Advanced Reference: Relates to the transfer of heat and patient heat loss during anaesthesia and surgery, as with transmission via air currents moving from warm to cooler area.

Convulsion   **Quick Reference:** A fit or seizure.

Advanced Reference: Involuntary, spasmodic muscular contractions, as seen in patients with epilepsy.

COPD   **Quick Reference:** Chronic obstructive pulmonary disorder (or disease). Also termed chronic obstructive airway disease (COAD).

Advanced Reference: Involves a group of chronic conditions that result in air-flow blockage in the lungs and breathing-related problems, i.e. bronchitis and chronic bronchitis and emphysema.

Coproxamol   **Quick Reference:** A compound analgesic.

Advanced Reference: It is a combination of the narcotic dextro-propoxyphene and paracetamol.

Cornea   **Quick Reference:** Transparent part of the eyeball.

Advanced Reference: The cornea lies over the pupil and iris. If it becomes scarred by injury or disease, it can cause a disturbance to or loss of vision.

Coronary arteries   **Quick Reference:** Arteries which supply the heart muscle itself.

Advanced Reference: The right and left coronary arteries branch off the aorta as it leaves the heart. The left divides into an anterior interventricular branch which passes downwards between the ventricles to the apex of the heart. There is also a left circumflex branch which runs round between the left atrium and ventricle. The right coronary artery runs round between the right atrium and ventricle and supplies the right ventricle and the sinoatrial node.

Corpuscle   **Quick Reference:** A small body or cell.

Advanced Reference: Generally used to describe the red blood cells.

Corpus luteum   **Quick Reference:** The yellow mass of cells that fills the ovarian *follicle* after the ovum has been shed.

Advanced Reference: One of its products is *progesterone*, which prepares the lining of the uterus for the implantation of a fertilised ovum. Another secretion is the hormone *relaxin*.

Corrosion   **Quick Reference:** The process in which metals and *alloys* are attacked chemically by moisture, air, *acids* or *alkalis*.

Advanced Reference: If left to continue the affected substance will be worn away.

Corrugated tubing   **Quick Reference:** Refers to a type and design of tubing used in anaesthetic and ventilator tubing.

Advanced Reference: Originally referred to the black antistatic rubber design but now includes various plastic and disposable varieties. So designed in the corrugated manner as it allowed for lengthwise stretching, collection of exhaled vapour and reduced resistance.

Cortex   **Quick Reference:** The outer layer.

Advanced Reference: The outer layer of an organ or other structures such as bone, brain, kidney and adrenal gland.

Cortical (bone)   **Quick Reference:** Dense compact bone of the shaft that surrounds the medullary cavity.

Advanced Reference: Forms a layer around softer spongy bone in a similar manner to the *enamel* of teeth.

Cortical blindness   **Quick Reference:** Loss of or injury to the visual pathways in the brain.

Advanced Reference: Involves loss of sight due to an organic lesion in the visual cortex.

Corticosteroid   **Quick Reference:** Steroid hormone.

Advanced Reference: Produced and secreted by the cortex of the adrenal glands, also produced synthetically. Best known is hydrocortisone, which is used primarily as an anti-inflammatory.

Cortisol   **Quick reference:** Major glucocorticoid synthesised in the adrenal *cortex*.

Advanced Reference: Its action has an influence on the *metabolism* of *glucose*, *protein* and *fats*. In pharmacology it is referred to as *hydrocortisone*.

Coryza   **Quick Reference:** (cor-e-zar) Inflammation of the nasal *mucous membrane*.

Advanced Reference: Produces a runny nose. Catarrh (excessive secretion of mucus in the nasal passages and related structures).

COSHH   **Quick Reference:** Control of Substances Hazardous to Health.

Advanced Reference: Regulation brought out under the Health and Safety at Work Act. It concentrates on the control and use of substances which may be harmful to health and therefore require the monitoring and assessment of their use. The regulations are updated regularly as and when needed. In relation to hospitals it covers such everyday substances as cleaning and sterilising fluids, gases and solvents.

Cough CPR   **Quick Reference:** Self-administered form of CPR.

Advanced Reference: Said to be useful for someone who is alone and suspects they are having a cardiac arrest. Based on the theory that coughing, like chest compressions, increases intrathoracic pressure and results in increased blood flow. Not a front-line technique with any of the resuscitation bodies but always mentioned as an alternative in specific and related situations.

Counter shock   Quick Reference: *Defibrillation.*

Advanced Reference: Indicates the high-intensity direct current delivered during defibrillation.

Cox-2 inhibitors   **Quick Reference:** Group of anti-inflammatory drugs.

Advanced Reference: As with other *NSAIDs* they reduce the production of *prostaglandins* but in a more specific manner. Used commonly in the symptomatic treatment of *osteo* and *rheumatoid arthritis* and other causes of acute pain.

CPAP   **Quick Reference:** Continuous positive airway pressure.

Advanced Reference: Indicates the application of positive airway pressure throughout all phases of (spontaneous) ventilation. Designed to reduce airway collapse and so increase oxygenation.

CPR   **Quick Reference:** Cardiopulmonary resuscitation.

Advanced Reference: Involves providing artificial ventilation and/or chest compressions as well as further necessary actions (defibrillation, IV therapy) to a patient who has ceased breathing and has no cardiac output.

Craniotomy   **Quick Reference:** Opening of the skull.

Advanced Reference: Surgical opening of the cranium.

Cremophor®   **Quick Reference:** Solubilising (emulsifying) agent used in drug preparations.

Advanced Reference: The use of Cremophor® was highlighted when suspected of being responsible for certain adverse effects of the now withdrawn induction agent althesin.

Crepitus   **Quick Reference:** A grating noise or sensation.

Advanced Reference: The crackling sound heard with a *stethoscope* over inflamed lungs or the sounds made by broken-bone ends moving against each other.

Cricoid cartilage   **Quick Reference:** The uppermost ring of cartilage around the trachea.

Advanced Reference: Ring-shaped cartilage at the lower end of the larynx which forms the only complete ring within the trachea. All others are C-shaped, with the space towards the rear intended to facilitate movement and expansion of the oesophagus.

Cricothyrotomy   **Quick Reference:** Emergency access to the upper respiratory tract.

Advanced Reference: An emergency procedure which involves gaining access from the exterior to the respiratory tract via the cricothyroid membrane using a variety of devices.

Critical care **Quick Reference:** Refers to specific areas and departments of hospitals.

Advanced Reference: Term used to indicate areas involved in emergency work, i.e. A&E, ICU, Operating theatres.

Critical incidents **Quick Reference:** Indicates an event or set of events/ actions that are considered of such serious nature that they must be highlighted and formally reported upon.

Advanced Reference: An increasingly used process which deals with once common and almost taken for granted occurrences, which are now formally investigated, reflected and feedback provided in an attempt to instigate action for improvement and change. May involve personnel, equipment and processes.

Crohn's disease **Quick Reference:** (crones) An inflammatory condition of the digestive tract.

Advanced Reference: Can affect anywhere throughout the digestive tract. Symptoms may mimic acute appendicitis with chronic diarrhoea and weight loss.

Cross-matching **Quick Reference:** Indicates establishing the compatibility of the patient's blood with donor blood. Also referred to as X-match.

Advanced Reference: Intended to identify a blood group (A, B, AB, O) plus the Rhesus factor (Rh+ and Rh−) when blood replacement is considered probable. If the need is assessed as only a possibility most centres have a policy of only grouping and saving serum (GSS), which reduces waste and cost as it cuts out a full cross-match process. The full process involves grouping the patient's blood using serum containing anti-A and anti-B followed by incubation of both donor and recipient samples in order to detect signs of *agglutination*. The A, B, AB and O *antigens* are the most important with reference to blood donation and it is possible for one or the other to be

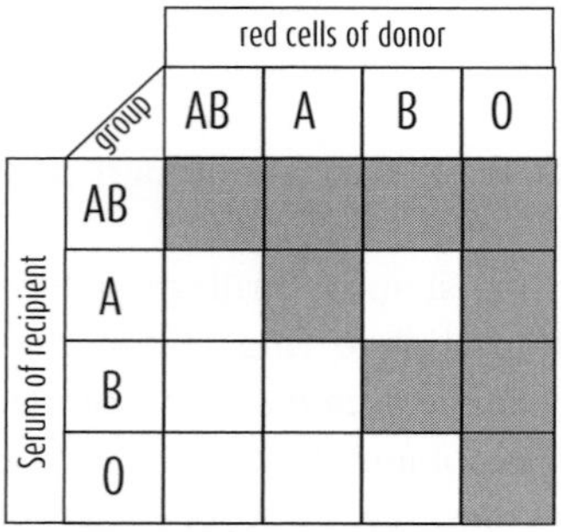

	red cells of donor			
group	AB	A	B	O
AB				
A				
B				
O				

Fig. 5. Blood compatibility (shaded areas show compatibility)

present, or for both together or for neither to be present. The determining of compatibility also involves many minor *agglutinogens*, D (Rhesus factor) being the most significant. Samples with Factor D are said to be Rh-positive; those without, Rh-negative. In the absence of time to do a full X-match or where none is available, the universal donor blood, O-negative, may be used.

Croup **Quick Reference:** A harsh cough and strained noisy breathing in children.

Advanced Reference: Causes vary from retarded growth of the *larynx* to *allergy* and both viral and bacterial infection. Croup scoring systems are employed to assess the condition using criteria such as breath sounds, *strido*r, cough, flaring and cyanosis.

Cruciate **Quick Reference:** (croosh-e-ate) Anterior and posterior ligament in the knee.

Advanced Reference: Gives stability to the knee. The cruciate ligament limits forward movement of the tibia on the femur. Commonly ruptured in sporting activities by a sharp twisting movement.

Crush syndrome **Quick Reference:** Condition brought on following trauma.

Advanced Reference: Involves the trapping and compression of a limb and the build up of toxins, i.e. histamine, lactic acid, carbon dioxide, and then the effects when they are released into the circulation causing toxic shock. The time for which a limb is trapped is critical in terms of release and availability of advanced care. Different protocols cite various guidelines on release time, with some saying never release if a limb has been trapped for 10 minutes without advanced help while others cite 30 minutes.

Cryo (surgery) **Quick Reference:** Destruction of tissues by freezing.

Advanced Reference: Cryo is from the Greek meaning cold. Involves a number of agents, i.e. liquid nitrogen and nitrous oxide. Utilised in ophthalmic procedures, urology and dermatology.

Cryogenic **Quick Reference:** Pertaining to or bringing about the production of lower temperatures.

Advanced Reference: Cryonics is the practice of freezing a dead diseased human with the aim of restoring life in the future when a cure is found.

Cryptosporidium **Quick Reference:** A protozoan parasite found in contaminated water.

Advanced Reference: They are parasitic when present in the intestinal tract.

Crystalloid **Quick Reference:** (cris-tal-oid) Refers to clear intravenous solutions.

Advanced Reference: More correctly, refers to solutions which may pass through a semi-permeable membrane, as opposed to colloids, which, because of the large molecules in solution, cannot pass through the tissues.

Crystapen® **Quick Reference:** A proprietary antibiotic.

Advanced Reference: Used to treat many forms of infection, an important one in the past being that associated with rheumatic fever which caused heart valve injury.

CSF   **Quick Reference:** Cerebrospinal fluid.

Advanced Reference: The fluid which bathes the central nervous system, contained by the meninges, which are the covering membranes.

CSSD   **Quick Reference:** Central Sterile Services Department.

Advanced Reference: At one time a hospital-based sterilising and supply department. Organisational changes have meant that these services are more likely now to be provided by either a central/regional department or external contractor. Some theatres however do still maintain a TSSU (Theatre Sterile Services Unit).

Cuffed oropharyngeal airway   **Quick Reference:** (COPA) Modified oral airway.

Advanced Reference: It has an inflatable cuff positioned on the distal end.

Culture   **Quick Reference:** The growing of micro-organisms and cells in the laboratory.

Advanced Reference: The process of growing (culturing) micro-organisms or other living cells artificially on suitable nutritional substances such as agar, mixed with blood or broth. A culture swab, also referred to as swab on a stick, is used for bacteriology specimens (e.g. pus).

Curette   **Quick Reference:** A surgical instrument used for scraping the walls of a cavity in order to remove unwanted materials.

Advanced Reference: The most common procedure that utilises a curette is a *D&C* (dilatation and curettage) of the uterus.

Cushing's syndrome   **Quick Reference:** A condition resulting from excess amounts of **corticosteroid** hormones in the body.

Advanced Reference: Symptoms include weight gain, reddening of the neck, excess growth of body and facial hair, raised blood pressure, *osteoporosis*, raised blood glucose levels and, sometimes, mental disturbance. May be due to over-stimulation of the adrenal glands, usually because of tumours.

Cut-down   **Quick Reference:** To make access to a blood vessel via incision through the skin and underlying tissues.

Advanced Reference: Procedure used when venous access is not possible via direct cannulation, as in emergency situations when the casualty is peripherally shut down.

Cutting needle   **Quick Reference:** Type of suture needle.

Advanced Reference: A cutting needle is triangular in cross-section and has its cutting edge directed towards the wound and its flat surface away from the wound. Used for suturing tough or dense tissues, e.g. fascia and skin.

CVP   **Quick Reference:** Central venous pressure.

Advanced Reference: CVP is the pressure created by the circulating blood volume. Measured in cmH_2O (centimetres of water) with a manometer or transducer via a catheter inserted through a central vein and with the tip of the catheter lying just outside of the right atrium.

Cyanide **Quick Reference:** (symbol – CN). A poisonous salt derived from hydrocyanic acid (HCN). Identified by giving off a smell of bitter almonds.

Advanced Reference: Produces unconsciousness by inactivating cellular respiration, which is followed by convulsions and death. If inhaled as hydrogen cyanide, it can be fatal within less than a minute. Taken orally as sodium or potassium cyanide, it will also kill within minutes. It can also be absorbed by splashes on the skin. Cyanides are used in the production of synthetic rubbers and insecticides, and are liberated by burning polyurethane foam which is used in furniture upholstery. A common antidote is *amyl nitrite*.

Cyanosis **Quick Reference:** (sigh-a-nosis) Blue tint to the skin and mucous membranes.

Advanced Reference: Due to insufficient oxygenation of the blood.

Cyclimorph® **Quick reference:** Proprietary form of morphine combined with cyclizine.

Advanced Reference: The combination of narcotic analgesic, antiemetic and antihistamine used to treat moderate to severe pain.

Cyclizine **Quick Reference:** An antihistamine and antiemetic.

Advanced Reference: Used in the treatment of motion sickness and general nausea and vomiting.

Cyclopropane **Quick Reference:** Gas used as an inhalation anaesthetic. Chemical formula C_3H_6.

Advanced Reference: Now withdrawn from use but was suitable for both induction and maintenance of anaesthesia. However, it had the disadvantage of being highly explosive. Because of this, it was not suitable in proximity to diathermy so was mostly used for induction only.

Cyclotron **Quick Reference:** An apparatus for accelerating charged particles.

Advanced Reference: This includes protons, deuterons and ions, which are propelled by an alternating electrical field in a constant magnetic field.

Cyst **Quick Reference:** (sist) A swelling containing fluid. A bladder.

Advanced Reference: They appear often in the skin and ovaries, but can develop in many other body sites. Cystic means pertaining to a cyst.

Cystectomy **Quick Reference:** Removal of urinary bladder but may also refer to removal of a *cyst*.

Advanced Reference: Most commonly indicates total or partial excision of the urinary bladder, usually due to cancer. Also referred to as neo-bladder. Various procedures are carried out to create a false or replacement bladder using segments of bowel (*urinary diversion*) or stomach, into which the ureters are implanted; the alternative is the creation of a urinary *stoma*.

Cystic fibrosis **Quick Reference:** (CF) Hereditary disease affecting mainly the lungs but also the liver, pancreas and intestines.

Advanced Reference: A significant sign of the disease is repeated infection of the lungs as the bronchioles become blocked with thick secretions, therefore limiting full expansion of the alveoli. Bacteria thrive in this environment so leading to infection. Treatment is with antibiotics and continual physiotherapy and, in worsening cases, lung transplantation is carried out.

Cystitis   **Quick Reference:** (sist-it is) Inflammation of the urinary bladder.

Advanced Reference: Usually due to bacterial infection and, because of the shorter urethra, it is more common in women as this allows easier access for ascending infection.

Cystocele   **Quick Reference:** (sist-o-seal) Herniation of the bladder into the vagina.

Advanced Reference: Commonly due to overstretching of the vagina walls during childbirth.

Cystoscope   **Quick Reference:** Instrument for examining the interior of the bladder.

Advanced Reference: An endoscopic procedure which involves the passage of a telescope via the urethra into the bladder.

Cystostomy   **Quick Reference:** Opening of the bladder and making access to the exterior.

Advanced Reference: A surgical procedure which involves making an opening into the bladder via the abdominal wall. Usually carried out when the normal exit (urethra) is obstructed. Cystotomy indicates opening the bladder by surgical incision.

Cystourethrogram   **Quick Reference:** X-ray/test of the urinary bladder and urethra.

Advanced Reference: Taken while voiding following injection of contrast media into the bladder. Carried out to determine causes of incontinence, strictures and infections. A retrograde cystourethrogram is a radiograph taken as the contrast media is being injected back down the urethra into the bladder.

Cytology   **Quick Reference:** The study of cells under the microscope.

Advanced Reference: The study of the function and structure of cells. An example is a cervical smear of the cervix.

Cytomegalovirus   **Quick reference:** A commonly occurring virus of the herpes virus group. The name, cytomegalo = large cell, is derived from the swollen appearance of infection.

Advanced Reference: Usually asymptomatic but can remain latent in the body causing recurrent infections. During acute infection the virus is excreted in the saliva, urine and vagina. May also be passed on via blood transfusion and organ transplantation and from mother to *fetus* either in the uterus or during vaginal delivery, sometimes proving fatal or causing liver disease and motor disability.

Cytotoxics   **Quick Reference:** Drugs used in the treatment of cancer.

Advanced Reference: Anticancer agents that have the essential property of preventing normal cell replication and so inhibiting the growth of tumours.

D

Dacron® **Quick Reference:** Relates to vascular surgery grafts. Made of *polyethylene terephthalate* fibre.

Advanced Reference: Dacron® grafts are of either the knitted or woven type, comprising of polyethylene, which are elastic in nature and kink resistant. Some are impregnated with *gelatin* or *collagen*, which helps seal the graft. Knitted grafts require pre-clotting with the recipient's blood.

Dacron® cuff **Quick Reference:** A sheath of Dacron® surrounding an arterial or venous catheter.

Advanced Reference: Fixed to the upper length of catheters and intended to adhere to surrounding tissue before it exits the skin and to prevent accidental displacement. Found in intravenous feeding lines and used in combination with tunnelling of the catheter, which further acts as an anchor as well as reducing catheter infection.

Damping **Quick Reference:** Term related to recording and monitoring devices (CVP, invasive arterial) indicating a reduction in amplitude (size) and therefore interference of the trace.

Advanced Reference: Most commonly seen in invasive arterial monitoring systems when the trace reading is affected by air bubbles in the flushing fluid, blood clots or kinking of the manometer tubing.

Dantrium® **Quick Reference:** Proprietary skeletal muscle relaxant, e.g. dantrolene sodium.

Advanced Reference: Used in the treatment of *malignant hyperthermia (hyperpyrexia)*. The preparation contains *mannitol*, which acts as a preservative.

D&C **Quick Reference:** Dilatation and curettage. A gynaecological procedure.

Advanced Reference: Involves dilatation of the os of the cervix and a curette being used to remove endometrium for examination.

Dead space **Quick Reference:** Area of the anatomy or circuitry where no gas exchange takes place.

Advanced Reference: Anatomical dead space includes the mouth, nose, pharynx and large airways. Equipment dead space involves anaesthetic masks and circuits. Insertion of an endotracheal tube reduces dead space as it bypasses the anatomical dead space. Mask anaesthesia greatly increases dead space but should be of limited duration and not have too detrimental an impact. The issue of equipment dead space is of greater importance when dealing with paediatric circuits.

Debridement   **Quick Reference:** Thorough cleansing/clearing of a wound.

Advanced Reference: Involves cleaning and removal of foreign materials and damaged, dead tissue, usually following traumatic injury.

Decadron®   **Quick Reference:** A proprietary corticosteroid.

Advanced Reference: A preparation of dexamethasone used to replace steroid deficiency and in the treatment of shock.

Decapitation   **Quick Reference:** Literally, removal of the head.

Advanced Reference: Often used to indicate removal of either the entire or only the top of the skull.

Decapsulation   **Quick Reference:** Surgical incision and removal of a fibrous capsule.

Advanced Reference: Renal decapsulation is the freeing and removal of the capsule surrounding the kidney.

Decibel   **Quick Reference:** (symbol dB) Unit for comparing sound level or loudness of sound.

Advanced Reference: The decibel is a logarithmic unit used to describe a ratio and also used to express the relative difference in power or intensity. One decibel equals approximately the smallest difference in acoustic power the human ear can detect. The bel (B) is used to quantify the reduction in audio level over one mile (1.6 km). The decibel (dB) = 0.1 bel.

Decidua   **Quick Reference:** (des-id-ua) The *mucous membrane* that lines the uterus during pregnancy. It is shed at *parturition* with the *placenta*.

Advanced Reference: It is formed under the influence of *progesterone* and represents the maternal portion of the *placenta*.

Deciduous   **Quick Reference:** Temporary. Shedding at a specific stage of growth.

Advanced Reference: As teeth, first or primary set in childhood, referred to as milk teeth.

Decilitre   **Quick Reference:** (symbol dl) Metric unit of volume.

Advanced Reference: Equal to one-tenth of a litre.

Decompression   **Quick Reference:** To reduce internal pressure. A surgical procedure designed to release pressure on an organ or structure.

Advanced Reference: An example would be drilling into or removing a section of the skull to relieve intracranial pressure or removal of a vertebra to prevent it pressing on the spinal cord.

Decubitus   **Quick Reference:** In Latin indicates to lie down. The position of a patient in bed.

Advanced Reference: Decubitus ulcer is another name for *bed sore*.

Defence mechanism   **Quick Reference:** An immunological mechanism by which the body resists invasion by pathogens.

Advanced Reference: Also used to indicate a psychological means of coping with conflict and anxiety.

Defibrillation   **Quick Reference:** The application of an electric shock across the heart using a defibrillator.

Advanced Reference: An attempt to restore normal rhythm to the heart when in fibrillation, either ventricular or atrial, by applying energy in the form of an electric shock. The shock depolarises the cardiac cells and allows the sino-atrial node to take over and institute normal sinus rhythm. Ventricular fibrillation requires a more powerful shock to be effective than that needed to correct atrial fibrillation (*cardioversion)*.

Deflagration   **Quick Reference:** To burn with great heat and intense light.

Advanced Reference: The process of combustion that propagates via the thermal conductivity (hot burning material that heats the next layer of cold material and ignites it).

Defunctioning colostomy   **Quick Reference:** A surgical intervention for disease of the lower colon and rectum.

Advanced Reference: Carried out when there is a need to either rest the colon following anastomosis or to have a permanent bypass in order to keep the contents (faeces) away from the diseased portion. A loop of colon is brought out onto the skin surface so that the faeces is discharged into a *colostomy* bag attached to the skin.

Degenerative   **Quick Reference:** Degeneration. To decline in quality. May involve physical or moral qualities.

Advanced Reference: The *morbid* impairment of any structural tissue or organ. A degenerative disease; one in which function declines and deteriorates.

Deglove   **Quick Reference:** Injury to extremities, i.e. fingers, toes and sometimes buttocks.

Advanced Reference: Involves the peeling off of tissue down to the bone, including neurovascular bundles and tendons, usually due to trauma.

Deglutition   **Quick Reference:** Swallowing.

Advanced Reference: A reflex action initiated by touch receptors in the *pharynx* that triggers the tongue to move a food bolus backwards towards the *oesophagus*.

Dehiscence   **Quick Reference:** Splitting open.

Advanced Reference: Term applied to the breakdown of surgical incisions in the postoperative period. Usually due to infection. Relates to the slang term 'burst abdomen'.

Dehydration   **Quick Reference:** A reduction in the total water content of the body.

Advanced Reference: Excessive fluid loss may be due to reduced or lack of intake, sweating, persistent vomiting and diarrhoea. Signs and symptoms include thirst, muscle cramp, muscle weakness and a low urine output of less than 400 ml in 24 hours (oliguria).

Delirium   **Quick Reference:** Disturbance of brain function causing confusion, excitement and other symptoms of disorganised mental activity.

Advanced Reference: Due to injury, fever and poisoning, among other things.

Delorme's procedure   **Quick Reference:** Surgical repair of the perineal area involving a complete thickness rectal prolapse.

Advanced Reference: A full thickness rectal prolapse protruding from the anus. Comprised of two layers of the rectal wall and occurs most commonly in older adults, with females more affected, and is associated with weak pelvic and anal muscles.

Deltoid   **Quick Reference:** Triangular. The deltoid muscle.

Advanced Reference: This muscle lies on the anterior border and upper surface of the outer third of the clavicle and enables the arm to abduct, flex and rotate.

Demand pacemaker   **Quick Reference:** Device used to stimulate the heart.

Advanced Reference: Used when the heart and impulses are not sufficient. Functions on the principle of measuring the interval between beats and if the normal value is exceeded the pacemaker delivers a stimulating pulse.

Dementia   **Quick Reference:** (dem-en-sure) Loss of intellectual function.

Advanced Reference: Resulting in deficient memory and concentration. The condition is progressive although it can also be due to thyroid disturbance or infection, but most cases are due to the degenerative processes of ageing.

Dendrite   **Quick Reference:** Filament of a nerve cell.

Advanced Reference: Carries electrical signals from the synapse to the cell body. Each neurone (nerve cell) has many dendrites.

Denervate   **Quick Reference:** (de-nerve-ate) To remove nerves or their function.

Advanced Reference: Indicates without nerve supply. As happens in some conditions and surgical procedures, i.e. following cardiac transplantation.

Density   *Quick Reference:* The mass of a substance, per unit volume. Measured in kilograms per cubic metre (kg/m^3) or grams per cubic centimetre (g/cm^3). Density $= \frac{mass\ (m)}{Volume\ (V)}$

Advanced Reference: Density varies slightly with temperature in the case of solids and liquids, which expand and become less dense, however with gases the density varies depending upon the container and surrounding pressure.

Dentition   **Quick Reference:** The arrangement of teeth in the mouth.

Advanced Reference: The 20 deciduous teeth, incisors, canines and molars, comprise the teeth of young children, and the permanent or adult teeth consist of up to 32 made up of *incisors*, *canines*, premolars and *molars*.

Deoxygenate   **Quick Reference:** To deprive of oxygen.

Advanced Reference: To become depleted of oxygen. *Desaturate*.

Depilation   **Quick Reference:** Removal of body hair with chemicals.

Advanced Reference: An alternative to preoperative shaving and clipping but has the potential to cause skin irritation and allergic reactions.

Depolarisation **Quick Reference:** The neutralisation of an electric charge.

Advanced Reference: A depolarising block involves skeletal muscle paralysis associated with the loss of polarity of the motor end-plate, as occurs following the administration of a cholinergic antagonist.

Depo-medrone® **Quick Reference:** Proprietary corticosteroid.

Advanced Reference: Used in the treatment of inflammation and to relieve allergic disorders such as rheumatoid arthritis, hayfever and asthma. It is a preparation of the steroid methyl prednisolone.

Dermatitis **Quick Reference:** Inflammation of the skin.

Advanced Reference: The dividing line between dermatitis and *eczema* is not clear but generally the former can be used when the skin is injured by an external agent and the latter when the cause is from within the body.

Dermatology **Quick Reference:** Speciality dealing with skin disorders.

Advanced Reference: The dermis is the connective tissue underlying the epithelium of the skin.

Dermatome **Quick Reference:** The area of the skin innervated by the branch of a single spinal nerve. Dermatomes form into bands around the trunk of the body but have a different arrangement in the limbs. Dermatone is regularly used to indicate the same meaning.

Advanced Reference: Has relevance in relation to regional anaesthesia in determining the extent of the block as areas of the skin are supplied by particular spinal nerves. Dermatomes are named according to the spinal nerve which supplies them. Dermatome is also a surgical instrument used for cutting slices of skin in preparation for grafting and an alternative version, also termed a mucotome is used, for cutting strips of mucous membrane for grafting.

Dermoid cyst **Quick Reference:** A type of cyst.

Advanced Reference: Formed by a collection of cancerous cells that contain one or more of the three primary embryonic layers, i.e. skin, hair and teeth.

Desaturate **Quick Reference:** Indicates the desaturation of oxygen from the red cells.

Advanced Reference: Used generally to indicate an inadequate supply of oxygen in the haemoglobin and tissues.

Desflurane **Quick Reference:** Volatile anaesthetic agent.

Advanced Reference: Requires an elaborate vaporiser which is heated and pressurised. A relatively insoluble agent making for rapid induction and recovery.

Desiccation **Quick Reference:** The act of drying up.

Advanced Reference: Indicates creating a state of dryness by removing water.

Detached retina **Quick Reference:** Can be the result of trauma or may happen spontaneously.

Advanced Reference: The retina, or part of it, separates from the choroids and the patient complains of a gradual decline in their field of vision.

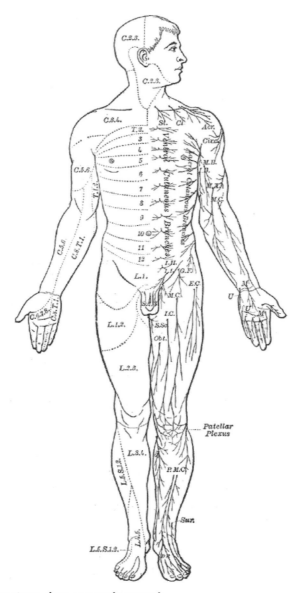

Fig. 6a. Dermatome chart. www.nda.ox.ac.uk

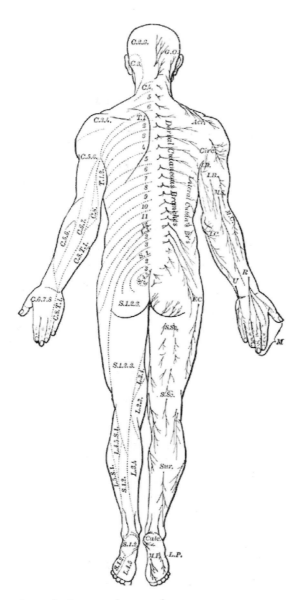

Fig. 6b. Dermatome chart. www.nda.ox.ac.uk

Detergent   **Quick Reference:** Cleaning agent.

Advanced reference: Detergents work by lowering surface tension, which enables water to penetrate more effectively and remove grease by forming an emulsion.

Detritus   **Quick Reference:** Dead epithelial tissue.

Advanced Reference: Common to the skin surface.

Detrusor   **Quick Reference:** A muscle that has the action of expelling a substance.

Advanced Reference: The detrusor muscle in the urinary bladder provides a muscular coat and dysfunction of this muscle can lead to urinary incontinence.

Dettol™   **Quick Reference:** Antiseptic and disinfectant.

Advanced Reference: Used to treat abrasions and minor wounds as well as disinfecting instruments. It is a preparation of chloroxylenol.

Deuteranomaly   **Quick Reference:** Type of colour blindness.

Advanced Reference: It is the most common colour-vision deficiency affecting approximately 5% of white males and 0.25% of females.

Dextran   **Quick Reference:** An intravenous plasma substitute/expander.

Advanced Reference: A carbohydrate consisting of glucose units. Used as a plasma expander in haemorrhage or shock due to burns. Can interfere with cross-matching of blood. Two major preparations are available: Dextran 40, a 10% solution in glucose or saline and used to improve blood flow and prevent thrombosis; and Dextran 70, a 6% version in glucose or saline, used to expand blood volume.

Dextrocardia   **Quick Reference:** Abnormal position of the heart.

Advanced Reference: A rare congenital heart condition involving unusual positioning, i.e. usually rotated to the right. The patient may not even be aware of the abnormality until connected to an ECG where the trace will show an inversion of activity, i.e. the P-wave will be completely opposite to its normal position. Those affected by this condition lead a normal life as the heart functions as normal.

Dextrolyte®   **Quick Reference:** Proprietary sodium solution.

Advanced Reference: Used to treat mild to moderate sodium depletion, as in dehydration. Produced in an oral preparation containing sodium chloride, potassium chloride, glucose and sodium lactate.

Dextro-saline   **Quick Reference:** Intravenous solution.

Advanced Reference: A preparation of 0.18% saline and 4.3% dextrose. This equates to 0.18 g of sodium and 4.3 g of dextrose per 100 ml.

DF 118   **Quick Reference:** A synthetic opioid analgesic. Dihydrocodeine. Also referred to as DHC.

Advanced Reference: Used to treat moderate to severe pain. Available in tablet, elixir and ampoule for injection. Said to be approximately one-sixth as potent as morphine. Is produced as paracodeine, a combination of codeine and *paracetamol*. In some countries used as an alternative to *methadone*.

Diabetes **Quick Reference:** A general term but characterised by excessive urine production (*polyuria*).

Advanced Reference: Diabetes insipidus is a rare form in which the kidney tubules do not reabsorb sufficient water. This can be due to inadequate production of antidiuretic hormone (ADH) by the pituitary gland, leading to excessive production of dilute urine. This can be because ADH receptors in the renal tubules are defective. Diabetes mellitus involves a relative or absolute lack of insulin due to deficiency in its secretion from the pancreas, which can in turn lead to uncontrolled carbohydrate metabolism. Signs and symptoms of the latter form are lassitude and debility, weight loss, pruritis and a lowered resistance to infection.

Diabetic retinopathy **Quick Reference:** Retinal changes that occur in long-term *diabetes*.

Advanced Reference: Leads to blurred and deteriorating vision due to blood vessel damage caused by over-accumulation of glucose and fructose. Characterised by small haemorrhages, microaneurysms and exudation.

Diagnosis **Quick Reference:** The determination of the nature of a disease.

Advanced Reference: Diagnosis refers to determining the cause of an illness or disorder and differential diagnosis distinguishes between conditions with similar symptoms.

Dialysis **Quick Reference:** To separate, to filter. Process that performs the filtering function of the kidneys in renal failure. The two main types are *haemodialysis* and peritoneal dialysis.

Advanced Reference: Dialysis utilises the principle of selective *diffusion* through a membrane, as applied in the artificial kidney machine. The membrane divides a stream of the patient's blood from a prepared solution of salts and glucose (dialysis fluid – dialysate), and waste material, usually removed by the kidneys, passes from the bloodstream into the fluid. In peritoneal dialysis (CAPD – continuous ambulatory peritoneal dialysis) dialysis fluid is perfused into and drained out of the abdominal cavity intermittently utilising the peritoneum as the membrane through which the filtering takes place.

Diaphragm **Quick Reference:** (die-a-fram) Sheet of muscle separating the thorax from the abdomen.

Advanced Reference: The diaphragm arises from the lumbar vertebrae, the lower ribs and the lower end of the sternum. It converges on a flat sheet of dense fibrous tissue and the whole structure forms a sort of dome. A diaphragmatic hernia is a protrusion of a part of the stomach through the oesophageal opening in the diaphragm.

Diaphysis Quick Reference: The shaft of a long bone.

Advanced Reference: Consists of compact bone enclosing the medullary cavity.

Diarrhoea Quick Reference: (die-or-ea) Frequent passage of loose motions.

Advanced Reference: Prolonged diarrhoea can lead to excess loss of fluids, nutrients and salts and is due to a number of causes including irritable bowel syndrome, intestinal inflammation or infection, anxiety and absorption irregularities.

Diastole Quick Reference: Resting phase of the heart.

Advanced Reference: Diastole precedes the systole phase and indicates the period when the ventricles are filling with blood.

Diathermy Quick Reference: A high-frequency alternating current (AC) which produces heat.

Advanced Reference: The heat is generated not by the electric current but by the oscillation of the ions in the tissues. A pulsed high-frequency AC model coagulates the tissues with minimal disruption whereas a blended current of cutting and coagulation improves haemostasis. Monopolar diathermy is most commonly used in the operating room and consists of the electro-surgical generator, active electrode, patient return electrode and the patient. The return electrode, sometimes wrongly referred to as the *earth-plate*, forms an important component of the whole unit and if improperly applied can lead to burns. It should be positioned on a well-vascularised area and as close to the operating site as possible while also being away from bony prominences and any prosthesis as this could interfere with conductivity. Bipolar diathermy does not require an earthing plate as the circuit consists of the generator and coaxial lead which conveys and returns the current.

Diazemuls® Quick Reference: Proprietary anxiolytic drug.

Advanced Reference: Used to treat anxiety and to provide sedation for minor surgery. Also used as a premedication as it has some skeletal-muscle-relaxant properties. Produced as an emulsion for injection. Is a preparation of the benzodiazepine diazepam.

DIC Quick Reference: Disseminated intravascular coagulation (clotting).

Advanced Reference: Associated with many conditions, e.g. severe haemorrhage, pancreatitis, major surgery and cardiopulmonary bypass. Abnormal coagulation occurs within the micro-circulation using up clotting factors and reducing peripheral flow. This results in reduced clotting efficiency and profuse bleeding. Treatment is with heparin as it prevents the further using up of coagulation factors, permitting normal clotting function.

Dicrotic notch Quick Reference: A double beat.

Advanced Reference: Evident when an artery expands a second time giving rise to a dicrotic beat, as seen on an invasive arterial trace. Happens when the output from the heart is strong and the tension of the pulse is low.

Didelphys Quick Reference: (di-del-fis) Double uterus.

Advanced Reference: Malformation of the uterine structure. Can be accompanied by a double cervix and vagina.

Diethyl ether Quick Reference: An agent used in general anaesthesia.

Advanced Reference: Anaesthetic ether. It is flammable and explosive in the presence of oxygen. Causes nausea and vomiting.

Diethylstilbestrol Quick Reference: (DES) Synthetic *oestrogen*.

Advanced Reference: Developed for women with a low oestrogen level during pregnancy who are at risk of *miscarriage* and *premature birth*.

Difficile Quick Reference: Member of the *Clostridium* bacteria group. Also known as C-Dif.

Advanced Reference: Commonly found in the intestinal tract but in the right circumstances and environment, i.e. during or after antibiotic therapy, can be a cause of enterocolitis.

Difficult intubation Quick Reference: Broad-meaning term indicating problems with normal laryngoscopy and intubation.

Advanced Reference: May be due to numerous factors including stiff jaw, small mouth, receding jaw, cervical spine deformity, *TMJ syndrome*, Pierre Robin, Treacher-Collins and Goldenhar syndromes, large *epiglottis*, large or swollen tongue, deviated larynx, pharyngeal oedema, short neck and large/barrel chest/breasts. Numerous devices and procedures are in use for dealing with difficult intubation scenarios, e.g. *Polio*-bladed and *McCoy* laryngo-scopes, *cricothyrotomy* and *retrograde intubation*. Differs as a term and in meaning from *failed intubation*. There are a number of *airway classification* systems in use intended to prevent or reduce the severity of this situation.

Difficult mask ventilation (and oxygenation) Quick Reference: (abbre-viation – DMV) Indicates being able to maintain an adequate airway and deliver oxygen using mask ventilation.

Advanced Reference: The five predictors of difficult bag/mask ventilation are said to be OBESE: (1) obese, (2) bearded, (3) elderly, (4) snorers, (5) edentulous. Additionally there are the four Ds of difficult airway manage-ment: (1) dentition, (2) distortion, (3) disproportion, (4) dysmobility.

Diffuse Quick Reference: Scattered or widespread.

Advanced Reference: The opposite to diffuse is being in close proximity, localised.

Diffusion Quick Reference: Spontaneous movement of molecules in a liquid or gas.

Advanced Reference: The distribution leads to an equalising out with the intention of reaching a uniform concentration. As with gas, exchange in the lungs between oxygen and carbon dioxide.

Digestion Quick Reference: The process of breaking down food in the stomach and intestines.

Advanced Reference: The food is broken down into soluble and diffusible products capable of being absorbed by the blood.

Digestive tract **Quick Reference:** Digestive system. Responsible for breaking down food into compounds that can be absorbed into the body.

Advanced Reference: Begins at the *mouth* and ends at the *rectum/anus*.

Digoxin **Quick Reference:** A heart/cardiac medication.

Advanced Reference: Derived from the *digitalis* (Foxglove) plant. Regulates and strengthens the heartbeat.

Dilatation **Quick Reference:** The process of stretching a constricted passage.

Advanced Reference: Strictures occur in the urethra which have to be dilated. Anal dilatation involves stretching of the muscle fibres of the anal ring. There are numerous instruments termed dilators, i.e. urethral, anal, oesophageal, all specific to their intended need.

Dilated cardiomyopathy **Quick Reference:** Occurs when the left ventricle becomes enlarged leading to heart failure.

Advanced Reference: The effect is that the ventricle cannot pump effectively.

Diltiazem **Quick Reference:** Vasodilator and calcium antagonist drug. Tildiem®.

Advanced Reference: Used in the prevention and treatment of angina pectoris, especially when beta-blockers have not proven effective.

Dioxin **Quick Reference:** An organic chemical compound.

Advanced Reference: It is a carcinogen and can cause genetic changes leading to congenital abnormalities. The incomplete or inefficient burning of plastics (PVC) in hospital incinerators was highlighted as a potential source. Also referred to as agent orange, a defoliant used in wartime.

Diplopia **Quick Reference:** Double vision.

Advanced Reference: Awareness of two images of the one object. Often due to problems with the muscle coordination that is responsible for eye movement.

Diprivan® **Quick Reference:** Anaesthetic induction agent.

Advanced Reference: Proprietary form of propofol. Also used as a maintenance agent in an infusion. Has a rapid recovery and fast excretion time so is recommended for day-case surgery.

Disarticulation **Quick Reference:** Separation of a limb at the joint.

Advanced Reference: An example is disarticulation of the leg, separated at the hip joint. Sometimes referred to as hind-quarter.

Disc **Quick Reference:** A flattened circular structure.

Advanced Reference: Intervertebral disc is a fibrous cartilage pad that separates the bodies of the two adjacent vertebrae. Discectomy indicates excision of part or the entire disc. The optic disc is a white spot in the retina where the optic nerve enters.

Discard-a-pad® **Quick Reference:** Pad used by the scrub practitioner to safely dispose of sharps.

Advanced Reference: Besides being used for the disposal of needles, sutures and blades, it can also be an aid to efficient checking of the needles.

Disinfectant **Quick Reference:** Surface cleaning fluid.

Advanced Reference: An agent that disinfects, applied particularly to agents used on inanimate objects, whereas an antiseptic is an agent that is capable of destroying micro-organisms and is used on bodily tissue.

Dislocation **Quick Reference:** Term that indicates moving out of position.

Advanced Reference: The displacement of any part, more especially a bone, from its natural position. Involves the joint in such instances as shoulder, hip and elbow.

Disproportion **Quick Reference:** A lack of proportion, usually between two elements of the same item.

Advanced Reference: Term applied to a fetus that has a large head in proportion to the body and has trouble passing through the mother's pelvis.

Dissect **Quick Reference:** To cut, as used in anatomy.

Advanced Reference: Tissues are dissected during surgery. Usually to separate tissues according to natural lines of structure.

Dissecting forceps **Quick Reference:** A surgical instrument used for holding tissues.

Advanced Reference: They come in many shapes and sizes and are used primarily for holding tissue. They may be toothed or non-toothed. Some of the more common in use are Lane's, McIndoe, Gillies, DeBakey, Bonny's.

Dissipate **Quick Reference:** To disperse, scatter.

Advanced Reference: Can be used in relation to the spread of a drug or dispersal of a gas.

Dissociation **Quick Reference:** The act of separating.

Advanced Reference: The oxygen dissociation curve is a graph representing the normal variation in the amount of oxygen that combines with haemoglobin as a function of the partial pressure of oxygen.

Distal **Quick Reference:** Furthest from central.

Advanced Reference: Remote, further away from a set point of reference. Opposite to proximal. In dentistry the term is used to designate a position on the dental arch farther from the median line of the jaw. Situated away from the centre of the body or point of origin.

Distention **Quick Reference:** Enlargement. Also spelt distension.

Advanced Reference: Abdominal distension is the result of swelling due to gas in the intestines or fluid in the abdominal cavity.

Distillation **Quick Reference:** The separation of a liquid mixture into its components.

Advanced Reference: The liquid is first heated to vapour, which is then cooled so that it condenses and can be collected as a liquid. The mixture can then be separated if the component liquids have different boiling points, each one vaporising at a different temperature.

Diuresis **Quick Reference:** More urine production than normal.

Advanced Reference: Increased excretion of urine.

Diuretic **Quick Reference:** (die-your-etic) Drug or substance which increases the flow of urine.

Advanced Reference: Some diuretics act on the distal tubule of the kidney while others stimulate the Loop of Henle and are termed loop diuretics. A common example of this latter group is frusemide (Lasix®). *Mannitol* also brings about an increase of urine output but this is due to the action of osmotic pressure.

Diverticulitis **Quick Reference:** Inflammation or infection of one or more diverticula.

Advanced Reference: Affects especially colonic diverticula and can involve perforation or can be abscess formation. Sometimes referred to as left-sided *appendicitis.*

Diverticulum **Quick Reference:** Plural = diverticula. A pouch or sac.

Advanced Reference: Can occur normally or can be created by herniation of the mucous membrane through a defect in a muscular coat.

Division of adhesions **Quick Reference:** The surgical separating of fibrous bands to which organs and various parts of anatomy have adhered.

Advanced Reference: Adhesions usually occur following previous surgery and can cause internal obstruction.

DMARDs **Quick Reference:** Disease-modifying antirheumatic drugs. A classification of antirheumatic agents.

Advanced Reference: They modify the course of the disease as opposed to just treating the symptoms, by acting on the immune system itself.

DNA **Quick Reference:** Deoxyribonucleic acid.

Advanced Reference: The material of which the chromosomes and genes are composed. It is present in the nucleus of each cell and contains all the instructional information needed to determine the structure and function of that cell.

Donor **Quick Reference:** One who gives. Donator. Opposite of recipient.

Advanced Reference: In relation to the health-care setting, it can indicate blood or organs to someone who is histocompatible. The universal donor refers to someone with the blood group O (negative).

Donor transplant coordinator **Quick Reference:** Health professional involved in the coordination of organs for transplantation.

Advanced Reference: In the early days of the development of this role they dealt primarily with renal transplantation. This has now developed into dealing with the patient and relatives involving all possible organs for harvesting and transplantation.

Dopamine **Quick Reference:** A neurotransmitter and sympathomimetic, e.g. intropin.

Advanced Reference: Used in the treatment of cardiogenic shock following heart attack or during surgery to support a falling blood pressure. Sometimes used in a small dosage regime to dilate the renal artery following the transplant of a kidney.

Doppler **Quick Reference:** A machine that works by relating the drop in pitch of a note when a moving source of sound passes the recording source.

Advanced Reference: Doppler is used to detect flow in blood vessels, i.e. for CVP insertion and placement with the use of a surface probe.

Dopram® **Quick Reference:** Proprietary preparation of doxapram.

Advanced Reference: A respiratory stimulant used to relieve severe respiratory difficulties such as postoperative respiratory depression. Side-effects include a rise in blood pressure and heart rate and dizziness.

Dorsal **Quick Reference:** Indicates towards the back of the body.

Advanced Reference: Can also be used in relation to the *posterior* of an organ.

Dorsalis pedis **Quick Reference:** Refers to the artery in the upper foot above the toes.

Advanced Reference: Used to take a pulse and is palpable between the first and second metatarsal bones on top of the foot. Sometimes used as a site for arterial cannulation.

Dorsiflexion **Quick Reference:** Bending backwards of the fingers or toes.

Advanced Reference: Indicates bending backwards but in many cases actually upwards, e.g. the great toe.

Dorsum **Quick Reference:** The back or posterior surfaces.

Advanced Reference: Example is the back of the hand. Dorsal relates to the back or posterior region.

Dosimetry **Quick Reference:** The calculation of dosages to treat a condition.

Advanced Reference: Used most commonly when calculating radiation dosages in cancer treatment. A dosimeter is a piece of equipment used to record the amount of radiation being received by workers, usually in the form of a small badge.

Double-glove **Quick Reference:** To don two pairs of gloves to give extra protection to the patient.

Advanced Reference: Used regularly in orthopaedics as an extra safeguard, especially when working within a joint.

Draffin suspension rods **Quick Reference:** Surgical instrument used during tonsillectomy or surgery on the mouth.

Advanced Reference: Made of stainless steel and placed in a holder on either side of the patient's head. The tongue plate of the mouth-gag fits into the rings on the rods allowing the mouth to stay open while freeing-up both hands of the surgeon.

Drain Quick Reference: A device used in surgery for draining fluid, blood and pus from a cavity or wound, usually in the immediate postoperative period.

Advanced Reference: There are many types of drains available to suit the site and need, from a simple corrugated drain to an underwater seal drain. All are either passive or active, which means they are allowed to flow freely or make use of suction or vacuum.

Drape Quick Reference: Refers to a sterile covering used to cover and protect the operative site.

Advanced Reference: Drapes are manufactured from waterproofed paper and fabric and are available in various sizes and shapes designed to suit the site and type of surgery.

Dressings Quick Reference: Sterile covering placed over a wound.

Advanced Reference: Applied with the intention of protecting the wound and incision, mainly from infection, especially following surgery.

Drip Quick Reference: Slang term used to indicate an intravenous infusion.

Advanced Reference: Although at times used to indicate the fluid itself, it generally applies to the entire configuration of fluid, giving set and cannula. A drip stand is used to hold or hang the IV bag and can be free-standing or attached to the table, and it can have an adjustable height facility.

Dromoran® Quick Reference: A narcotic analgesic.

Advanced Reference: A preparation of the opiate and narcotic levorphanol tartrate. Used to relieve severe pain.

Droperidol Quick Reference: Powerful tranquilliser. Droleptan®.

Advanced Reference: Often used in conjunction with fentanyl in neuroleptic techniques and as an antiemetic. No longer widely used or available in the UK.

Dry gangrene Quick Reference: Tissue death that occurs as a result of compromised circulation. Notable for the absence of bacterial contamination.

Advanced Reference: Commonly affects the extremities, turning them black and leathery. Also known as mummification.

Dual block Quick Reference: Also known as Phase II block.

Advanced Reference: If depolarising agents are given repeatedly, the nature of the neuromuscular block eventually changes and increasingly displays the properties of a non-depolariser making it possible for an anticholinesterase to bring about a degree of reversal. If intermittent suxamethonium infusion is being used, the recommendation is to allow the block to wear off at intervals.

Dual sensory impairment Quick Reference: Deaf-blindness.

Advanced Reference: A condition of ageing in which both visual and hearing impairment and degeneration manifest concurrently. The definitive cause is not known but such factors as *diabetes* and *atherosclerosis* are known to contribute to the condition.

Duct **Quick Reference:** A tube or channel.

Advanced Reference: A channel with well-defined walls for the passage of excretions or secretions.

Duodenum **Quick Reference:** The first portion of the intestine.

Advanced Reference: Lies between the stomach and the jejunum and measures approximately 20–25 cm in length. The pancreatic and common bile ducts open into it.

Dupuytrens **Quick Reference:** (dupe-ya-trons) Painless thickening of the connective tissue of the palm.

Advanced Reference: Involves the palmer fascia and the contracture can cause permanent bending and fixation of one or more fingers. Can be due to many causes including trauma. Surgical correction involves a palmer *fasciectomy*.

Dura **Quick Reference:** The dura mater.

Advanced Reference: The outermost and toughest of the three meningeal membranes which surround the brain and spinal cord.

Dural tap **Quick Reference:** Relates to puncture of the *dura* during epidural anaesthesia.

Advanced Reference: Happens when the anaesthetist overshoots the dural space during an *epidural* and punctures the dura leading to *CSF* leak. This leads to post-dural puncture headache (PDPH) and if it does not correct spontaneously or the patient continues to suffer, an *epidural blood patch* (EBP) procedure is performed.

DVT **Quick Reference:** Deep vein thrombosis. Formation of a thrombus (blood clot) in the veins, e.g. the inner thigh or calf.

Advanced Reference: Becomes dangerous if and when it moves from the original site and travels (embolus) in the circulation to another site, such as the lungs (pulmonary embolism). Many measures are utilised to reduce the potential for DVT, i.e. preoperative heparin, TED (thromboembolic deterrent) stockings, heel pads, intermittent leg massage devices.

Dynamic hip screw **Quick Reference:** (DHS) A metal internal fixation device used to stabilise certain proximal fractures of the femur.

Advanced Reference: Designed to provide strong and stable internal fixation for a variety of fractures to the neck of the femur.

Dynamo **Quick Reference:** The generation of power or strength.

Advanced Reference: Commonly a device that generates electricity.

Dys **Quick Reference:** Prefix denoting bad.

Advanced Reference: In medical terms it implies difficult.

Dysaesthesia **Quick Reference:** (dis-a-thesia) Distortion of any sense.

Advanced Reference: Refers especially to sense of touch. Also referred to as dysesthesia and hypoaesthesia.

Dysarthria **Quick Reference:** Speech disorder resulting from neurological injury.

Advanced Reference: Due to weakness or lack of coordination of the muscles involved in speech. Signified by speech being slow, weak and imprecise. Although it can be congenital, it is most often the result of cerebral palsy, or muscular dystrophy.

Dysentery   **Quick Reference:** (dis-en-tree) Disorder marked by inflammation of the intestines.

Advanced Reference: Affects most commonly the colon, displaying signs and symptoms that include abdominal pain, frequent motions, sometimes containing blood and mucus. Can be due to *bacteria*, *protozoa* and parasitic worms as well as chemical irritation.

Dyskaryosis   **Quick Reference:** Abnormal changes in cells.

Advanced Reference: An example would be the changes in epithelial cells of the cervix during pregnancy.

Dyslexia   **Quick Reference:** (dis-lex-ea) Defect in development in which there is an inability to read but not accompanied by intellectual impairment.

Advanced Reference: Cause is not fully understood and often comes to light in childhood but even in cases where reading is mastered, spelling remains erratic.

Dysmorphia   **Quick Reference:** (dis-more-fea) Body dysmorphic disorder. Classified as a mental disorder.

Advanced Reference: A preoccupation with a self-perceived defect in appearance or being overly concerned with a very slight physical anomaly.

Dyspepsia   **Quick Reference:** Discomfort in the process of digestion.

Advanced Reference: Due to many reasons ranging from over-eating to *peptic ulcer*, intestinal disorders and *gall bladder* disease.

Dysphagia   **Quick Reference:** (dis-fage-ea) Difficulty in swallowing. From the Greek dys (= difficulty) and phagia (= to eat).

Advanced Reference: Difficulty in the passage of solids or liquids from the mouth to the stomach. Can be a symptom of blockage or muscle spasm of the *oesophagus*.

Dysphasia   **Quick Reference:** (dis-faze-ea) Impediment in speaking and verbal comprehension. Also referred to as aphasia.

Advanced Reference: It is mostly a difficulty in understanding speech and is commonly accompanied by difficulties in reading and writing.

Dysplasia   **Quick Reference:** Abnormal development of tissue.

Advanced Reference: Can involve skin, bone or a wide range of tissues.

Dyspnoea   **Quick Reference:** (dis-p-nea) Difficulty in breathing.

Advanced Reference: Undue shortness of breath or laboured breathing.

Dysrhythmia   **Quick Reference:** (dis-rith-mea) Abnormal heart rhythm.

Advanced Reference: Term used to indicate disordered or disorganised heart rhythms.

Dystocia **Quick Reference:** (dis-toe-shea) Abnormal or difficult *labour*.

Advanced Reference: Fetal dystocia can be caused by the shape, size or position of the *fetus*; placental dystocia indicates difficult delivery of the placenta; and shoulder dystocia is when one shoulder of the fetus lodges on the mother's pubic bone.

Dystonia **Quick Reference:** Dystonic. Abnormal *tonicity* of muscle.

Advanced Reference: Characterised by prolonged and repetitive muscle contractions that may cause twisting and turning of body parts.

Dystrophy **Quick Reference:** (dis-trof-e) Wasting condition brought about by defective nutrition.

Advanced Reference: Dys = difficult, abnormal. Commonly applied to muscular conditions, e.g. muscular dystrophy.

E

Early warning scores Quick reference: Method of assessing unwell hospitalised patients.

Advanced Reference: A simple physiological scoring system that utilises five parameters: mental response, pulse rate, systolic blood pressure, respiratory rate and temperature. A sixth, urine output, is also often included with postoperative patients.

Earth plate Quick Reference: Term and description commonly but wrongly applied to the patient electrode of a *diathermy* machine.

Advanced Reference: More correctly termed inactive electrode, indifferent electrode or grounding pad, or even diathermy plate. Usually gel covered as a contact medium on the skin side and placed in an area of thick tissue such as the thigh.

ECG Quick Reference: Electrocardiograph.

Advanced Reference: A recording or visual display (electrocardiogram) of the electrical changes in the heart muscle taken via electrodes attached to the external chest. During routine anaesthesia three leads are used as rhythm and rate are adequate for this setting; however, for a diagnostic reading a 12-lead ECG tracing is preferable offering a more in-depth view of heart function, viewing it from multiple angles.

If a permanent print-off is desired it is useful to know that ECG paper consists of small and large squares and the standard speed for a printer is 25 mm/s. The small squares measure 1 mm (therefore paper travels at 25 small squares per minute). To roughly assess rate, count the number of large squares between two R waves and divide 300 by the number of large squares and this will provide the rate, i.e. $300 \div 5 = 60$ beats per minute.

Echocardiography Quick Reference: A diagnostic test of the heart.

Advanced Reference: Uses ultrasound waves to form images of the chambers and valves of the heart as well as surrounding structures. Can also be used to measure cardiac output and detect inflammation (pericarditis).

Echogenic Quick Reference: Relates to echoes of ultrasound waves.

Advanced Reference: In ultrasonography indicates giving rise to reflections (echoes).

Eclampsia Quick Reference: (e-clamp-see-a) Convulsions during pregnancy due to *toxaemia*.

Advanced Reference: Pre-eclampsia precedes the crisis. Eclampsia produces fits/convulsions and possible coma and is characterised by oedema,

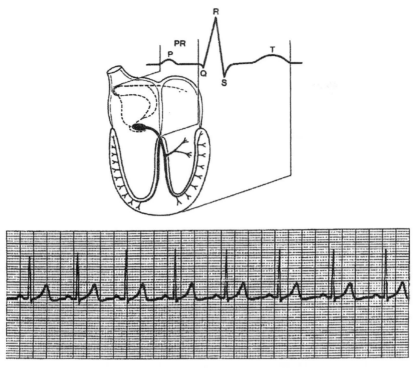

Fig. 7. Relation of an electrocardiogram to the anatomy of the cardiac conduction system

hypertension and protein in the urine (proteinuria). Immediate treatment is delivery of the baby as the condition can be fatal to both mother and fetus.

ECMO **Quick Reference:** Extracorporeal membrane oxygenation. Technique for providing cardiac and respiratory support. Most regularly used in intensive care medicine and neonatal intensive care units (NICU).

Advanced Reference: Utilised with those patients whose heart and lungs are so severely diseased that they fail to carry out their intended function. Works in a similar manner to a *heart–lung machine*, where large blood vessels are cannulated and blood is continuously diverted to an external oxygenator. Commonly used in conjunction with a *ventricular assist device* (VAD), especially with those awaiting heart transplantation.

Eco **Quick Reference:** Refers to ecology, ecological. Also termed bionomics.

Advanced Reference: The science of the relationships between organisms and their environment.

ECT **Quick Reference:** Electroconvulsive therapy.

Advanced Reference: Used in the treatment of mental illness by applying a small electric shock to the external scalp via electrodes. This passes through the frontal lobes of the brain and brings about a brief period of unconsciousness followed by convulsion. It is used in the treatment of depression and schizophrenia in patients who do not respond to other treatment regimes.

-ectomy　**Quick Reference:** Surgical removal of part or all of an organ.

Advanced Reference: A suffix which indicates to excise or remove surgically, e.g. appendicectomy (removal of the appendix), gastrectomy (removal of the stomach).

Ectopic　**Quick Reference:** Outside of or away from the normal site.

Advanced Reference: Indicates an abnormal anatomical situation or position. Examples being ectopic pregnancy (when a pregnancy starts to develop in the Fallopian tube instead of uterus), also ectopic heartbeat (a beat that originates from an area other than the normal conduction pathway).

Ectropion　**Quick Reference:** Turning outwards of the eyelid.

Advanced Reference: The margin of the eyelid becomes averted and requires surgery to shorten the lower lid. Most commonly seen in the elderly, those suffering nerve palsy or if the skin of the lower eyelid has been scarred following trauma or previous surgery.

Eczema　**Quick Reference:** A skin inflammation in which there is the formation of small vesicles with subsequent weeping, scaling and crusting.

Advanced Reference: There is an *hereditary* form (*atopic*) due to an immunological defect and it is often accompanied by *asthma* and *hayfever*.

Edinburgh tray system　**Quick Reference:** A system/process devised for surgical tray layout.

Advanced Reference: Designed to make the location of instruments more functional and safer. Involves the layout, grouping, accessibility and accountability of instruments when in use on the surgical tray in theatres.

EEG　**Quick Reference:** Electroencephalogram.

Advanced Reference: A recording of the electrical activity in the brain taken through electrodes attached to the scalp.

Efcortesol®　**Quick Reference:** Proprietary preparation of hydrocortisone.

Advanced Reference: A corticosteroid used as an anti-inflammatory for allergy, in the treatment of shock and to restore a deficiency of steroid hormone in the body.

Efferent　**Quick Reference:** Leading away from the centre towards the periphery.

Advanced Reference: Efferent arterioles exit via the glomerulus of the kidney after entering as an afferent vessel. Efferent motor nerves leave the brain to supply muscles.

Effusion　**Quick Reference:** An outpouring of fluid into the tissues or a cavity.

Advanced Reference: Examples where this is common are the knee and pleural space and can involve blood and serum. Causes can be due to inflammation or congestion.

Elasticity   Quick Reference: The property that allows any material to recover after stretching.

Advanced Reference: Elast(o) denotes flexibility.

Elastic stockings   Quick Reference: Refers to support devices worn throughout the perioperative period to prevent DVT.

Advanced Reference: Correct term is *TED* stockings (thromboembolism deterrent).

Elastin   Quick Reference: Protein that forms the major constituent of elastic tissue fibres.

Advanced Reference: Constituent of yellow elastic *connective tissue*. It is brittle when dry but flexible and elastic when moist.

Elastomer   Quick Reference: A rubber-like *polymer* (elastic = ability to return to original shape; -mer = many parts).

Advanced Reference: Used in dentistry as an impression material and for various prostheses in such specialities as *maxillofacial* surgery.

Elective   Quick Reference: Chosen when to do. Used to differentiate between a scheduled and an emergency procedure.

Advanced Reference: Common example is an elective Caesarean section as opposed to an emergency. The former indicates a planned event for its own reasons, whereas the latter involves a decision due to maternal and/or fetal complications.

Electrode   Quick Reference: A conductive point of delivery or return for an electrical charge.

Advanced Reference: ECG electrodes are commonly referred to within the theatre as dots for applying a 3-lead ECG to the patient (chest). Each electrode provides a connection between the patient and the machine interpreting the electrical activity of the heart. Further examples of electrodes include those used for *EEG*, *ECT*, nerve stimulation and the diathermy earth plate.

Electrolysis   Quick Reference: (elec-trol-a-sis) Chemical changes brought about by means of electricity.

Advanced Reference: An example is the passing of electricity through water which decomposes/separates into oxygen and hydrogen. Also refers to the process of removing body hair.

Electrolyte   Quick Reference: A solution that is capable of conducting electricity. A substance that forms a solution through which an electric current can be passed as the molecules involved separate into ions, i.e. groups of atoms with an electrical charge, the cations being attached to the negative electrode and the anions to the positive.

Advanced Reference: Ions are formed when a compound dissociates in a solution, e.g. $NaCl > Na^+ + Cl^-$. The most common are *sodium*, *potassium*, *calcium* and *magnesium*. The resultant solutions have the ability to conduct electricity, hence the term electrolyte.

Electromagnetic **Quick Reference:** Pertaining to magnetism that is induced by an electric current.

Advanced Reference: Involves radiation such as microwaves, x-rays and radiowaves.

Elephantiasis **Quick Reference:** Gross swelling of the legs and/or genitalia due to blockage of the *lymphatic* vessels.

Advanced Reference: Also known as lymphatic filariasis, caused by parasitic worms invading the lymphatic system. The worms are passed on by mosquitoes.

Emaciation **Quick Reference:** (em-ace-e-a-shun) Indicates extreme wasting of body tissue.

Advanced Reference: Extreme loss of body weight, malnourishment. Seen in patients suffering chronic disease and elderly patients admitted for treatment who are depleted of fluids and nourishment.

Embolisation **Quick Reference:** The process or condition of becoming an *embolus*. Embolotherapy.

Advanced Reference: The process by which a vessel or organ is obstructed by an embolus. Also, the surgical introduction of various substances into the circulatory system to obstruct specific blood vessels.

Embolism **Quick Reference:** Blocking of a blood vessel by material carried in the blood stream that can lead to remote blockages within the vascular system, i.e. embolism.

Advanced Reference: The material (embolism) can be a blood clot, fat, air and, less commonly, amniotic fluid and even a sheared off fragment from an IV cannula or catheter. Removal is termed an embolectomy, usually carried out with a long catheter inserted into the vessel which has an inflatable balloon at its tip designed to pass the obstruction when deflated, which is then drawn back when inflated and so withdraws the obstruction.

Embryo **Quick Reference:** (em-bre-o) The stage in the development of a plant or animal that follows the fertilisation of an egg by a sperm.

Advanced Reference: In humans, it is the stage from two weeks after fertilisation until two months, after which period it is termed the *fetus*. Embryology is the scientific study of the growth of embryos.

EMD **Quick Reference:** Electromechanical dissociation, also termed pulseless electrical activity (PEA).

Advanced Reference: Indicates an absence of sufficient cardiac output while displaying a normal or near-normal ECG trace. Can be due to pulmonary embolism, pneumothorax, hypovolaemia and hypercarbia.

Emesis **Quick Reference:** Indicates vomiting.

Advanced Reference: Often incorporated with other medical terms, i.e. *haematemesis* (vomiting of blood). An emetic is any substance that can induce vomiting. An *antiemetic* is a drug administered to prevent vomiting.

EMG   Quick Reference: Electromyogram. A recording of muscle contraction when stimulated by a nerve impulse.

Advanced Reference: Involves the responses of the muscles in the diagnosis of nerve conduction defects and muscle contraction.

Emphysema   Quick Reference: (em-fa-seem-a) Abnormal presence of air or gas in the tissues, e.g lungs and subcutaneous tissues.

Advanced Reference: Term normally applied to the lungs in which the alveoli are grossly enlarged and can eventually be destroyed. Found in those suffering from asthma, bronchitis and is associated with smoking and air pollution. The main symptom is breathlessness. The alveoli can become so damaged that air exchange is barely adequate for bodily needs.

Empyema   Quick Reference: (em-pie-ema) An internal abscess.

Advanced Reference: With empyema the pus occupies a natural cavity within the body, e.g. pleura. Treatment involves drainage and antibiotics.

Emulsion   Quick Reference: Dispersion of one liquid in another.

Advanced Reference: Indicates a preparation in which droplets of one liquid are dispersed into another. Many medicines are prepared in this way.

Enamel   Quick Reference: A protective, hard glossy outer covering.

Advanced Reference: The hard outer covering of the teeth.

Encapsulated   Quick Reference: Contained within a capsule.

Advanced Reference: The eye can be described as being within a capsule, i.e. the orbital space within the skull. There are other situations where sebaceous cysts form within a fibrous capsule.

Encapsulectomy   Quick Reference: Removal of the capsule and contents.

Advanced Reference: Often performed during removal of sebaceous cysts. Removing the entire capsule minimises the re-occurrence of the cyst.

Encephalo(n)   Quick Reference: (en-cef-alo) Relating to the brain.

Advanced Reference: Encephalopathy indicates any disease of the brain, especially involving physical changes. Encephalitis is inflammation of the brain usually due to viral infection. Encephalography is a radiological examination of the brain. An encephalocele involves protrusion of the brain through a hole in the skull.

Endarterectomy   Quick Reference: Unblocking of a vessel.

Advanced Reference: Commonly refers to an artery (carotid) and the removal of *intima* and *plaque* which are causing a blockage. Also referred to as disobliteration.

Endemic   Quick Reference: Indicates a disease which is always present in a population.

Advanced Reference: As opposed to epidemic, which describes a disease which arrives, spreads and then disappears.

Endobronchial   Quick Reference: Indicates to enter the bronchus.

Advanced Reference: Endobronchial tubes and blockers are inserted into the bronchus via the trachea. Both are used in thoracic surgery, however blockers are rarely used now whereas endobronchial tubes such as the *Robert-Shaw* and Carlens tubes continue to be the design of choice for *one-lung anaesthesia*.

Endocarditis   **Quick Reference:** Inflammation of the membrane lining the heart (endocardium), the innermost layer of the heart.

Advanced Reference: Especially affects the valves of the heart. Acute endocarditis is often the result of rheumatic fever. A number of bacteria can also be involved, e.g. *Staphylococcus aureus, Staphylococcus pneumoniae, Staphylococcus viridans*. Depending on the severity, treatment can range from antibiotics to surgical replacement of valves.

Endocrine   **Quick Reference:** Term indicating internal secretion.

Advanced Reference: An endocrine gland is one which releases its secretion (hormone) directly into the bloodstream to act upon another part of the body.

Endogenous   **Quick Reference:** Growing within the body.

Advanced Reference: Produced from internal causes, as with disease.

Endometriosis   **Quick Reference:** Condition in which *endometrium* (lining of the uterus) is found in abnormal sites throughout the body.

Advanced Reference: The commonest alternative sites are the surface of the ovaries, *peritoneum* covering the bladder and pelvic colon as well as on the uterus and round ligaments in the pelvis. These ectopic fragments pass through the same monthly cycle as the normal uterine membrane, becoming swollen before a period (*menstruation)* and then bleeding. As there is then no outlet for this blood, pain can develop during the days prior to onset of menstrual bleeding.

Endometrium   **Quick Reference:** Inner layer of the uterus.

Advanced Reference: Endometrium is a highly vascular structure that has two distinctive layers. The first layer is the superficial one within the uterine cavity and sheds itself during menstruation, i.e. stratum functionalis. The deeper layer is permanent and carries the vascular supply that helps re-form the outer layer after each menstrual cycle.

Endorphin   **Quick Reference:** (en-door-fin) A class of chemical substances found throughout the nervous system. They are produced in response to painful stimuli. More correctly termed endomorphine.

Advanced Reference: Most abundant in the spinal cord, they are concerned with sensation and appear to modify the feeling of pain. It is thought that the painkilling action of narcotics may be due to their imitating the natural effect of endorphins, to which they are chemically related.

Endoscope   **Quick Reference:** Instrument for examining the interior of the body.

Advanced Reference: Examples are gastroscope and cystoscope. Can be of rigid or flexible design and may incorporate a light source, all modern versions using a fibre-optic light source. Endoscopy is the overall term used to indicate the examination and inspection of body parts and cavities without the need in many cases for invasive surgery.

Endothelin   Quick Reference: Naturally produced vasoconstrictor.

Advanced Reference: Originally produced in endothelial cells as well as other areas of the body, it is a very potent vasoconstrictor which circulates in the blood. In excess it may be the cause of *pulmonary hypertension*.

Endotoxins   Quick Reference: A poison forming part of the bacterium and damaging only tissues in a localised area.

Advanced Reference: Found inside of bacteria and liberated into the tissues when the organism disintegrates, whereas exotoxins are secreted by the intact bacteria.

Endotracheal   Quick Reference: Indicates within the trachea. Abbreviated to ET.

Advanced Reference: Most commonly refers to the insertion of an endotracheal tube (ETT) into the trachea during anaesthesia or to provide ventilatory support in various situations, such as emergency resuscitation, and in the ICU for long-term ventilation.

End-plate   Quick Reference: Indicates the motor end-plate of the nervous system.

Advanced Reference: Located at the terminal membrane of an axon and the post-junctional membrane of the adjoining muscle tissue.

End-tidal   Quick Reference: Applies to gas readings taken at the end of the expiratory cycle.

Advanced Reference: End-tidal carbon dioxide indicates the reading by a capnometer/capnograph at expiration and is an indication of alveolar carbon dioxide levels.

End-to-side anastomosis   Quick Reference: Involves anastomosing one end of a vessel/structure to the side of another.

Advanced Reference: Examples include jejunum to stomach and donor renal artery to recipient internal iliac artery as in renal transplant.

Enema   Quick Reference: Substance (usually liquid preparation) injected in to the lower bowel.

Advanced Reference: Used to evacuate faeces from the rectum, or in radiography, when the enema contains barium, to outline the rectum and colon.

Enflurane   Quick Reference: Volatile anaesthetic agent. Ethrane®.

Advanced Reference: Anaesthetic supplement delivered via a calibrated vaporiser (colour-coded yellow/orange). Only a small proportion is metabolised, making it particularly safe for repeated use. There is some evidence that it is not suitable for those with a history of epilepsy.

ENT   Quick Reference: Ear, nose and throat. Surgical/medical speciality.

Advanced Reference: Although grouped together as a speciality, practitioners are tending to specialise in certain areas of each. Also termed otorhino-laryngology.

Enteral   Quick Reference: The intestine. The prefix entero denotes the intestine.

Advanced Reference: Indicates via the intestinal tract, especially with reference to feeding which may also be provided via the *parenteral* and intravenous routes.

Enteritis   Quick Reference: Inflammation of the intestine.

Advanced Reference: Usually applied to the small intestine.

Enterobacter   Quick Reference: Gram-negative aerobic bacteria.

Advanced Reference: A member of the normal gut *flora* but outside of this environment causes severe infections, mainly of the respiratory and urinary tracts. Known as an opportunistic bacteria as it attacks debilitated and immuno-suppressed people. ITU patients are commonly at risk of the bacterial *pneumonitis* it causes.

Enterovirus   Quick Reference: A virus which infects the gastrointestinal tract and then the central nervous system.

Advanced Reference: The virus produces specific diseases elsewhere in the body, i.e. polio, after entering through the alimentary tract.

Entomology   Quick Reference: The study of insects. A branch of zoology.

Advanced Reference: A medical entomologist deals with insects that cause disease.

Entonox   Quick Reference: A mixture of oxygen and nitrous oxide.

Advanced Reference: A mixture of 50% oxygen and 50% nitrous oxide. Colour coding is a blue cylinder with a blue and white quartered shoulder. During storage, cylinders must be laid flat, especially in cold environments, in order to avoid the liquid nitrous oxide settling in the lower half of the cylinder, leaving pure oxygen in the upper half. Consequently if used the patient would be receiving only oxygen until this was used up and then later pure nitrous oxide. Therefore, it is recommended that the cylinder is shaken and inverted a number of times prior to use.

Entropion   Quick Reference: A condition involving the eyelid turning inwards.

Advanced Reference: Mostly affects the lower lid, allowing the lashes to make contact with the eye resulting in irritation and inflammation. Surgical intervention may include the excision of a triangle-shaped piece of skin, muscle and tarsus. The edges are then sutured together to avert the lid margin.

Enucleation   Quick Reference: To shell out, enucleate.

Advanced Reference: Involves the removal of a structure, tumour, or gland, for example, as a whole. As with removal of the eye.

Enuresis   **Quick Reference:** Involuntary passing of urine.

Advanced Reference: Nocturnal enuresis is referred to as bed wetting.

Enzyme   **Quick Reference:** A substance produced by living cells which promotes chemical change.

Advanced Reference: An enzyme is a biological catalyst responsible for metabolism both inside and outside the cells. They are proteins and are specific for one reaction or a well-defined group of similar reactions.

Epanutin®   **Quick Reference:** Anticonvulsant drug.

Advanced Reference: Used to treat grand mal epileptic seizures. A preparation of phenytoin.

Ephedrine   **Quick Reference:** (ef-e-dreen) Vasoconstrictor and bronchodilator.

Advanced Reference: Used mainly in the treatment of asthma, chronic bronchitis and hypotension, especially during spinal anaesthesia when sudden falls in blood pressure are possible.

Epicardium   **Quick Reference:** Outer surface lining of the heart.

Advanced Reference: Often referred to as the visceral layer of the serous pericardium. This is a transparent layer with delicate connective tissue that creates a smooth but glossy surface, which prevents fibrosis and friction between the adjacent structures within the mediastinum.

Epidemic   **Quick Reference:** The occurrence of a number of cases of similar illness in excess of normal expectation.

Advanced Reference: Disease attacking many people at the same time in a community or region.

Epidemiology   **Quick Reference:** Study of factors determining disease.

Advanced Reference: Purpose is to establish programmes to prevent and control the development and spread of disease by looking at the influences, frequency and distribution of disease, injury and other health-related events as well as their causes in relation to a defined population.

Epidermis   **Quick Reference:** The outer part/layer of the skin.

Advanced Reference: The thin layer of epithelium that is closely connected to the dermis. Cutaneous = in relation to the skin.

Epididymis   **Quick Reference:** (epi-did-i-miss) A comma-shaped structure attached to the testis.

Advanced Reference: Its function is to aid the changes within the spermatozoa. It is a 6-m length of tubing tightly packed into the comma shape, which forms the proximal end of the vas deferens. Research suggests that spermatozoa can be stored within the epididymis potentially for 30 days or longer. After this period, the spermatozoa are likely to begin degeneration and become dysfunctional and following this reabsorption takes place.

Epidural   **Quick Reference:** Indicates a regional anaesthetic technique.

Advanced Reference: Refers to the administration of a local anaesthetic injected outside of the dura, in the thoracic, lumbar or sacral levels of the spinal cord. Used commonly in obstetrics during labour and delivery. Usually involves the insertion and placement of an indwelling catheter which is used to top up the levels of analgesia when needed.

Epidurography   Quick Reference: Radiographic investigation of the spine.
Advanced Reference: Involves the injection of a *radiopaque* medium into the *epidural* space.

Epigastrium   Quick Reference: A region of the abdomen.
Advanced Reference: The upper part of the abdomen in the angle of the ribs over the stomach.

Epiglottis   Quick Reference: A leaf-shaped cartilage that lies at the back of the pharynx.
Advanced Reference: The epiglottis covers the opening from the pharynx into the larynx and so prevents food from entering the trachea.

Epilepsy   Quick Reference: The falling sickness as it is sometimes called.
Advanced Reference: A convulsive attack due to an abnormality of brain function, which may result in a momentary loss of attention or consciousness.

Epiphysis   Quick Reference: (epif-y-sis) Expanded articular end of a long bone.
Advanced Reference: Separated from the shaft during growth by a plate of cartilage laying down new bone. When an individual is fully grown the cartilage disappears and the epiphysis fuses with the shaft.

Episiotomy   Quick Reference: An incision in the perineum.
Advanced Reference: The cut is made during childbirth to prevent tearing when the vaginal opening needs to be widened to enable free passage of the baby. Following delivery, the cut is sutured.

Epistaxis   Quick Reference: Bleeding from the nasal cavity.
Advanced Reference: May be the result of infection or injury. Can be a life-threatening condition if bleeding is excessive and not treated.

Epithelial   Quick Reference: Refers to epithelium, i.e. the tissue that covers parts of the body, both internally and externally.
Advanced Reference: It is classified as simple when it is one cell thick and stratified when there is more than one cell making up the layers.

Epontol®   Quick Reference: Anaesthetic induction agent. Propanidid.
Advanced Reference: A non-barbiturate anaesthetic induction agent which has been superseded by newer agents. Dissolved in the same solvent (Cremophor) as Althesin® (another agent now withdrawn) making it difficult to inject due to its oily nature. It has a history of producing hypotension, apnoea and bronchospasm.

Epoxy   Quick Reference: Group of resins capable of forming tough polymer structures. Also referred to as polyepoxide.
Advanced Reference: Epoxy resins are heat and chemical resistant and popularly used in the production of adhesives, when they are mixed with a

catalysing agent (hardener). They can instigate *endocrine* disorders and the agents used as *catalysts* can cause allergic reactions.

ERCP   **Quick Reference:** Endoscopic retrograde cholangiopancreatography.

Advanced Reference: Involves a combination of endoscopy and contrast *radiology* and is used to demonstrate the biliary and pancreatic ducts.

Erectile   **Quick Reference:** Upright, to stand vertical.

Advanced Reference: The *penis* and *clitoris* are composed largely of erectile tissue which enables them to become 'erect' during sexual stimulation.

Ergometrine   **Quick Reference:** Uterine stimulant drug.

Advanced Reference: Used during childbirth in the third stage to assist delivery of the placenta and to prevent postnatal bleeding. Commonly used to bring about uterine contraction during termination of pregnancy and evacuation of products of conception. Ergot is a fungus which is a parasite of rye and contains numerous alkaloids used in medicine, one action being that it directly stimulates involuntary muscle.

Ergonomics   **Quick Reference:** The study of the efficiency of people in relation to their working environment.

Advanced Reference: Vital in lifting and handling in regard to health and safety.

Erosion   **Quick Reference:** The breaking down of tissue usually by ulceration.

Advanced Reference: Can refer to a tumour eroding into neighbouring tissues and erosion of the cervix caused by the replacement of the normal squamous epithelium by columnar epithelium.

Erythema   **Quick Reference:** (erith-eem-ea) Reddening of the skin.

Advanced Reference: An increased blood flow in the capillaries that may be caused by infection, exposure to cold or an allergic reaction.

Erythrocyte   **Quick Reference:** (ereeth-ro-site) A mature red blood cell.

Advanced Reference: The red blood cell contains haemoglobin, the substance that transports oxygen from the lungs to the tissues and carbon dioxide from the tissues to the lungs.

Erythromycin   **Quick Reference** (earth-row-my-sin) An antibiotic.

Advanced Reference: Used in the treatment of pneumonia, Legionnaire's disease and as an alternative to penicillin in patients who are allergic.

Eschar   **Quick Reference:** Dry *slough* or scab produced by a thermal burn.

Advanced Reference: An escharotomy is the surgical incision of constricting eschar in order to permit the cut edges to separate and restore blood flow to unburned tissue distal to the eschar.

Escherichia coli   **Quick Reference:** An organism commonly found in the intestines.

Advanced Reference: Mostly harmless in its normal environment but can be the cause of serious infection if found in other parts of the body.

Eschmarch bandage   **Quick Reference:** (es-kark) A rubber bandage that is rolled onto an arm or leg to produce a bloodless field.

Advanced Reference: The bandage is applied from the distal end of the limb, making sure it is fully stretched and overlapping itself, and once it reaches the pre-fitted tourniquet, this is inflated to the required pressure. Originally functioned as a tourniquet itself but produces unknown pressures.

Esmolol **Quick Reference:** An antiarrhythmic.

Advanced Reference: Used for the short-term treatment of supraventricular arrhythmias, namely atrial fibrillation, atrial flutter and perioperative tachycardia.

ESR **Quick Reference:** Erythrocyte sedimentation rate.

Advanced Reference: Measures the rate at which red cells settle when a column of blood is left for an hour.

Ester **Quick Reference:** A class of chemical compounds formed by the bonding of an alcohol and an organic acid.

Advanced Reference: A compound formed by mixing alcohol and an acid resulting in the elimination of water. Fats are esters produced by the bonding of fatty acids with the alcohol. An esterase is any enzyme that splits esters.

Ethanol **Quick Reference:** Ethyl alcohol.

Advanced Reference: Form of alcohol present in alcoholic drinks and produced from fermentation of sugar and yeast.

Ethics **Quick Reference:** Relates to rules or principles. Correct conduct.

Advanced Reference: Clinical ethics involves the ethical analysis of decision making in the care of patients.

Ethmoid **Quick Reference:** Sieve-like. Small bone of the skull.

Advanced Reference: Forms the roof of the nose. Its name comes from the structure which is pierced with many small holes through which the olfactory nerves pass.

Ethyl chloride **Quick Reference:** Inhalation anaesthetic agent.

Advanced Reference: Originally a volatile agent with a rapid onset and highly inflammable. No longer used as an anaesthetic agent but still functional as a cold indicator when measuring the extent of spread during regional anaesthetic techniques. Sometimes used as a topical local anaesthetic to freeze areas.

Ethylene **Quick Reference:** A colourless inflammable gas derived from petroleum. (Chemical formula – C_2H_4).

Advanced Reference: Has been used as an inhalational anaesthetic.

Ethylene glycol **Quick Reference:** Antifreeze.

Advanced Reference: Used as a substitute for alcohol as an intoxicating liquor, usually with fatal results.

Ethylene oxide **Quick Reference:** A gas used for its sterilisation properties.

Advanced Reference: It can penetrate inaccessible parts and areas of a piece of equipment not able to be sterilised by other methods or treated with steam sterilisation. However, it is explosive and potentially carcinogenic so its use is controlled and also requires a lengthy aeration period as well as a specialised area for use. Due to these adverse actions and necessary controls it is now seldom used in the hospital setting.

Ethyl violet **Quick Reference:** Substance added to carbon dioxide absorbents as an indicator.

Advanced Reference: Chemical formula $C_{31}H_{42}N_3Cl$. Known to develop a yellow tinge when used with *Barium lime*.

Etomidate **Quick Reference:** Anaesthetic induction agent.

Advanced Reference: The proprietary form of it is Hypnomidate®, a non-barbiturate used mainly because of its lack of cardiovascular depressant effects.

Eucalyptus **Quick Reference:** (you-cal-ip-tus) Oil obtained from the eucalyptus tree.

Advanced Reference: Used as a remedy for coughs and colds. Applied externally as a rub or inhaled as a vapour.

Eusol **Quick Reference:** (you-sol) Chlorine-based antiseptic.

Advanced Reference: Contains hypochlorous and boric acids.

Eustachian tube (canal) **Quick Reference:** (you-station) A narrow tube (canal) that connects the middle ear with the naso*pharynx*.

Advanced Reference: Its function is to equalise pressure between the middle ear and the atmosphere.

Evacuator **Quick Reference:** A surgical instrument/device used in urology. Example is Ellick's evacuator.

Advanced Reference: Designed to flush out small fragments of stone or tissue shavings [from transurethral resection of the prostate or bladder tumour (TURP/TURT), etc.] from the bladder.

Evaporation **Quick Reference:** Pertaining to evaporation of a liquid into a vapour.

Advanced Reference: Applicable especially with reference to patient heat loss via large incisions during surgery when heat is lost with fluid evaporation. Alcohol-based skin preps also utilise evaporation, as the water in which they are diluted holds them on the skin surface until evaporation of the alcohol occurs, this being long enough to lower bacterial count.

Exchange transfusion **Quick Reference:** Used in the treatment of severe cases of *haemolytic* disease of the newborn.

Advanced Reference: Involves replacing the whole of the baby's blood with Rhesus-neg blood of the correct group for the baby.

Excise **Quick Reference:** To remove by cutting out.

Advanced Reference: Surgical excision is the cutting away of a structure or diseased/unwanted tissue.

Excretion **Quick Reference:** Elimination of by-products of digestion and metabolism.

Advanced Reference: The main organs of excretion are the kidneys (water, salts, acids, nitrogen compounds), lungs (carbon dioxide and water), skin (water, salt) and liver (bile pigments, salts, toxins).

Exenteration **Quick Reference:** Surgical removal of inner organs.

Advanced Reference: Commonly used to indicate excision of the contents of the pelvis. Also, in ophthalmic surgery it refers to the removal of the entire contents of the orbit.

Exfoliation **Quick Reference:** Peeling/removing of a surface layer.

Advanced Reference: Commonly used to mean the flaking and peeling of a surface layer of skin, as witnessed in patients with psoriasis.

Exocrine **Quick Reference:** A gland that discharges its secretion by means of a duct.

Advanced Reference: Examples are salivary glands and the pancreas. Opposite to endocrine, which indicates a gland without a duct.

Exogenous **Quick Reference:** Of external origin.

Advanced Reference: A condition that is caused by external factors and/or the environment.

Exotoxin **Quick Reference:** A poisonous substance.

Advanced Reference: A soluble poisonous substance produced during the growth of a micro-organism and released into the surrounding medium.

Expiratory reserve volume (ERV) **Quick Reference:** The maximum volume of air expired beyond or at the end of normal expiration.

Advanced Reference: The quantity of air that can be expired with effort after normal expiration has been achieved.

Expiratory valve **Quick Reference:** Adjustable pressure-limiting valve found as part of an anaesthetic circuit.

Advanced Reference: The valve opens to allow the passage/release of expired gas and then closes to prevent the drawing in of air. A common example is the *Heidbrink* valve which has a thin disc held in place by a spring attached to a screwed adjuster, which opens and closes the valve.

Expulsion **Quick Reference:** To force out, squeeze under pressure.

Advanced Reference: The act of expelling something, as with the *fetus* or *placenta* from the *uterus*.

Extended endocardial resection procedure **Quick Reference:** (EERP) Surgical removal of endocardial fibrosis around the base of a left ventricular *aneurysm*.

Advanced Reference: Done to relieve *ventricular tachycardia* in patients with *ischaemic* heart disease.

Extension **Quick Reference:** To extend. Unbend. To straighten a limb.

Advanced Reference: Most commonly applies to the movement of muscles when bringing about the straightening of a limb. An extensor muscle is one that causes straightening of a limb or other body part.

External counter-pulsation **Quick Reference:** A non-invasive technique used to increase blood flow to the heart and reduce its workload.

Advanced Reference: A multi-session treatment where pressure cuffs are placed on the lower legs and inflated sequentially gently compressing leg blood vessels and assisting blood back to the heart. The benefit is that it lowers the pressure the heart normally pumps against and increases return volume. Used in the treatment of angina while helping to reduce the need for medication.

Extracellular **Quick Reference:** Situated or occurring outside of the cells.

Advanced Reference: An example is extracellular fluid, which indicates all body fluids situated outside of the cells, i.e. intravascular and interstitial.

Extracorporeal **Quick Reference:** Situated outside of the body.

Advanced Reference: Commonly relates to situations when blood is diverted outside of the body, e.g. *cardiopulmonary bypass* and *renal dialysis* but also to procedures where treatment is non-invasive such as *lithotripsy* (extracorporeal shock-wave lithotripsy – ESWL).

Extradural **Quick Reference:** Situated or occurring outside of the dura mater.

Advanced Reference: Epidural indicates placing local anaesthetic outside of the dura and within the epidural space.

Extrasystole **Quick Reference:** (extra-sis-toe-lee) Indicates extra beats seen on an *ECG* trace.

Advanced Reference: *Ectopic* beats are an example of extrasystoles.

Extravasation **Quick Reference:** Escape or leakage of fluid from a blood vessel into the tissues.

Advanced Reference: Occurs when a needle or cannula 'tissues'. Should the drug or medicine being injected have the potential for harm, there are agents which can help disperse or speed up absorption, e.g. *hyaluronidase*.

Extremity **Quick Reference:** Indicates the distal point.

Advanced Reference: Could indicate the foot or hand but more usually individual fingers and toes.

Extubation **Quick Reference:** The removal of an endotracheal tube from the trachea.

Advanced Reference: General term for removal of all types and designs of tube from the trachea.

Exudate **Quick Reference:** A discharge of serous fluid.

Advanced Reference: Composed of fluid, cells and debris which, due to inflammation, have escaped from the blood vessels and into the tissues.

F

Fabry disease **Quick Reference:** Caused by a missing or faulty *enzyme* needed to process oils, waxes and fatty acids.

Advanced Reference: Often present in patients suffering a *stroke.* The inactivity of the enzyme allows the build-up of *lipids* to a harmful level going on to have a detrimental effect on the eyes, kidneys, nervous and cardiovascular systems.

Face mask **Quick Reference:** Masks that connect the patient to breathing systems, including anaesthetic circuits, oxygen and gas-air delivery systems.

Advanced Reference: Anaesthetic models were traditionally malleable, of low dead space and made from black (antistatic) rubber, but are now available in a range of sizes, shapes and are manufactured from plastic/PVC, rubber and silicone. Whatever the design or material, they are intended to contour the face, giving a snug, leak-proof and comfortable fit, helped by the inflatable cuff around the edge of most models. They have a standard 22-mm fitting to connect direct to the circuit tubing or via an angled connector. Face masks also include those designed to fit over the nose as used in dental anaesthesia, the Goldman being a popular model. The original design for children most commonly used was the Rendell-Baker (rubber) version but numerous variations are now available and all adhere to the shallow (low dead space) design and comfort fit. Use of a face mask is not without its inherent risks, with pressure being the foremost, causing injury to a branch of the trigeminal and/or facial nerve, while an ill-fitting and too large a mask can be a risk to the eyes. Masks used in recovery are mostly of the transparent PVC oxygen-delivery type and include the MC model and Venturi (Mix-O-Mask). Those attached to gas-air delivery systems tend to be of similar design to anaesthetic and resuscitation types (Ambu), some with incorporated *Heidbrink* and demand valves.

Faciomaxillary **Quick Reference:** Refers to the surgical speciality dealing with the correction of facial injury and correction.

Advanced Reference: Also referred to as maxillofacial or in slang terms as max-fax. Involves and incorporates aspects of dentistry, orthodontics, plastic, orthopaedic and ENT surgery.

Factor VIII **Quick Reference:** Antihaemophilic factor.

Advanced Reference: A clotting factor, the absence of which leads to coagulation disorders such as *haemophilia.*

Faeces Quick Reference: (fee-sees) Waste material eliminated via the anus.

Advanced Reference: Consists of undigested food, *cellulose*, water, *mucus*, *fibre* and dead cells from the lining of the intestine and *bile* pigments which form the colour of the waste matter.

Fahrenheit Quick Reference: (far-en-hite) Temperature-measuring scale. Symbol F.

Advanced Reference: Sets the freezing point of water at 32 °F and boiling point at 212 °F. Body temperature using this scale is 98.4 °F.

Failed intubation Quick Reference: Indicates a failure to intubate a patient following a certain number of attempts.

Advanced Reference: Often confused with *difficult intubation* but whereas the latter involves the reasons that may lead to the difficulty, failed intubation usually involves a policy or guidance of what should be done in this situation. Commonly involves aspects such as how many attempts should be made before considering alternatives. In the emergency setting, this would also involve a statement about the anaesthetic assistant's maintaining cricoid pressure until the airway is protected or the patient is again conscious.

Falciform Quick Reference: Sickle-shaped ligament within the hepatic system.

Advanced Reference: A fold of peritoneum connected to the anterior abdominal wall and diaphragm which separates the two lobes of the liver.

Fallopian tubes Quick Reference: Tubes which run from the ovaries to the upper corners of the uterus on either side.

Advanced Reference: They are lined with ciliated epithelium which collects the egg from the ovaries and helps propel it down the tube toward the uterus. If fertilisation happens but the ovum does not travel to the uterus, an *ectopic* pregnancy can occur within the Fallopian tube.

Fallot's tetralogy Quick Reference: *Congenital* heart condition.

Advanced Reference: The condition involves four component defects, i.e. an opening in the interventricular septum, a narrowing of the pulmonary valve, over-development of the right ventricle and displacement of the aorta to the right. A child suffering this condition is cyanosed because the circulating blood is not adequately oxygenated.

Faradic stimulation Quick Reference: Applying an electric current to stimulate muscle. Faradism.

Advanced Reference: Physiotherapy technique where muscles are made to contract by the application of an intermittent electric current. Intended to activate or strengthen flaccid and/or lax muscle. Utilised in obstetrics to stimulate the pelvic muscles which have lost tone due to childbirth.

Fascia Quick Reference: (fash-ea) Fibrous tissue wrapped around muscles and organs.

Advanced Reference: Referred to as the packing material of the body. Found throughout the body, e.g. periosteum covering bones, which merges facial sheaths of neighbouring muscles and lies just under the skin as the superficial and deep fascia. The superficial fascia houses fat, nerves and blood vessels while the deep fascia is densely fibrous.

Fasciculation   Quick Reference: (fas-ic-you-lay-shun) Twitching or flickering of muscle.

Advanced Reference: The reaction produced when the muscle relaxant suxamethonium (*scolene*) is injected. Fasciculation occurs as the drug produces *depolarisation*.

Fasciectomy   Quick Reference: (fash-ee-ectomy) Removal of fascia.

Advanced Reference: The most common procedure involving this is palmer fasciectomy which is carried out to relieve contracture of fingers (*Dupuytren's*).

Fasciotomy   Quick Reference: (fas-she-otomy) Surgical incision or transection of fascia.

Advanced Reference: Carried out to relieve pressure on muscles and nerves in such areas such as the calf, as it could lead to tissue necrosis due mainly to lack of oxygen.

FASIER   Quick Reference: Follicle Aspiration Sperm Injection and Assisted Rupture. Form of fertility treatment.

Advanced Reference: Carried out under ultrasound guidance to remove the egg directly from the follicle. Next, the sperm and egg are mixed inside the syringe and then inserted into the uterus, by injection.

Fasting blood sugar   Quick Reference: (FBS) Measured blood glucose after not eating for at least 8 h.

Advanced Reference: It is often the first test done to check for *diabetes.*

Fat embolism   Quick Reference: Fatty deposit entering and travelling within the blood circulation.

Advanced Reference: Common after orthopaedic procedures such as hip replacement when reaming out of the bone has been carried out.

Fats   Quick Reference: A group of naturally existing compounds known as *lipids.*

Advanced Reference: Composed of a combination of one molecule of a substance called glycerol and three of *fatty acids*. There is a layer of fat beneath the skin and around certain organs which acts as a cushion and as insulation, as well as an energy reserve store since fat has twice the number of calories as carbohydrates. It is also stored at deeper layers as *adipose* tissue.

Fatty acids   Quick Reference: Any of the saturated or unsaturated acids.

Advanced Reference: Organic compound, components of *lipids* essential in the diet. Some are synthesised by the body while others must be obtained from the diet.

Fatty liver disease   Quick Reference: Also called steatosis. A build-up of fat in liver cells.

Advanced Reference: Caused by long-term alcohol abuse. Along with hepatitis and cirrhosis, it is one of the three primary types of alcohol-induced liver disease.

Fazadinium® **Quick Reference:** Non-depolarising neuromuscular blocking drug.

Advanced Reference: Has a rapid onset of action of approximately 1 min, hence it has been considered as an alternative to suxamethonium.

Febrile **Quick Reference:** Refers to *fever*. To be hot, suffering fever.

Advanced Reference: Associated with *pyrexia*, febrile convulsions in children are caused by fever.

Feeding tube **Quick Reference:** Refers to invasive catheters inserted into the body to provide nutrition.

Advanced Reference: The term most commonly refers to *TPN* lines (Nutri-cath®), inserted into a central vein rather than direct *gastrostomy* tubes. Inserted when a patient is unable to take food through the enteric route because of obstruction, following surgery on the gastrointestinal tract or when on long-term ventilation.

Femero-popliteal bypass **Quick Reference:** Vascular surgery procedure.

Advanced Reference: Involves the restoration of blood flow to the leg with a vascular graft bypassing an occluded section of the femoral artery.

Femoral **Quick Reference:** Relating to the femur.

Advanced Reference: Usually indicates the femoral artery or nerve.

Femur **Quick Reference:** The thigh bone.

Advanced Reference: Said to be the largest and strongest bone in the human body. At the upper end its rounded head fits into the acetabulum (cup-shaped socket) of the pelvis to form a ball and socket joint. At its lower end it forms a joint at the knee.

Fenestra **Quick Reference:** A window or opening.

Advanced Reference: A common example is the opening between the middle and inner ear.

Fenestrated tracheostomy tube **Quick Reference:** A standard tracheostomy tube but has fenestrations which allow the patient to speak.

Advanced Reference: Ordinary tracheostomy tubes are used for temporary access to the trachea due to obstruction or when long-term ventilation is required. They are comprised of the tube itself with an introducer and securing side flaps and they incorporate an inflatable tracheal cuff and a standard connection to link up with circuits. The fenestrated tube allows the patient to speak by channelling air upwards to the vocal cords.

Fenestration **Quick Reference:** An opening or window.

Advanced Reference: An ENT procedure intended to assist hearing when deafness is due to otosclerosis. Involves making an opening in the bony labyrinth of the ear.

Fentanyl **Quick Reference:** (fen-tan-ill) A narcotic analgesic. *Sublimaze*®.

Advanced Reference: Synthetic analgesic derived from pethidine. Used as a supplement during anaesthesia and is a powerful respiratory depressant.

Fentazin® **Quick Reference:** Perphenazine. Used in the treatment of psychosis.

Advanced Reference: Used to treat anxiety or as an antiemetic prior to surgery.

Fermentation **Quick Reference:** Process carried out by certain micro-organisms, e.g. *yeasts*, bacteria and moulds, which break down organic substances that contain carbon, hydrogen and oxygen into simpler molecules.

Advanced Reference: Besides being used in the production of alcohol, bread, cheese and yoghurt, drugs such as antibiotics also utilise the process.

Ferric **Quick Reference:** Ferrous or indicates iron.

Advanced Reference: Ferrous sulphate is used to treat iron-deficiency anaemia.

FESS **Quick Reference:** Functional Endoscopic Sinus Surgery. Endoscopic examination of the sinus cavity within the skull.

Advanced Reference: The insertion of a fine telescope into the nasal or other skull cavity to determine the cause of blocked sinuses.

Feticide **Quick Reference:** Also referred to as fetocide.

Advanced Reference: Destruction of a fetus (or embryo) in the uterus.

Fetal circulation **Quick Reference:** The system vessels and structures through which blood moves in the fetus. The specific circulation as opposed to the maternal (mother's) circulation and link between the two.

Advanced Reference: Before birth the *fetus* is dependent on the mother's blood for its oxygen and nourishment and exchange takes place through the *placenta* although there is no direct connection between the blood supplies of the mother and fetus. However, there is free *diffusion* between the maternal and fetal circulations across the thin membrane (barrier) in the placenta.

Fetus **Quick Reference:** Unborn offspring developing in the uterus.

Advanced Reference: Also often spelt foetus. From conception up until the 8th week it is termed an embryo but between the 8th week and the end of pregnancy, it is referred to as the fetus.

Fetus in foeto **Quick Reference:** Indicates when one twin grows inside the other.

Advanced Reference: Also termed 'inclusion twin'. A situation when instead of growing independently, one twin has formed and begun to develop inside the other within the womb and is discovered later in life, usually existing within the abdomen or pelvis.

Fever **Quick Reference:** A state in which the body temperature is above normal.

Advanced Reference: Often caused by bacterial and viral infection and can accompany any infectious illness. Generally accompanied by shivering, nausea, headache and diarrhoea.

Fibre   **Quick Reference:** Refers to dietary fibre or roughage.

Advanced Reference: It is that part of food that cannot be digested and assists the passage of waste through the bowel.

Fibre optics   **Quick Reference:** Refers to the light-carrying system used in fibrescopes.

Advanced Reference: Utilises glass or plastic fibres to carry images and light. As compared to rigid scopes, the nature of fibre optics allows for a degree of flexibility when carrying out an examination.

Fibrillation   **Quick Reference:** Rapid uncoordinated contractions of the heart muscle.

Advanced Reference: May be atrial (AF) or ventricular (VF) in nature. Whichever, fibrillation produces an ineffective pumping action of the heart muscle.

Fibrinogen   **Quick Reference:** An enzyme involved in the clotting of blood.

Advanced Reference: Fibrinogen is a soluble protein dissolved in the plasma and converted into threads of an insoluble protein, fibrin, which forms a mesh and eventually becomes a clot after serum has been squeezed out.

Fibrinolysis   **Quick Reference:** (fibrin-ol-a-sis) The dissolution of fibrin by enzymatic action.

Advanced Reference: Digestion of fibrin within a clot by the *enzyme plasmin*. Fibrinolytic = causing fibrinolysis. Antifibrinolytic agents are substances that inhibit fibrinolysis.

Fibrin sealant   **Quick Reference:** Biological tissue glue composed of thrombin and fibrinogen. Used to prevent air and blood leaks.

Advanced Reference: Applied topically to help stop bleeding. The main active ingredient is fibrinogen and it works by forming a flexible covering over the oozing blood vessel.

Fibroadenoma   **Quick Reference:** Solid benign lump in the breast.

Advanced Reference: Mostly painless and mobile. However, may cause discomfort and become larger, especially during pregnancy. Removed surgically if necessary.

Fibroid   **Quick Reference:** Overgrowth of muscle and connective tissue in the wall of the uterus.

Advanced Reference: Described as smooth muscle tumours, usually benign and can vary in size. Can cause pain, pressure on adjacent structures, vaginal bleeding and infertility. May be treated conservatively or with surgery.

Fibroma   **Quick Reference:** *Benign neoplasm.*

Advanced Reference: Tumour composed mainly of fibrous connective tissue and can grow in all organs.

Fibromyalgia Quick Reference: A rheumatic syndrome causing pain in the joints as well as related tissues, e.g. muscles, tendons.

Advanced Reference: The condition is characterised by fatigue, morning stiffness, numbness in the hands and feet as well as headaches, sleep problems, depression and anxiety.

Fibroplasia Quick Reference: Production of fibrous tissue.

Advanced Reference: Commonly found during wound healing but can be found in other situations such as fibrosis of the retina, which can occur in the newborn who have been given too high a percentage of oxygen levels and can lead to blindness.

Fibrosarcoma Quick Reference: Type of soft-tissue sarcoma.

Advanced Reference: A malignant tumour of fibrous tissue which grows relatively slowly often in muscles near the surface of the body. Can invade neighbouring tissue and metastasise to the lungs.

Fibrosis Quick Reference: Growth of scar tissue.

Advanced Reference: Common conditions include cystic fibrosis and pulmonary fibrosis. Fibrositis is inflammation of fibrous tissue, often the back and neck, and involves pain and stiffness.

Fibrous tissue Quick Reference: Body tissue laid down by fibroblast cells.

Advanced Reference: It is composed of *proteins, collagen* and *elastin* and may be loose or dense depending on the proportions of the individual components.

Filters Quick Reference: Devices used to remove bacteria and unwanted particles from fluids and gases.

Advanced Reference: Most commonly filters are used within breathing and intravenous systems to prevent cross-infection and remove unwanted particles, i.e. micro-aggregates during blood transfusion which have built up during the storage period and can be a cause of pulmonary (micro) embolism. With reference to breathing circuits, they are usually positioned as close to the patient as possible or, depending on the circuit in use, sited so as to prevent exhaled gases contaminating beyond the circuit of an anaesthetic machine or ventilator. Other examples of filter use are in drawing up needles, especially those used during epidural and spinal procedures to prevent glass particles from being injected; filters are also fitted to the ends of continuous epidural catheters.

Fissure Quick Reference: A cleft or groove in a structure.

Advanced Reference: A common example is an anal fissure, which is a crack in the mucous membrane of the anus often caused by hard faeces.

Fistula Quick Reference: A passage or tube. Plural is fistulae.

Advanced Reference: An abnormal junction between the cavity of one organ with another or the surface of the body. Examples include vesico-vaginal (urinary bladder and vagina), fistula in ano (anal canal and surface) and arterio-ventricular (AV) fistula (artery and a vein).

Fitzpatrick   **Quick Reference:** System for classifying skin types by their colour and response to sunlight.

Advanced Reference: Involves the amount of melanin a person has in their epidermis. The classification covers six types, from those who always burn in the sun to those with dark/black skin types who do not burn.

Fixation   **Quick Reference:** To render something stable or immovable.

Advanced Reference: Usually applied to the repair and stabilisation of bones and joints.

Fixator   **Quick Reference:** Orthopaedic-related device that produces rigid immobilisation of bones following repair.

Advanced Reference: An external frame that connects to pins inserted into bones and is used for immobilisation or systematic bone lengthening.

Flagyl®   **Quick Reference:** Antibacterial preparation.

Advanced Reference: Proprietary form of the amoebicidal drug metronidazole which is used when dealing with anaerobic bacteria. Available as an infusion for intravenous use.

Flail chest   **Quick Reference:** Chest injury involving broken ribs and/or sternum.

Advanced Reference: The fracture causes disruption of the normal functioning of the thorax in that the broken section becomes detached and no longer moves outwards on inspiration but is drawn inwards by negative pressure and is pushed outwards during expiration while the rest of the thorax contracts.

Flamazine®   **Quick Reference:** Proprietary antibacterial cream.

Advanced Reference: Used to treat wounds, burns, ulcers, bedsores and skin graft donor sites. It is a preparation of silver sulphadiazine in a water-soluble base.

Flap   **Quick Reference:** Usually refers to a section of tissue used for grafting.

Advanced Reference: The flap is left attached with its blood supply intact and can be used to repair defects within functional range.

Flash point   **Quick Reference:** The lowest temperature at which certain liquids give off sufficient flammable vapour to produce a brief flash when a flame is applied.

Advanced Reference: The term usually applies to substances that vaporise very easily such as alcohols and petrol.

Flavonoids   **Quick Reference:** Any of a group of *metabolites* produced by plants.

Advanced Reference: They are nutritionally beneficial. Also referred to as bio-flavonoids.

Flexion   **Quick Reference:** Indicates bending.

Advanced Reference: The movement of bending a joint. Opposite to extension. A flexor muscle is any muscle that causes the bending of a limb or other body part.

Floating ribs Quick Reference: Refers to the last (lower) pairs of ribs.

Advanced Reference: These are connected only to the vertebrae but not the sternum as are the rest of the ribs.

Flora Quick Reference: The resident micro-organisms of the body.

Advanced Reference: Refers to the micro-organisms that usually occupy a particular area of the body, e.g. the gut and mouth.

Flowmeter Quick Reference: A flowmeter measures the flow of gas on an anaesthetic machine.

Advanced Reference: It measures the flow rate of a gas in litres per minute and is individually calibrated to the gas in question. Consists of a flow control valve, a tapered tube (wider at the top) and a bobbin. When the needle valve is opened gas enters and pushes the bobbin up the tube by passing around it so that it is in fact floating. Readings are taken against the markings on the glass tube and level with the top of the bobbin.

Floxapen® Quick Reference: Proprietary antibiotic. Flucloxacillin.

Advanced Reference: Used in the treatment of skin and ENT-related infections, especially those caused by the *Staphylococcus* group and have become resistant to penicillin.

Fluid balance Quick Reference: Relates to the intake and output of fluids usually referring to a daily basis.

Advanced Reference: Average adult daily intake is approximately 1500 ml daily but can vary with climate. Output involves the fluid in urine, faeces, sweat and evaporation. Patients undergoing surgery (especially major procedures) should have their fluid balance monitored by also including loss from preoperative fasting, bleeding and evaporation from the open wound. Input during surgery is mainly via intravenous infusion.

Fluid logic Quick Reference: Operating system utilised by some gas-driven *ventilators*.

Advanced Reference: Ventilators which derive their energy from compressed gases are considered to be either pneumatically driven or fluid-logic devices. Within *pneumatic* devices there are moving parts, but with fluid-logic systems there are none, therefore reducing the likelihood of (mechanical) failure.

Fluid overload Quick Reference: Occurs when fluids are given in larger volumes and at faster rates than can be absorbed and excreted.

Advanced Reference: Can lead to pulmonary oedema, heart failure and hypertension.

Fluid retention Quick Reference: Failure to excrete excess or a build-up of fluid from the body.

Advanced Reference: May be due to renal failure, cardiovascular or metabolic disorders.

Fluke   Quick Reference: Denotes a group of parasitic worms.

Advanced Reference: Occur in the liver, gut, lungs and blood vessels of humans and attach to the host using suckers.

Flumazenil   Quick Reference: Benzodiazepine antagonist.

Advanced Reference: Also known as Anexate®. Reverses the sedative effects of the benzodiazepine group of drugs.

Fluorescence   Quick Reference: The property of producing light when acted upon by radiant energy.

Advanced Reference: Fluorescent = giving off a bright light. A fluorescent lamp is a glass tube coated with a fluorescent substance that emits light when acted upon by *ultraviolet* light.

Fluorine   Quick Reference: A chemical (*halogen*) element. A non-metallic pale greenish-yellow corrosive gas. Chemical symbol = F.

Advanced Reference: Taken in excess it is poisonous but is a normal constituent of bones and teeth and is added to water supplies (as fluoride) as a measure to reduce dental caries. Fluoride is a salt containing fluorine. Fluoridate = to add fluoride to drinking water. Fluorinate = to treat or mix with fluorine.

Fluorocarbons   Quick Reference: Organic *inert* compounds consisting of *carbon* and *fluorine.* Used in the manufacture of lubricants and non-stick coatings.

Advanced Reference: They dissolve *oxygen* and *carbon dioxide* and this property is utilised to replace red blood cell preparations in the treatment of *ischaemia* and they are considered to be an important component in the development of artificial blood.

Fluoroscope   Quick Reference: Viewing screen used in radiology/radiography.

Advanced Reference: It is a fluorescent screen that enables images to be viewed directly rather than by taking X-ray films.

Flutter   Quick Reference: Refers to an irregular heartbeat, an arrhythmia.

Advanced Reference: Atrial flutter, referred to as saw-tooth when viewed on an *ECG* trace, is due to rapid atrial discharge and can be up to 300 beats per minute. In relation to theatre it can be caused by insertion of a *CVP* catheter, as well as hypovolaemia and pulmonary embolism. Treated with cardioversion, pacing and drug therapy (digoxin, amiodarone, verapamil).

Folate   Quick Reference: Folic acid. Member of the B *vitamin* complex.

Advanced Reference: Involved in many bodily functions including red-cell formation and growth. Recommended during pregnancy as it is thought to assist in preventing *premature births*, *Spinal Bifida* and low birth weight.

Foley   Quick Reference: Urinary (bladder) catheter.

Advanced Reference: Made from PVC, latex, silicone (or silicone coated). Classified as an indwelling catheter as its primary use is following such procedures as transurethral resection of the prostate (TURP) when the most popular version is the three-way model, which has a drainage channel, irrigating channel and a third containing a valve for inflating the ballooned tip, designed to prevent retrograde slippage and/or inadvertent removal. The range includes various gauges, different balloon-tip volume and a pre-formed model.

Follicle   **Quick Reference:** A very small secreting gland.

Advanced Reference: In the ovary the ovum develops in a small cystic space filled with fluid called a Graafian follicle. Follicle-stimulating hormone (FSH) is one of the hormones of the anterior pituitary gland, and stimulates the formation of the ovum in the ovary and spermatozoa in the testis.

Fontanelle   **Quick Reference:** Space between the cranial bones of an infant.

Advanced Reference: When first born, a baby's skull bones have not completely come together and there are six places where the gaps are closed by a membrane. The largest is on the top of the head where the frontal bone and the two parietal bones at the sides leave a gap of approximately a square inch and this is called the anterior fontanelle. The gap usually closes by about 18 months of age.

Fontan procedure   **Quick Reference:** Palliative surgical procedure used in children with severe heart defects.

Advanced Reference: Involves diverting venous blood from the right atrium to the pulmonary arteries (bypassing the right ventricle). Originally a treatment for congenital tricuspid atresia. Generally a treatment for abnormality of the heart's pumping ability.

Foramen   **Quick Reference:** An opening or hole.

Advanced Reference: A natural opening especially into or through bone for the passage of blood vessels or nerves. The largest is the foramen magnum at the base of the skull through which the spinal cord passes into the vertebral column.

Forced expiratory volume (FEV)   **Quick Reference:** The volume of air exhaled under force in a given duration.

Advanced Reference: The capacity or volume of air forcibly exhaled in a given time, usually one second from the commencement of expiration. Any reduction in volume exhaled can be measured against normal volumes expected and any obstruction to air flow is easily detected. Treatment includes realignment and immobilisation.

Forceps delivery   **Quick Reference:** Extraction of the fetus from the uterus.

Advanced Reference: Forceps are used during the second stage of labour for a number of reasons including delayed delivery, maternal and/or fetal distress, or avoidance of maternal effort due to an existing condition in the mother. The forceps are formed by two parts which lock together when in place round the baby's head.

Foreign accent syndrome   Quick Reference: Condition where sufferers speak with a different accent following a brain injury due to trauma or stroke for example.

Advanced Reference: Involves damage to areas of the brain that affect speech. Sufferers often speak with an accent from a place they may never have visited and are usually unaware of this until pointed out by listeners.

Foreign body   Quick Reference: Anything found within the body which is not naturally there.

Advanced Reference: Can be within the digestive tract or lungs, either swallowed or inhaled. Many need to be removed surgically.

Foreskin   Quick Reference: Skin covering the end of the penis.

Advanced Reference: The prepuce. Covers the glans of the penis and its inner surface secretes a lubricating fluid.

Formaldehyde   Quick Reference: A pungent gas soluble in water and used for sterilisation of surgical instruments.

Advanced Reference: Used as a powerful disinfectant and for sterilising instruments that cannot withstand heat. Available in tablet form which gives off a strong irritant vapour. Also used in a water solution as formalin for transporting and preserving specimens in a laboratory.

Forrester spray   Quick Reference: Throat spray used in anaesthesia.

Advanced Reference: A design of throat spray used in anaesthetics for delivering local anaesthetic to the pharyngeal region.

Fortral®   Quick Reference: Proprietary narcotic analgesic.

Advanced Reference: The active constituent is the opiate èntazocine.

Fossa   Quick Reference: A depression or hollow area.

Advanced Reference: Many are found in or are related to bones, such as the *iliac fossa*, which is the depression on the inner surface of the iliac bone. The cubital fossa is the triangular depression at the front of the elbow where veins are sometimes used for IV cannulation or blood collection.

Four Cs   Quick Reference: Term associated with food hygiene.

Advanced Reference: The four Cs are: cleanliness, cooking, chilling and cross-contamination. All relate to avoidance of food poisoning and its consequences.

Fothergill's operation   Quick Reference: Gynaecological operation.

Advanced Reference: An operation carried out to correct prolapse of the uterus. Involves amputation of the cervix with anterior and posterior *colporrhaphy.*

Fracture   Quick Reference: Breakage of a skeletal bone.

Advanced Reference: May involve a complete or incomplete break. Various names apply depending on the site and nature of the break. Fractures in already diseased bones are termed pathological. When a broken bone pierces the skin there is a chance of developing *osteomyelitis*.

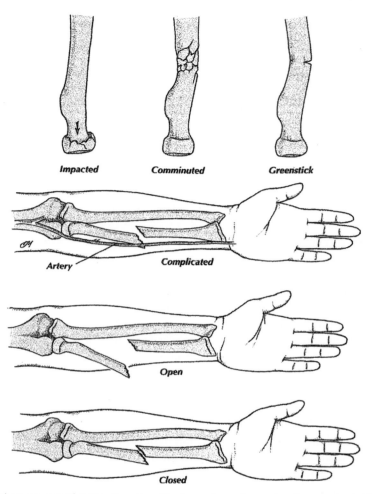

Impacted   *Comminuted*   *Greenstick*

Artery   *Complicated*

Open

Closed

Fig. 8. There are several major categories of fractures, depending on the site and extent of injury.

Fraternal **Quick Reference:** Comradeship, brotherly, to be close, have a
fraternal tie to someone.
   Advanced Reference: Also, fraternal twins as opposed to identical twins. Of
or relating to twins developed from two separate fertilised ova.

Frenulum **Quick Reference:** Section of tissue which limits the movement of
an organ.
   Advanced Reference: A fold of mucous membrane as in the fold under the
tongue or that at the underside of the penis where it meets the glans.

Frequency **Quick Reference:** The number of complete wavelengths of a wave
motion per second.

Advanced Reference: Represented by the symbol f and is measured in hertz (Hz). In the electromagnetic spectrum there is a large range of frequencies from low-frequency radiowaves to very high frequency gamma rays.

Fresh frozen plasma   **Quick Reference:** FFP.

Advanced Reference: Frozen plasma is rich in factor VIII and fibrinogen. Used during multiple transfusions to try to replace or balance clotting factors.

Friable   **Quick Reference:** Indicates that a substance (tissue) crumbles easy.

Advanced Reference: Term used in relation to tissues which, due to their texture, are difficult to repair or diathermise, as with the liver, and so bleeding is difficult to control.

Frozen section   **Quick Reference:** Tissue biopsy sample taken during surgery for examination.

Advanced Reference: When a frozen section is needed pre-arrangements are made with the laboratory. Immediately the specimen is taken it should be transported in a dry container to the laboratory. Results take about 20 min and are phoned back through to the surgeon.

Fuel cell   **Quick Reference:** A cell that generates electricity by the conversion of fuels through electrochemical reactions.

Advanced Reference: The two components needed for this to happen are a fuel and an oxidant. Common fuels involved are hydrogen and methanol and the oxidant is oxygen or air.

Fulguration   **Quick Reference:** Cautery.

Advanced Reference: The application of diathermy to destroy unwanted areas of, for example, tissue, warts, growths and skin tags.

Full blood count   **Quick Reference:** FBC. Blood screening carried out to ascertain the (normal) state of a patient's blood chemistry.

Advanced Reference: Involves blood grouping, cross-matching, clotting factors/times, Hb, urea and electrolytes (U&Es).

Fulminating   **Quick Reference:** Sudden.

Advanced Reference: With reference to a disease or condition, indicates sudden onset and rapid progress. An aggressive cancer.

Fumigation   **Quick Reference:** Process of burning or violating substances.

Advanced Reference: Utilising necessary vapours which destroy infective organisms and vermin.

Functional residual capacity (FRC)   **Quick Reference:** Lung volume at the end of normal expiration.

Advanced Reference: The volume of air remaining in the lungs after a normal expiration. FRC is the sum of *residual volume* (*RV*) and *expiratory reserve volume* (*ERV*).

Fundoplication   **Quick Reference:** Nissen fundoplication is the wrapping of the fundus of the stomach around the oesophagus at the gastric–oesophageal junction.

Advanced Reference: Indicated for severe gastro-oesophageal reflux. Common in children who have an inadequate anti-reflux barrier.

Fundus   **Quick Reference:** The part of a hollow remote or furthest from its opening. Latin for bottom.

Advanced Reference: The top of the uterus furthest from the cervix; fundus of the stomach, bladder and eye.

Fungus   **Quick Reference:** A simple kind of plant life.

Advanced Reference: Closely related to bacteria, they are parasites that live on other plants and animals. The cause of fungal diseases, e.g. usually superficial infections of skin (ringworm) and mucous membranes (thrush). Moulds and yeasts are examples.

Fusarium infection   **Quick Reference:** Causes inflammation of the cornea.

Advanced Reference: Symptoms include redness, pain, discharge, swelling, blurred vision and light sensitivity. Severe cases can lead to blindness.

Fuse   **Quick Reference:** Protective device for electric circuits.

Advanced Reference: Intended to interrupt excessive current flow which could lead to circuit damage, overload and fire. More recently they are being replaced by circuit breakers, which automatically trigger a switch and break a circuit in the event of overload and can be reset when the fault is rectified.

Fusiform   **Quick Reference:** Indicates spindle-shaped, tapering at both ends.

Advanced Reference: *Fusiformis* are a genus of **anaerobic** bacteria normally present in the mouth and intestine.

Fusion   **Quick Reference:** Surgical fixation of a joint.

Advanced Reference: An example is spinal fusion which involves bridging adjacent vertebrae with a bone graft to prevent movement.

G

Gadolinium **Quick Reference:** Symbol Gd. A malleable metallic element.

Advanced Reference: Used as a paramagnetic contrast agent in *magnetic resonance imaging* (MRI).

Gag reflex **Quick Reference:** Retching caused by contact of a foreign body with the mucous membrane of the throat.

Advanced Reference: It is an attempt by the body to prevent objects from entering the back of the throat which could lead to choking.

Gallamine **Quick Reference:** Non-depolarising muscle relaxant. Flaxedil.

Advanced Reference: Rarely used now, causes tachycardia and not suitable for obstetrics as it readily crosses the placenta, also not suitable for renal failure patients as it is excreted from the body almost entirely by the kidneys.

Gall bladder **Quick Reference:** Small bag/pouch attached to the underside of the liver.

Advanced Reference: Pear-shaped with muscular walls, it stores and concentrates bile then discharges it to the duodenum via the cystic duct.

Gallipot **Quick Reference:** A small pot for holding lotions etc. during surgery.

Advanced Reference: Often used in conjunction with kidney bowls (receivers) to hold prepping solutions, sutures, small swabs and other small items on the surgical trolleys which could become easily misplaced. Originally made of metal but now available in plastic and other materials.

Gallstones **Quick Reference:** Stones found in the gall bladder and related structures.

Advanced Reference: Found generally in the biliary tract, there are three types, i.e. cholesterol, bile pigment and mixed stones containing both of these plus calcium.

Galvonometer **Quick Reference:** Instrument for detecting and measuring small electric currents.

Advanced Reference: Works on the principle of an interaction between an electric current and a magnetic field.

Gamma globulin **Quick Reference:** Type(s) of blood protein.

Advanced Reference: They are antibodies responsible for immunity against specific infections.

Gamma rays **Quick Reference:** Ionising radiation. Electromagnetic rays.

Advanced Reference: This form of radiation has rays of shorter wavelength and greater penetration than X-rays. Used in both radiotherapy and sterilisation processes of medical products and devices.

Ganglion **Quick Reference:** A cystic swelling or a collection of nerve cells.

Advanced Reference: Refers to a network of nerves outside of the central nervous system. Alternatively, a painless cyst-like swelling found in a tendon sheath or joint capsule, often at the wrist.

Gangrene **Quick Reference:** Death of tissue.

Advanced Reference: Usually due to inadequate blood supply because of arterial disease or injury, which is commonly referred to as dry gangrene, whereas wet gangrene is more often caused by bacterial infection.

Garamycin® **Quick Reference:** Type of antibiotic.

Advanced Reference: Used primarily in the form of drops to treat bacterial infections of the eye and ear.

Gardasil® **Quick Reference:** Drug used as a vaccine against cervical cancer.

Advanced Reference: It works by combating the human papilloma virus (HPV) which is responsible for a high percentage of *cervical* cancers.

Gargle **Quick Reference:** To wash out the mouth and throat, usually during infection and irritation.

Advanced Reference: Normally carried out with an *antiseptic* or medicated solution. Ordinarily, the solution is spat out and not swallowed.

Gas laws **Quick Reference:** Refers to the laws and principles related to physiology and related equipment.

Advanced Reference: There are four main laws: (1) Boyle's Law, which states that at a constant temperature, the volume of mass of gas is inversely proportional to the pressure; (2) Dalton's Law, which states that the pressure exerted by a fixed amount of a gas in a mixture equals the pressure it would exert if alone, thus pressure exerted by a mixture of gases equals the sum of the partial pressure exerted by each gas; (3) Charle's Law, which states that the volume of a fixed mass of gas is directly proportional to its absolute temperature at a constant pressure; (4) Henry's Law, which states that the amount of gas dissolved in a solvent is proportional to its partial pressure above the solvent at a constant temperature.

Gastrectomy **Quick Reference:** Partial or total removal of the stomach.

Advanced Reference: Partial gastrectomy involves excision of various parts depending on the site and type of lesion or spread of disease. The common procedures are Billroth types 1 and 2 and Polya.

Gastric **Quick Reference:** Pertaining to the stomach.

Advanced Reference: Used in relation to the stomach, e.g. gastric juice, gastric ulcer.

Gastric stasis **Quick Reference:** Reduced or absent emptying of the stomach. Alternative term is gastroparesis, which indicates a mild gastro-paralysis.

Advanced Reference: Gastric stasis is seen in patients in late pregnancy or labour and those suffering shock following a road traffic accident (RTA).

Gastrin **Quick Reference:** Hormone released into the body by the stomach.

Advanced Reference: Released by the lower end of the stomach in response to the presence of protein-rich foods and stimulates acid release from the upper stomach.

Gastroenteritis **Quick Reference:** Inflammation of the stomach and intestine.

Advanced Reference: Characterised by vomiting, diarrhoea and pain.

Gastroenterostomy **Quick Reference:** Surgical opening between the stomach and small intestine.

Advanced Reference: Usually performed because of obstruction of the *pylorus*.

Gastro-oesophageal reflux **Quick Reference:** A backflow of stomach contents into the oesophagus.

Advanced Reference: Caused by relaxation of the lower oesophageal *sphincter*. Also called gastric *reflux*.

Gastrojejunostomy **Quick Reference:** Opening made between the stomach and upper loop of jejunum.

Advanced Reference: Performed usually because of pyloric obstruction so that food can pass directly from the stomach into the upper part of the small intestine. Gastroduodenostomy is the surgical creation of an anastomosis between the stomach and the duodenum.

Gastroparesis **Quick Reference:** Paralysis of the stomach.

Advanced Reference: Also called delayed gastric emptying. Can be due to impaired nerve supply to the stomach.

Gastroplasty **Quick Reference:** Plastic surgery of the stomach and/or lower oesophagus.

Advanced Reference: The term has become synonymous with procedures carried out on those said to be suffering morbid obesity and involves a range of approaches, e.g. gastric stapling, gastric partitioning and gastric bypass. All usually involve the reduction of the stomach's capacity and signalling a feeling of satiety (fullness) and therefore reducing food intake.

Gastroschisis **Quick Reference:** (gastro-sky-sis) Congenital *fissure* on the anterior abdominal wall.

Advanced Reference: Often accompanied by the protrusion of small intestine and part of the large intestine. Also referred to as schistocoelia.

Gastroscope **Quick Reference:** Illuminated tube passed down the oesophagus for examination and diagnosis.

Advanced Reference: A flexible instrument as opposed to a rigid oesophagoscope.

Gastrostomy **Quick Reference:** Opening between the stomach and the overlying abdominal wall.

Advanced Reference: Used when the oesophagus is blocked or the patient is unable to swallow. A self-retaining feeding tube is introduced into the opening.

Gauge   Quick Reference: Measuring system used for various pieces of medical and related items.

Advanced Reference: Standard Wire Gauge (SWG) is a British (Imperial) measurement and is mostly used in classification of needles. French (also termed Charriere) Gauge (FG) is the measuring system for cannulae and catheters, i.e. 5 FG = 1.6 mm = 0.66 in. There is also an American system, American Wire Gauge (AWG).

Gelatin   Quick Reference: Colourless, transparent substance made from animal collagen.

Advanced Reference: Used mostly in medicine in the manufacture of drug capsules or suppositories.

Gelofusine®   Quick Reference: Intravenous plasma expander.

Advanced Reference: A form of *gelatin* (animal protein), used to increase blood volume but is known to cause allergic reactions.

Gender alignment   Quick Reference: Sex change (operation).

Advanced Reference: Refers mainly to surgery, more commonly male to female, carried out because of sexual identity problems and involves changing anatomical sex. Almost always done in conjunction with psychotherapy and hormonal regimes.

Gene   Quick Reference: A factor which controls the inheritance of a specific characteristic.

Advanced Reference: One of the hereditary factors in the chromosome and helps determine the physical and mental make-up.

Generic   Quick Reference: The official name of a drug or product.

Advanced Reference: This is opposed to the brand or ***proprietary*** name given by a particular manufacturer. The term non-proprietary name (rINN) was introduced by the EEC in 2001. However, to avoid mix-ups with drug names, both rINN and BAN (British approved name) may appear on labelling.

Genetics   Quick Reference: The study of inheritance, heredity.

Advanced Reference: Heredity is the biological process involved in the similarities between parents and offspring.

Genital   Quick Reference: Refers to the organs of reproduction.

Advanced Reference: The genitalia.

Genomic   Quick Reference: Pertaining to the genome (i.e. the complete ***gene*** complement of an organism).

Advanced Reference: Involves the study of the structure and function of the genome.

Gentamicin   Quick Reference: A broad-spectrum antibiotic.

Advanced Reference: Used to treat many forms of infection, namely urinary tract, meningitis, endocarditis and septicaemia. Can be given intravenously or as a topical agent but not orally as it is not absorbed by the digestive system.

Gentian violet   **Quick Reference:** (gen-shun) An antiseptic dye.

    Advanced Reference: Used to treat bacterial and fungal skin infections, abrasions, etc. Also available as a skin preparation/cleanser for surgery and used to stain specimens for microscopic examination.

Genus   **Quick Reference:** Term used in the classification of animals and plants.

    Advanced Reference: A genus refers to any closely related or similar species.

GERD   **Quick Reference:** Gastro-(o)esophageal reflux disease.

    Advanced Reference: Also termed reflux oesophagitis. Indicates a back-flow of acid from the stomach into the oesophagus.

Geriatrics   **Quick Reference:** Branch of medicine that deals with disease and treatment of the aged.

    Advanced Reference: Also involves the problems associated with aging and the causes and nature of disease unique to this group.

Gerstmann Straussier syndrome   **Quick Reference:** An inherited autosomal-dominant disease. Has links with *CJD*.

    Advanced Reference: Involves progressive and chronic *ataxia* leading to terminal *dementia*.

Gestation   **Quick Reference:** Period between conception and birth.

    Advanced Reference: Gestation is calculated from the beginning of the last menstrual period and has a duration of approximately 40 weeks.

Gestational diabetes   **Quick Reference:** Condition which affects women solely during pregnancy. Defined as *glucose* intolerance during pregnancy.

    Advanced Reference: Becomes apparent around the 24th to 28th week of pregnancy and occurs because the pregnant woman's body cannot produce enough *insulin*, resulting in a high blood sugar. Treatment involves a combination of diet and exercise measures but if that is not possible it is treated with insulin.

Ghrelin   **Quick Reference:** Hormone produced by stomach cells.

    Advanced Reference: Stimulates the feeling of hunger, increases insulin release from the pancreas and controls growth hormone release from the pituitary gland.

Gingiva   **Quick Reference:** Indicates the soft tissue of the gums.

    Advanced Reference: Gingivitis is inflammation of the gums due to bacterial infection.

Girdlestone   **Quick Reference:** Operation performed for osteoarthritis.

    Advanced Reference: Involves excision of the head of the femur and part of the *acetabulum* followed by the suturing of a mass of muscle between the bone ends.

Girth   **Quick Reference:** Circumference.

    Advanced Reference: Can be related to the abdomen when girth measurements are important following trauma, i.e. an increasing measurement could indicate internal haemorrhage.

Giving-set **Quick Reference:** Standard term for an intravenous blood-transfusion set.

Advanced Reference: Also termed drip-set, which again is a general term whereas giving-set refers to the particular design for blood transfusion as opposed to a fluid administration set.

Glabellar **Quick Reference:** The smooth area between the eyebrows just above the nose.

Advanced Reference: Smooth prominence on the frontal bone and in the midline that is the most forward projecting point of the forehead.

Gland **Quick Reference:** An organ that forms and releases substances that act elsewhere in the body.

Advanced Reference: If the secretion is carried to the surface of the body or lining of a hollow organ it is termed exocrine (digestive and sweat glands) but if it is carried in the bloodstream it is termed endocrine (pituitary and thyroid).

Glans **Quick Reference:** Usually refers to the glans male *penis* but may also indicate the end of the female *clitoris*.

Advanced Reference: It is most commonly the acorn-shaped head of the penis.

Glasgow coma scale **Quick Reference:** Scale developed to assess head injury patients.

Advanced Reference: Although devised for head-injured patients, the scale is often applied to the recovery ward for assessing general consciousness state. It is also used to record the depth of coma, i.e. the lower the score the deeper the state of unconsciousness indicated.

Glaucoma **Quick Reference** (glore-coma) A disease of the eye.

Advanced Reference: Occurs usually after middle-age and involves an increase in pressure of the fluid inside the eye which damages the optic nerve and retina. Due to drainage of aqueous humour being blocked.

Gleason (score) **Quick Reference:** Scale or grading system used to evaluate prognosis for prostate cancer.

Advanced Reference: Evaluation is done via microscopic appearance from a tissue biopsy sample. The scale covers a grading of 2 to 10, with 4 or less being low, 5–7 intermediate and 8–10 indicating a more aggressive cancer.

Glioma **Quick Reference:** A tumour of the *brain* or *spinal cord*.

Advanced Reference: Arises from neurological tissue. Although regarded as malignant, these tumours do not spread outside of the nervous system but invade the tissue in which they lie so that there is no clear line between normal and new growth, therefore making surgical removal with any degree of certainty very difficult.

Global assessment functioning **Quick Reference:** (GAF) A rating system used in *psychiatry* to assess treatment effectiveness.

Advanced Reference: Assesses psychiatry status from 1 (lowest level of functioning) to 100 (highest level) in relation to psychological, social and occupational functioning.

Globulin(s)   **Quick Reference:** Class of *proteins*.

Advanced Reference: Those present in the blood are termed serum globulins. Immunoglobulins have functions as *antibodies* while others are involved in the transport of various blood constituents.

Glomerulonephritis   **Quick Reference:** Inflammation of the glomeruli of the kidney.

Advanced Reference: Formerly known as Bright's disease. An acute condition usually following streptococcal infection.

Glomerulus   **Quick Reference:** A tangle of minute blood vessels in the kidney.

Advanced Reference: The glomerulus is sited inside the *Bowman's capsule* and is involved in the filtration of the blood in the process of urine formation.

Glossal   **Quick Reference:** Of or relating to the tongue. Glosso is a prefix indicating the tongue. Hypoglossal is the portion of the mouth beneath the tongue, also referred to as sublingual.

Advanced Reference: Glossitis is inflammation of the surface of the tongue; glossoplegia indicates paralysis of the tongue; and surgical removal is termed a glossectomy.

Glossopharyngeal nerve   **Quick Reference:** The ninth cranial nerve.

Advanced Reference: Contains both motor and sensory fibres supplying muscles of the throat, parotid and salivary glands, while also relaying sensation from the throat, tonsil and back part of the tongue, including the sense of taste. Additionally carries sensation from the middle-ear and carotid body.

Glossoptosis   **Quick Reference:** Glosso refers to tongue and ptosis denotes a lowered position of an organ. Glossoptosis is the downward displacement or retraction of the tongue.

Advanced Reference: It is a condition evident in a number of syndromes (Pierre Robin) affecting children and a feature of *sleep apnoea*.

Glottis   **Quick Reference:** Part of the larynx.

Advanced Reference: The area which contains the vocal cords.

Glove powder   **Quick Reference:** Talc-like substance included with surgical gloves to aid donning and removal.

Advanced Reference: Suspected of being the cause of tissue inflammation and postoperative adhesions besides the respiratory effects on staff.

Glucagon   **Quick Reference:** Hormone secreted by the pancreas.

Advanced Reference: This hormone instigates a rise in circulating blood sugar by increasing the release of glucose from the liver.

Glucocorticoid   **Quick Reference:** Any of the *corticosteroids* that regulate carbohydrate, lipid and protein metabolism.

Advanced Reference: They also inhibit the release of corticotrophin.

Glucose   Quick Reference: A simple sugar.

Advanced Reference: Combustion of glucose and oxygen forms water and carbon dioxide and forms the principal source of energy in the body.

Glucose reagent sticks   Quick Reference: Product used to measure glucose concentration.

Advanced Reference: Usually made of plastic with a reagent tip, used to measure blood and/or urine glucose levels. Useful more as a guide than accurate measurement. Sometimes referred to by product name, i.e. Dextro-sticks, Lab-Sticks or Multi-Sticks.

Glue   Quick Reference: Indicates tissue/skin glue.

Advanced Reference: There are a growing number of bio-adhesives in use and development. At present those available are mostly intended for skin and superficial use.

Glue ear   Quick Reference: Otitis media.

Advanced Reference: Occurs in children and can lead to deafness as the middle ear becomes blocked by sticky thick material which interferes with the movement of the *ossicles*. Treatment involves placement of a grommet into the ear drum to allow ventilation of the middle ear.

Gluteal   Quick Reference: Pertaining to an area of the buttocks.

Advanced Reference: The fleshy area of the buttocks is formed by three muscles.

Gluten   Quick Reference: A protein found in cereals.

Advanced Reference: People with coeliac disease cannot tolerate gluten and should eat a gluten-free diet.

Gluteraldehyde   Quick Reference: A disinfectant and chemical sterilising agent.

Advanced Reference: Closely related to formaldehyde and referred to by its brand name of Cidex®. Used in the sterilisation of surgical instruments. Has been replaced by safer products as health and safety assessments have highlighted the respiratory and contact/skin hazards.

Glycaemic index   Quick Reference: Index that measures the ability of a food to elevate blood sugar.

Advanced Reference: Indicates how quickly carbohydrates are digested and thus how a food affects blood sugar levels.

Glycerol   Quick Reference: (glis-erol) Mixture of fat and oils. Also termed glycerin.

Advanced Reference: Used in many skin preparations, as a sweetening agent in medicines and as a laxative in rectal suppositories.

Glyceryl trinitrate   Quick Reference: Vasodilator drug also known as nitroglycerine (*GTN*).

Advanced Reference: Used in the relief of angina, it relaxes smooth muscle and dilates blood vessels. Available as sublingual tablets and skin patches as well as in ampoule form (*Tridil*®) for infusion during surgery to lower blood pressure.

Glycine   **Quick Reference:** Irrigating solution used in urological procedures.

Advanced Reference: Used as a 1.5% solution during transurethral resection of the prostate (*TURP*) and related procedures when diathermy is required.

Glycogen   **Quick Reference:** A carbohydrate starch.

Advanced Reference: Formed from glucose and stored in the liver and muscles as an energy reserve to be called upon as needed by the body. As glucose is used up, glycogen is converted at the same rate so that glucose levels remain constant.

Glycosides   **Quick Reference:** Naturally occurring sugar compounds used in medications.

Advanced Reference: Refers to the cardiac glycosides such as digitalis (digoxin), which is produced from the leaf of the foxglove plant and is used in the treatment of *congestive heart failure* and as an *antiarrhythmic*.

Glycosuria   **Quick Reference:** Condition related to diabetes mellitus in which there is a raised level of sugar in the urine.

Advanced Reference: Also referred to as osmotic diuresis, the condition leads to excretion of glucose in the urine. Occurs when blood glucose levels exceed 11 mmol/l causing renal receptors to become saturated.

Goitre   **Quick Reference:** (goy-ta) Enlargement of the thyroid gland.

Advanced Reference: Simple goitres are attributed to iodine deficiency and do not involve excessive over- or underactivity of the thyroid itself. Can be removed surgically if necessary.

Golden hour   **Quick Reference:** Term related to emergency medicine.

Advanced Reference: Refers to the first hour of injury when immediate advanced care is proven to improve survival rates. Introduced originally in connection with heart attack patients.

Goldman   **Quick Reference:** Name associated with a number of anaesthetic-related devices.

Advanced Reference: There is the Goldman draw-over vaporiser and Goldman nasal mask/inhaler used mainly in dental anaesthesia.

Goldman cardiac risk index   **Quick Reference:** Preoperative risk assessment.

Advanced Reference: Developed (and up-dated by Detsky) for the pre-operative identification of non-cardiac surgery patients at risk from major cardiovascular complications. The index takes such complications as age, recent *myocardial infarctions*, *angina*, pulmonary *oedema*, aortic stenosis, *arrhythmias* and poor general health status into account.

Gonadotrophin   **Quick Reference:** Hormone formed in the pituitary gland.

Advanced Reference: It acts on the gonads and in the form of chorionic gonadotrophin suppresses the mother's menstrual cycle during pregnancy.

Gonads   **Quick Reference:** Primary sex organs.

Advanced Reference: Indicates the ovaries or testis.

Gonorrhoea   **Quick Reference:** (gone-or-ear) A sexually transmitted venereal disease.

Advanced Reference: Caused by the *Gonococcus* bacteria which invade the mucous membranes of the urethra and can also invade the uterus. Can often be the cause of male urethral strictures.

Gordon-Greene tube   **Quick Reference:** Endobronchial tube.

Advanced Reference: The Gordon-Greene tube is significant by having a slot for the right upper lobe bronchus and a cranial hook.

Gouge   **Quick Reference:** Orthopaedic surgical instrument.

Advanced Reference: A type of chisel of curved design used for scooping out bone.

Gout   **Quick Reference:** High level of uric acid in the blood.

Advanced Reference: Causes painful inflammation of a joint, the big toe joints being commonly affected.

Graefe's knife   **Quick Reference:** Fine pointed knife used in ophthalmology.

Advanced Reference: Used to make an incision into the *limbus*, in order to aid removal of a cataract.

Graft   **Quick Reference:** Transfer of a body part from one site to another.

Advanced Reference: Can involve tissue alone or entire organs. Autograft indicates when the donor is also the recipient, e.g. skin graft; isograft means a graft between identical individuals; allograft, between dissimilar members of the same species; and xenograft, between different species. Orthotopic indicates a graft placed in the normal anatomical site and heterotopic is a graft placed in an anatomically abnormal site.

Gram   **Quick Reference:** Unit of weight used in the metric system.

Advanced Reference: 28 grams equates to 1 (one) ounce.

Gram's stain   **Quick Reference:** Method of staining and classifying bacteria.

Advanced Reference: The staining that enables the bacteria to be classified as either Gram-positive or Gram-negative. The method involves using crystal violet, and then iodine solution followed by ethanol or ethanol-acetone. The bacteria stained purple are called Gram-positive and those which have been decoloured and have taken up the counterstain (red dye) are Gram-negative.

Granulation tissue   **Quick Reference:** Tissue formed at the site of a wound.

Advanced Reference: Composed mainly of small blood vessels and fibres. Granulation is the first stage of wound healing.

Granulocytes   **Quick Reference:** Type of white blood cell.

Advanced Reference: White blood cells containing neutrophils, eosinophils and basophils.

Granuloma   **Quick Reference:** Mass of granulation tissue.

Advanced Reference: Usually formed at the site of localised infection.

Graphite   **Quick Reference:** A soft, black form of carbon.

Advanced Reference: Used in pencil 'leads' and lubricants.

Gravid Quick Reference: Refers to pregnancy.

Advanced Reference: A gravid (pregnant) uterus. Primigravida indicates the first pregnancy.

Gray's scan Quick Reference: A scan technique used in ultrasonography.

Advanced Reference: A television video-scan converter amplifies and processes echoes according to strength into a visual display, ranging from white for the strongest echoes through to varying shades of grey.

Great veins Quick Reference: Term used to denote the major veins.

Advanced Reference: Specifically the inferior and superior vena cava and pulmonary veins.

Greenstick fracture Quick Reference: Type of bone fracture (in children).

Advanced Reference: Found in the long bones of children. Is not a break where the bone separates completely: one side breaks while the other bends. This is due to the high level of connective tissue in children's bones as opposed to calcium (in adult bones) and makes the bones more flexible.

Grey matter Quick Reference: Cellular tissue in the nervous system.

Advanced Reference: The brain and spinal cord contain two kinds of tissue, grey matter and white matter, which are found in varying zones of these areas. In the spinal column, grey matter is gathered into a central column surrounded by white matter, and in the brain it is clumped into nuclei and over the surface of the cerebrum and cerebellum.

Grid-iron incision Quick Reference: Incision used to locate the appendix.

Advanced Reference: So named due to access being made via splitting the internal oblique and transverse muscles which have a grid iron or mesh appearance.

Groin Quick Reference: Area which includes the upper thigh and lower abdomen.

Advanced Reference: Used regularly but inaccurately in lay terms to indicate the genitalia.

Grommet Quick Reference: Tube inserted into the ear to assist drainage and drying.

Advanced Reference: A grommet is a small plastic tube used to dry up glue ear. It is inserted into the ear drum creating a vent and passage for drainage.

Guedel Quick Reference: Oropharyngeal airway.

Advanced Reference: Named after an American anaesthetist who introduced the design of oropharyngeal airway and who also devised the stages of anaesthesia.

Guillotine Quick Reference: Surgical instrument used in throat surgery.

Advanced Reference: Used for excision of the *tonsils*.

Gullet Quick Reference: The oesophagus.

Advanced Reference: Muscular tube connecting the throat to the stomach.

Guns Quick Reference: Slang term for early stapling instruments.

Advanced Reference: Many are now available for anastomosing and suturing various organs and tissues, both during open and minimally invasive surgery.

Gynaecology **Quick Reference:** Surgical/medical speciality dealing with the female reproductive system.

Advanced Reference: Gynaecology and obstetrics are considered as separate specialities though normally practised by the one specialist.

Gynaecomastia **Quick Reference:** Abnormal enlargement of the male breasts.

Advanced Reference: May happen around the time of puberty due to hormonal imbalance or can be associated with overactivity of the thyroid gland, liver disease and conditions which are treated with oestrogens.

Gypsum **Quick Reference:** *Plaster of Paris* (POP).

Advanced Reference: Calcium sulphate, chemical formula $CaSO_4$.

H

HAART Quick Reference: Highly active antiretroviral therapy.

Advanced Reference: Involves the aggressive use of extremely potent antiviral agents in the treatment of *human immunodeficiency virus* (HIV) infection.

Haem Quick Reference: A compound containing iron.

Advanced Reference: The protein globin combines with haem to form *haemoglobin* and enables the molecule to carry oxygen.

Haemaccel® Quick Reference: (heem-a-cel) Intravenous plasma expander.

Advanced Reference: A gelatin solution with a high molecular weight (30 000 Da) and therefore useful as a plasma expander. Due to its lengthy shelf-life it is used in major accident packs where storage may be required. Known to produce hypersensitivity reactions.

Haemangioma Quick Reference: Red birthmark, benign tumour involving blood vessels.

Advanced Reference: Often referred to as strawberry birthmark, which appears on the skin of newborns but in most cases disappears within the first year. Involves the abnormal multiplication of cells lining the blood vessels. Drug treatment can be used to block the formation of new blood vessels.

Haematemesis Quick Reference: (hem-a-tem-asis) Vomiting of blood.

Advanced Reference: Usually indicates bleeding from the stomach. If dark in colour, can indicate that it has been in the stomach for a lengthy time and been partially digested by gastric secretions and is often referred to as having a coffee-granule appearance.

Haematocrit Quick Reference: Total red cell count (volume).

Advanced Reference: Also referred to as packed cell volume (PCV) and is expressed as a proportion of blood volume.

Haematology Quick Reference: Indicates the study of blood.

Advanced Reference: The speciality that deals with the composition, function and diseases of blood.

Haematoma Quick Reference: A blood-filled swelling.

Advanced Reference: A swelling caused by bleeding into the tissues, usually as a result of injury or even after injection, i.e. intramuscular, intravascular or intra-arterial.

Haematuria Quick Reference: Blood in the urine.

Advanced Reference: Often a symptom of injury or disease to any part of the urinary tract. However, can also be witnessed short-term following unconnected surgery of the pelvis and lower abdomen.

Haemodialysis **Quick Reference:** A form of renal *dialysis.*

Advanced Reference: Used in chronic renal failure where the patient's blood is diverted through a dialysis machine for filtering via a *shunt* or arterio-ventricular (AV) *fistula.*

Haemodilution **Quick Reference:** An increase in the fluid content of blood.

Advanced Reference: A ratio decrease in the concentration of *erythrocytes*.

Haemodynamic **Quick Reference:** Haem = blood, dynamic = movement.

Advanced Reference: Pertaining to the movement of blood within the circulation.

Haemoglobin **Quick Reference:** The red pigment of the blood, carried by the erythrocytes. Abbreviated to Hb.

Advanced Reference: Composed of the protein globin and an iron compound (haem) it is the means of transporting oxygen from the lungs to the rest of the body.

Haemolysis **Quick Reference:** (heem-ol-a-sis) Breakdown of red blood cells.

Advanced Reference: The disintegration of red blood cells followed by the liberation of blood pigment into the circulation. Can occur in conditions of the newborn, following heart valve surgery, because of an allergy reaction or due to parasites such as those responsible for malaria.

Haemolytic **Quick Reference:** With association to destruction of red blood cells *(erythrocytes).*

Advanced Reference: Haemolytic *anaemia* is due to the destruction of red cells. Haemolytic disease of the newborn results from destruction of the red cells of the fetus by antibodies in the mother's blood passing through the placenta. Commonly happens when the fetus is Rhesus-positive but the mother is Rhesus-negative, i.e. the fetal cells are incompatible in the mother's circulation and therefore instigate the production of *antibodies.*

Haemophilia **Quick Reference:** Blood disease involving a deficiency of certain clotting factors.

Advanced Reference: An inherited disease affecting males but carried by females who remain symptom free. Those affected are unable to synthesise Factor VIII. This absence produces prolonged and repeated haemorrhage which can be external or internal, the latter due to no obvious cause.

Haemophilus influenzae **bacterial infection** **Quick Reference:** (Hib) Bacterial infection unrelated to influenza.

Advanced Reference: An infection that can lead to numerous serious illnesses including: *meningitis*, *blood poisoning* and *pneumonia.*

Haemoptysis **Quick Reference:** (heem-op-t-sis) Coughing up of or spitting of blood.

Advanced Reference: Can be due to bleeding within the mouth or nose or from the respiratory tract and lungs.

Haemorrhage Quick Reference: (hem-or-age) Bleeding. Escape of blood from a vessel.

Advanced Reference: Haemorrhage or bleeding can be internal or external, from an artery, vein or capillary. There are three stages of bleeding in relation to surgery: (1) primary – which occurs at the time operation, (2) reactionary – which happens within 24 hours, or (3) secondary – 7–10 days postoperatively.

Haemorrhoids Quick Reference: (hem-a-roids) Commonly referred to as piles.

Advanced Reference: Technically they are varicose veins found at the junction of the rectum and anal canal. May be internal or external to the sphincter. Causes include prolonged constipation and uterine pressure during pregnancy. Treatments include anal stretching, excision, banding, cryotherapy and cautery.

Haemostatic dressing Quick Reference: Refers to a range of dressings and agents used to stem external bleeding, developed initially for military use but being introduced into civilian practice.

Advanced Reference: Includes the HemCon® bandage which is impregnated with a positively charged agent produced from crustacean shells (chitosan) that works by attracting negatively charged blood cells and so creates a plug over the wound and adheres to tissue upon contact with moisture forming an antibacterial barrier. Other common examples are the Rapid Deployment Haemostat (RDH) bandage and Quick Clot®, which is composed of a mineral (zeolite) in granule form which is poured into a wound and absorbs the water content of blood creating a clot over the wound.

Hair removal Quick Reference: More specifically preoperative hair removal and methods, i.e. shaving, clipping or *depilation.*

Advanced Reference: Debate continues over preferred method, benefits and drawbacks. Evidence reveals that shaving leads to increased risk of infection, depilation has the potential for skin irritations and allergic reactions, and clipping may prove inadequate in some instances. Timing of hair removal and wet or dry techniques are related issues, with evidence that as close to surgery time as possible is the preferred option.

Halcion® Quick Reference: Tranquilliser and hypnotic drug.

Advanced Reference: A preparation of the benzodiazepine group, triazolam is used primarily to treat insomnia.

Haldane (chamber) Quick Reference: An air-tight chamber used for physiological studies.

Advanced Reference: Specifically utilised in the study of metabolic performance.

Half-life Quick Reference: Time taken for a substance (e.g. radioactive, pharmaceutical) to fall or reduce to half its original strength or value.

Advanced Reference: With regard to pharmaceuticals, it is a measure of how long it takes 50% of a drug to be excreted.

Hallux   **Quick Reference:** Indicates the big toe.

Advanced Reference: Hallux valgus refers to a bunion found on the big toe that is removed surgically if symptomatic. Causes include the wearing of tight, narrow shoes.

Halogen(s)   **Quick Reference:** Any of the five chemical elements: *fluorine, chlorine,* bromine, *iodine,* astatine.

Advanced Reference: Halogens are non-metals which occur naturally in salt deposits and as *ions* in sea water.

Halothane   **Quick Reference:** A volatile anaesthetic agent. Fluothane.

Advanced Reference: As with all volatile agents, it is colour-coded (red) and delivered to the patient via an agent-specific vaporiser. Said to be non-irritant and not to cause postoperative nausea and vomiting (PONV); however, one disadvantage is that repeated use can cause liver damage.

Hand–eye coordination   **Quick Reference:** Hand–eye coordination uses the eyes to direct attention and the hands to execute a task.

Advanced Reference: Relates to the increase in the use of minimally invasive surgery where the surgeon performs skilful moves indirectly by watching a screen rather than the traditional surgical method of direct vision and contact.

Happiness formula   **Quick Reference:** Theory put forward by the 'Positive' school of Psychology.

Advanced Reference: Pleasure = engagement + meaning = happiness. Putting forward that we need to be engaged and engrossed in what we do and have meaning to our lives.

Hard palate   **Quick Reference:** Bony portion of the roof of the mouth.

Advanced Reference: It is continuous posteriorly with the soft palate and bounded anteriorly and laterally by the gums.

Hard water   **Quick Reference:** Water that does not readily produce a lather with soap.

Advanced Reference: This is due to the presence of dissolved compounds of calcium, magnesium, sodium and iron. Also, the fatty acids in the soap and the metal ions produce a chemical reaction that leads to scum formation.

Harelip   **Quick Reference:** Congenital defect of the lip.

Advanced Reference: Is a failure of the two halves of the upper lip to join and is often associated with *cleft palate,* which is a failure of the two sides of the palate to fuse together.

Harness   **Quick Reference:** Device for holding an anaesthetic or airway equipment in place; face mask.

Advanced Reference: There are a number of designs; e.g. *Clausen*, Connell (three-tailed) and Hudson, which is popular in dental/oral surgery as it affixes the patient's airway tubing around the forehead.

Hartmann's procedure Quick Reference: Resection of a diseased or damaged part of the colon.

Advanced Reference: The proximal end of the bowel is brought out as a colostomy and the distal stump is closed by suturing. If necessary, bowel continuity can be restored later. Hartmann's pouch is the creation of an abnormal sack at the neck of the gallbladder, which quite often becomes the housing for a large stone.

Hartmann's solution Quick Reference: An isotonic intravenous solution.

Advanced Reference: Used for general fluid replacement and maintenance. Also referred to as lactated Ringer's solution and balanced salt solution.

Harvesting Quick Reference: Relates to the removal of organs for transplant.

Advanced Reference: Commonly used term indicating the surgical removal of kidneys, hearts, livers from a *cadaver* intended for transplantation.

HASAWA Quick Reference: Health and Safety at Work Act. UK legislation covering safety and health in the workplace.

Advanced Reference: Introduced in 1974 to replace loose and limited laws, rules and codes that governed individual workplaces and industries. It brought the safety of workers and others under one umbrella. An enabling act which allowed for adding and updating where and when necessary without having to pass each initiative through the full parliamentary process. The likes of *COSHH* and Manual Handling regulations added later are examples of the on-going nature of the law and are very applicable to the hospital setting.

Haversian canal Quick Reference: Longitudinal canal in bone.

Advanced Reference: The canal conveys blood vessels, nerves and in some instances lymph vessels.

Hayfever Quick Reference: A seasonal *allergy*.

Advanced Reference: A reaction to the pollen of certain grasses and plants characterised by runny nose (*rhinitis*) and sore eyes (*conjunctivitis*).

H_2-blocking drugs Quick Reference: Class of drugs that inhibit the manufacture of hydrochloric acid (HCl) in the stomach.

Advanced Reference: They actually work by inhibiting the receptors involved in acid production. Used to reduce gastric acid prior to induction of anaesthesia in an effort to limit the possibility of *Mendelson's syndrome*, should aspiration occur. Cimetidine is a common example.

Headlight Quick Reference: Operating light worn by the surgeon.

Advanced Reference: Popular within most specialities, it can be used to supplement overhead lighting or replace it, depending on the procedure and when close-up focusing is required. Usually of fibre-optic design and attaches to a static light source.

Head ring Quick Reference: Patient head support and stabiliser used during certain surgical procedures.

Advanced Reference: Traditionally made of sponge-rubber with a black antistatic rubber covering. However, numerous variations are now available made of gels and rubbers and of varying degrees of firmness and size.

Heart attack **Quick Reference:** A generalised term used to indicate cardiac irregularities.

Advanced Reference: Is more correctly an alternative for the more accurate *myocardial infarction*.

Heart block **Quick Reference:** Interruption in the conducting channels of the heart.

Advanced Reference: Usually indicates an interruption in conduction between the atria and ventricles, which can be due to fibrosis or lesions among other things. Described as first-, second- and third-degree heart block, indicating the level and severity, and causing significant changes visible on an ECG trace. Treatment depends on the degree and symptoms. With complete block, a pacemaker is often the answer. Trifascicular block is a triad of first-degree heart block, right bundle branch block and either left anterior or posterior hemi block. Infrahisian involves block of the distal conductive system.

Heart burn **Quick Reference:** Burning pain felt behind the sternum at oesophageal level.

Advanced Reference: Also known as pyrosis, it is a symptom of dyspepsia and *reflux*, where gastric acid enters the oesophagus and mouth causing a burning sensation. Can be due to such conditions as *hiatus hernia*. Relieved by alkaline preparations and those that reduce acid production in minor cases but in extreme situations surgery is often needed.

Heart failure **Quick Reference:** When the heart loses the capacity to produce sufficient output.

Advanced Reference: Can be acute or chronic in nature and affect or be due to either the right or left side of the heart. Can produce many signs and symptoms including breathlessness and oedema of the lungs and ankles, depending on the area of the heart affected.

Heart-lung machine **Quick Reference:** Used primarily during open heart surgery.

Advanced Reference: Consists basically of a pump and an oxygenator and takes over (bypasses) the function of the heart and lungs during open heart procedures, by diverting the blood out via the venous system through the oxygenator and returning it to the arterial circulation, while the heart is silent and in a suitable state to be operated upon.

Heat exchanger **Quick Reference:** Used to transfer heat from one fluid to another without the fluids coming into contact.

Advanced Reference: Utilised in many cooling systems.

Heat loss **Quick Reference:** Usually refers to patient heat loss while within the perioperative period.

Advanced Reference: Patients lose heat by conduction, convection, radiation as well as via evaporation. A number of heat-loss-preventative measures are employed including increasing room temperature, additional insulating clothing and coverings, warming of intravenous fluids and various designs of over and under heating blankets (water, warm-air, electric elements). Research has indicated the benefits of intraoperative warming, i.e. improved/shorter healing and postoperative recovery, and when it should be instituted, i.e. once within the operating room or prior to surgery and anaesthetic induction in a forward-waiting area.

Heel pad   **Quick Reference:** Pad placed under the heels of the patient during surgery when in the supine position.

Advanced Reference: Intended to relieve pressure on the calves and so blood vessels within, in an effort to prevent the formation of deep vein thrombosis (DVT).

Hegar's dilators   **Quick Reference:** (hay-gars) Dilator used in gynaecology.

Advanced Reference: Set of graduated dilators used during *D&C* or evacuation of uterus, to open up the cervix.

Heidbrink valve   **Quick Reference:** (hide-brink) A pressure-limiting valve.

Advanced Reference: An adjustable pressure-limiting valve used in a number of anaesthetic circuits, e.g. Water's, Magill.

Heimlich manoeuvre   **Quick Reference:** (hime-lick) Emergency treatment for upper airway obstruction.

Advanced Reference: A manoeuvre taught in first-aid and basic life support (BLS) courses, intended to remove a foreign body from the upper airway using compression of the upper abdomen. The principle being that squeezing the patient around their middle (between navel and lower sternum) region increases intrathoracic pressure and creates a force which expels the cause of the blockage.

Helicobacter pylori   **Quick Reference:** Bacteria found in the stomach. *H. pylori.*

Advanced Reference: Responsible for most ulcers and gastritis in the gastric tract. Its presence weakens the protective lining of the stomach and duodenum allowing digestive juices to irritate, leading to ulceration.

Helium   **Quick Reference:** Chemical symbol He, an inert gas.

Advanced Reference: Combined helium and oxygen mixture is used as a method of delivering alveolar oxygen to patients with airway constriction. The oxygen is carried by the helium, which, due to its low density, can more easily penetrate constricted areas. Available as an individual gas in brown cylinders or in a mixture with 21% oxygen in cylinders with a brown body and brown/white shoulder.

HELLP syndrome   **Quick Reference:** H = haemolytic anaemia, EL = elevated liver enzymes, LP = low platelet count. A life-threatening complication of *pre-eclampsia.*

Advanced Reference: Affects 10% of women suffering pre-eclampsia and mostly girls under 15 years and women over 35 years. Involves high blood pressure and protein in the urine.

Helmstein's procedure   **Quick Reference:** Bladder distension treatment. A urological procedure.

Advanced Reference: Method of using hydrostatic pressure to control severe bleeding of the bladder, usually due to tumours. A bladder catheter is inserted and an irrigation line attached followed by infusion of a controlled volume of fluid into the bladder which is then held there for set periods and repeated intermittently until bleeding stops.

Heloma   **Quick Reference:** A corn or callosity of the hands or feet.

Advanced Reference: Hard corns are commonly found on the outside of the small toe whereas a soft corn (clavus) occurs between the toes.

Hemianopia   **Quick Reference:** Loss of one half of the visual field.

Advanced Reference: Commonly involves the same half (right or left) in both eyes and may be inner or outer halves.

Hemi-arthroplasty   **Quick Reference:** Replacement of one half of the hip joint.

Advanced Reference: Involves replacing the head (and shaft) of the joint with a prosthesis.

Hemi-colectomy   **Quick Reference:** Surgical removal of a portion (approximately half) of the colon.

Advanced Reference: Also referred to as partial colectomy. Involves removal of the ascending section and a portion of the transverse colon. Usual to have a transverse colostomy created following the procedure.

Hemiplegia   **Quick Reference:** Paralysis of one side of the body.

Advanced Reference: One-sided paralysis sometimes the result of a cerebrovascular accident (CVA) when the opposite side to that affected has been injured. Anyone affected is referred to as a hemiplegic.

Hemisphere   **Quick Reference:** Half of a sphere.

Advanced Reference: One of the two halves of the *cerebrum* but which are in fact not exactly hemispherical but quarter-spherical.

HEPA (filter)   **Quick Reference:** High efficiency particulate air filter.

Advanced Reference: Extremely efficient design of filter that removes at least 97% of dust, pollen, mould, bacteria and any airborne particles with a size down to $0.3\,\mu$m, referred to as the most penetrating particulate size (MPPS).

Heparin   **Quick Reference:** An anticoagulant.

Advanced Reference: A naturally occurring anticoagulant formed in the liver. Used for general anticoagulant therapy and to prevent *thrombosis* and *embolism.* Has an immediate onset with a duration of action lasting approximately 4–6 h. Antagonised by *protamine* and inactivated naturally in the body by the *enzyme* heparinase, which prevents the action of ***thrombin*** on ***fibrinogen.***

Hepatitis   **Quick Reference:** Inflammation of the liver. Viral infection.

Advanced Reference: Type A (viral or infective), type B (serum) and type C (previously referred to as non-A and non-B). All due to differing causes, e.g. type A via food, infected water and cross infection; type B through infected blood and body fluids, type C from infected blood transfusions. There are further strains referred to as D and E. Both active and passive immunity can be attained via inoculation.

Hepatoxic   **Quick Reference:** Hepa = liver, toxic = poisonous.

Advanced Reference: Being injurious to the liver. As with alcohol and certain drugs or overdose thereof.

Hep flush®   **Quick Reference:** Proprietary ***anticoagulant,*** a mixture of ***heparin*** and ***sodium chloride***.

Advanced Reference: Used as a general anticoagulant rinse and to flush intravenous catheters and cannulae and as a hep-lock in the connecting tubing of these lines. Also available as Hepsal®.

Herceptin®   **Quick Reference:** (hair-sep-tin) Drug used to treat metastatic breast cancer. Also known as trastuzumab.

Advanced Reference: Herceptin® prevents the growth of specific proteins which can fuel the growth of breast tumours.

Hereditary   **Quick Reference:** Inherited. *Inherent*, implanted by nature.

Advanced Reference: Transmitted from parents to their children.

Hermaphrodite   **Quick Reference:** (herm-af-ro-dite) Condition in which both male and female characteristics are present.

Advanced Reference: Hermaphrodites have the primary sex organs (ovaries and testis) of one sex but accompanied by many secondary characteristics of the other.

Hernia   **Quick Reference:** The abnormal passing of one structure through another.

Advanced Reference: There are many types of hernia; for example, inguinal, umbilical, femoral, hiatus, incisional. They may be described as strangulated, incarcerated, irreducible, or sliding; some are congenital, others are caused through stress, strain and injury or disease. If any type becomes symptomatic they are usually treated by surgical repair.

Herniorrhaphy   **Quick Reference:** Repair of a hernia.

Advanced Reference: Involves the reinforcement of the weakened area with the patient's own tissues or synthetic material, i.e. mesh.

Heroin   **Quick Reference:** A narcotic analgesic.

Advanced Reference: Alternative name is diamorphine. A powerful synthetic derivative of morphine, prohibited in the USA but prescribed in the UK mainly for intractable pain and in palliative care. With reference to theatres, seen as an additive in spinal and epidural drugs.

Herpes zoster   Quick Reference: Shingles.

Advanced Reference A virus which also causes chicken pox. Irritates a nerve route, causing pain and redness over the affected site.

Herpetic   Quick Reference: Pertaining to herpes.

Advanced Reference: Relating to or caused by the *Herpes* viruses. There are two types of the herpes simplex virus (HSV): HSV1 and HSV2.

Hertz   Quick Reference: (hurts) The SI unit of frequency.

Advanced Reference: Symbol is Hz and is equal to one cycle per second.

Hespan®   Quick Reference: IV plasma expander. A proprietary form of Hetastarch. Also known as Pentaspan®.

Advanced Reference: A colloid solution presented in a 6% strength used for volume expansion. Has a high molecular weight (450 000 Da) and has a longer duration of action than many alternatives. Approximates in many aspects to human albumin.

Hg   Quick Reference: Symbol for mercury.

Advanced Reference: Witnessed in the theatre environment in blood pressure devices (sphygmomanometer) as the mercury column for taking pressure readings.

Hiatus hernia   Quick Reference: Protrusion of the upper part of the stomach through the oesophageal opening in the *diaphragm.* Hiatus indicates a space or opening.

Advanced Reference: Leads to movement of gastric acid into the oesophagus causing pain and heartburn. Worse after a heavy meal and when lying flat. There are various degrees of severity of the hernia, e.g. sliding hiatus hernia – in this type the herniated portion of stomach slides back and forth into and out of the chest. A fixed hiatus hernia involves the upper part of the stomach becoming caught up in the chest cavity, whereas the complicated hiatus hernia indicates when the whole of the stomach moves into the chest cavity.

Hibidil®   Quick Reference: Proprietary skin antiseptic.

Advanced Reference: Used also to treat wounds and burns. Produced in the form of a solution in sachets. It is a preparation of *chlorhexidine* gluconate.

Hibiscrub®   Quick Reference: Proprietary antiseptic and hand wash.

Advanced Reference: Used during the scrub-up procedure prior to surgery. It is a preparation of chlorhexidine gluconate in a surfactant liquid, such as detergent.

Hibisol®   Quick Reference: Proprietary antiseptic used to treat minor wounds and burns of the skin.

Advanced Reference: It is a preparation of chlorhexidine gluconate in iso-propyl alcohol together with emollients.

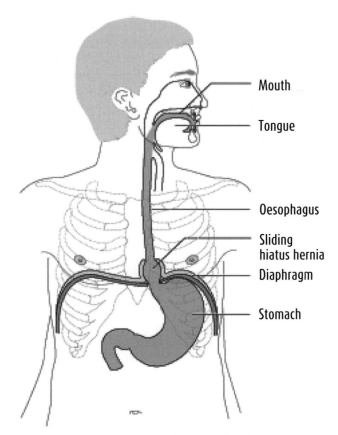

Mouth

Tongue

Oesophagus

Sliding
hiatus hernia

Diaphragm

Stomach

Fig. 9. Used with permission from BUPA: www.bupa.co.uk/health.

Hibitane®   **Quick Reference:** Form of antiseptic/disinfectant based on chlor-hexidine solution.

    Advanced Reference: A broad usage disinfectant derived from chlorhexidine solution and additional salts. Available as powder, creams, compounds and solutions, for both internal and external use.

Hiccup   **Quick Reference:** Involuntary inspiratory spasm involving muscles of respiration.

    Advanced Reference: Also spelt hiccough. Cause by a spasmodic contraction of the diaphragm and other respiratory organs, followed by sudden closure of the vocal cords, producing a characteristic sound.

Hidrosis   **Quick Reference:** Excessive production of sweat.

    Advanced Reference: Indicates the secretion of sweat.

Highland fling   **Quick Reference:** Colloquial name for a patient operating position.

Advanced Reference: Used for femoral bypass surgery, the patient is placed prone on the operating table with the operative leg angled at the knee and the lower leg placed over the other so that the toes point downwards towards the table end, supported by table attachments where necessary, with the surgeon working across the table from the opposite side.

Hilum **Quick Reference:** A point of attachment or entry.

Advanced Reference: A notch or hollow situated on the surface of an organ where blood vessels and nerves enter or leave. An example is the renal hilum at the pelvis of the kidney.

Hirschprung's **Quick Reference:** (hersh-prungs) Congenital condition involving abnormal enlargement of the colon.

Advanced Reference: Also referred to as megacolon, which involves a narrowed segment of bowel in the pelvic colon, causing a partial obstruction to the normal passage of faeces into the rectum. This results in dilatation of the bowel above the narrowing. The underlying cause is a failure of nerve cell development to the affected area. Technically termed as aganglionic megacolon.

Hirudin **Quick Reference:** Anticoagulant secreted from the salivary glands of leeches.

Advanced Reference: It prolongs coagulation by acting as an antithrombotic. Lepirudin is a recombinant form of hirudin used intravenously as an anticoagulant.

Hirudoid® **Quick Reference:** Proprietary vasodilator and anticoagulant.

Advanced Reference: Used to improve circulation in conditions such as varicose veins and deep bruises. Available as a cream or gel for topical application. Its active constituent is a derivative of *heparin.*

Histamine **Quick Reference:** A naturally occurring chemical released by body tissues.

Advanced Reference: Released when tissues are injured causing a sensitivity witnessed as redness (urticaria) leading to vasodilatation and hypotension.

Hist(o) **Quick Reference:** Prefix denoting tissue.

Advanced Reference: Also referred to as his and histo, all denote tissue, e.g. histopathology – study of the changes in tissue due to disease.

HME **Quick Reference:** Heat and moisture exchanger.

Advanced Reference: Device placed within the patient anaesthetic/ventilator circuit designed to provide humidification by recycling the patient's expired moisture and associated heat and incorporating a bacterial filter.

Hodgkin's disease **Quick Reference:** Disorder of the lymph nodes and spleen.

Advanced Reference: May also affect the bone marrow and other areas involved in the defence against infection. Causes cell proliferation and swelling combined with fever and general sickness while lowering resistance.

Hoffman prism   **Quick Reference:** Intubation aid.

  Advanced Reference: A prism that fits onto the laryngoscope blade to enhance visualisation during intubation.

Holistic   **Quick Reference:** Indicates an overall, multidisciplinary approach to patient care.

  Advanced Reference: A holistic approach to care involves not only attending to the current disease but also the entire physical, psychological and social factors affecting the patient.

Holter   **Quick Reference:** Refers to a monitor used in continuous ambulatory electrocardiography (CAE).

  Advanced Reference: The patient wears the monitor for 24 hours and it records their ECG during normal daily behaviour. Event monitoring (EM) is slightly different in that the device is activated by the user when symptoms occur.

Homeostasis   **Quick Reference:** Process by which the internal body systems remain within normal limits despite changes to the external environment.

  Advanced Reference: Refers to the maintenance and function of the body's physiological state and keeping within normal and desired parameters. Mainly involves temperature, acid–base balance, and blood pressure.

Homonymous hemianopia   **Quick Reference:** Loss of half the field of vision.

  Advanced Reference: Loss of vision on the same side in both eyes. Usually develops following a *stroke* or traumatic brain injury.

Hormone   **Quick Reference:** A chemical messenger secreted into the blood stream by an endocrine gland.

  Advanced Reference: A chemical released into the bloodstream by one organ (endocrine ductless gland) that has an effect on the function of other organs and tissues.

Horseshoe   **Quick Reference:** Patient head support used during surgery.

  Advanced Reference: A horseshoe-shaped head support/rest most suitable for when the patient is prone. Unlike the head ring, the gap in the horseshoe allows space for anaesthetic tubing and placement of the eye in order to avoid pressure injury.

Hot-line®   **Quick Reference:** IV fluid warmer.

  Advanced Reference: Brand name for a fluid warmer. Its benefit over a standard fluid warmer is that even at rapid infusion rates the fluid is warmed due to the tubing's configuration and higher temperatures of the hot-line.

HRT   **Quick Reference:** Hormone replacement therapy.

  Advanced Reference: The use of medication containing *oestrogen* and *progesterone* to reduce changes associated with the *menopause.* Can also protect against osteoporosis.

Hudson head harness   **Quick Reference:** Device used to fix/secure the endotracheal tube during surgery.

Advanced Reference: Fits around the forehead and holds the endotracheal tube and circuit tubing in place. Useful during oral surgery.

Human act-rapid® **Quick Reference:** Proprietary preparation of synthesised neutral human insulin.

Advanced Reference: Used to treat and maintain sugar levels in diabetes.

Human albumin solution **Quick Reference:** HAS. IV solution used as a plasma expander.

Advanced Reference: A form of pasteurised plasma heated to 60 °C and used as a volume expander.

Human immunodeficiency virus **Quick Reference:** HIV.

Advanced Reference: The virus responsible for AIDS (acquired immuno-deficiency syndrome).

Human papilloma virus **Quick Reference:** HPV. Member of the pap(o)virus group.

Advanced Reference: May be transmitted sexually and can be the cause of cervical and oral cancer. Also characterised by soft *wart*-like growths on the genitals.

Hyalase **Quick Reference:** Hyaluronidase. Used to increase the permeability of subcutaneous tissue or muscles.

Advanced Reference: Commonly used to disperse drugs when they have been inadvertently injected into the tissues (*extravasation)*. Also used as a dispersant in a number of topical creams and gels used to treat bruising and haematomas.

Hyaline **Quick Reference:** Substance that is clear or glass-like.

Advanced Reference: Hyaline cartilage is a type of elastic connective tissue composed of special cells in a translucent matrix.

Hydatid disease **Quick Reference:** Infection with a tape worm.

Advanced Reference: The disease usually forms cysts in the liver and lungs which require surgical removal. They are caused by a larvae of the tape worm and are passed on via dogs to other animals, e.g. sheep. The cysts may become infected or burst and set off an *anaphylactic* reaction.

Hydralazine **Quick Reference:** A vasodilator. Apresoline®.

Advanced Reference: Used in the treatment of both acute and chronic hypertension. Can be administered orally or intravenously.

Hydration **Quick Reference:** A chemical process in which water is added without disrupting the rest of the molecule. To hydrate is to provide fluid. To re-hydrate is to replace fluid.

Advanced Reference: Refers to the amount (adequate or otherwise) of water in the intracellular and extracellular compartments of the body.

Hydrocele **Quick Reference:** Collection of fluid surrounding the testicle.

Advanced Reference: The fluid collects in the tunica vaginalis (sac) with no obvious cause. Treatment can be through needle aspiration but as the incidence of re-occurrence is high, surgery for removal of the sac is the normal course.

Hydrocephalus   Quick Reference: Accumulation of cerebrospinal fluid in the ventricles of the brain.

Advanced Reference: Due to obstruction of a drainage route through the ventricles and into the arachnoid space or by failure in the absorption process. Causes can include meningitis and adhesions.

Hydrochloric acid   Quick Reference: Chemical formula HCl. Present in gastric juices in dilute form.

Advanced Reference: Formed from hydrogen gas and water.

Hydrocortisone   Quick Reference: Hormone secreted by the adrenal cortex.

Advanced Reference: A corticosteroid used for replacement therapy and suppression of allergic and inflammatory reactions.

Hydrogen   Quick Reference: Chemical symbol H.

Advanced Reference: A gaseous element, colourless, odourless and highly inflammable. Combines with oxygen to form water (H_2O). *Hydrogen ion concentration* indicates the acidity/alkalinity (pH) of a solution.

Hydrogen ion concentration   Quick Reference: Relates to pH (acid/alkali) status.

Advanced Reference: The number of hydrogen ions in a solution is a measure of the acidity of the solution.

Hydrogen peroxide   Quick Reference: Wound cleaning fluid. Chemical formula – H_2O_2.

Advanced Reference: A mild disinfecting and mainly cleaning fluid used usually in a 6% solution for flushing wounds of debris and dressing residue. Its cleaning action is due to the liberation of oxygen as it decomposes into water and oxygen as it makes contact with the tissues.

Hydrogen sulphide   Quick Reference: Colourless, flammable poisonous gas.

Advanced Reference: Formed by the decomposition of organic matter with a smell of rotten eggs. Used as an antiseptic and in bleaches. However its abilities to cool the body and slow down metabolism are being investigated for use in resuscitation.

Hydrogenation   Quick Reference: To combine with or treat with *hydrogen.*

Advanced Reference: Chemical reaction in which the net result is an addition of hydrogen (H_2).

Hydrolysis   Quick Reference: Splitting of a compound by the addition of water.

Advanced Reference: Separates into fragments of hydroxyl and hydrogen atom.

Hydrometer   Quick Reference: A calibrated hollow glass tube/chamber used for measuring the specific gravity or density of a liquid.

Advanced Reference: Works by comparing its weight with that of an equal volume of water.

Hydronephrosis   **Quick Reference:** Distension of the renal pelvis.

Advanced Reference: Caused by obstruction to urine flow usually because of stones, tumour, narrowing (often following tuberculosis) or congenital reasons. Treatment is dependent on cause to a great extent but a kidney badly affected usually requires surgery with the aim of preserving as much as possible.

Hydrophobia   **Quick Reference:** (hide-ro-fobe-ea) Hydro = water, phobia = fear. Repelling or unable to dissolve in water.

Advanced Reference: The viral infection rabies is often referred to as hydrophobia because sufferers develop a great fear of water in the later stages of the disease causing **convulsions.** The terms hydrophilic and hygroscopic indicate the opposite of hydrophobia, i.e. taking up and retaining water readily. Lipophilic indicates having affinity for lipids (fats).

Hydroponics   **Quick Reference:** Cultivation of plants without soil.

Advanced Reference: Involves replacing the soil with an inert material and feeding with a mineral-enhanced water solution.

Hydrosalpinx   **Quick Reference:** Abnormal condition of the Fallopian tubes.

Advanced Reference: In this condition the Fallopian tubes become cystically enlarged and filled with clear fluid and this is the result of infection which has sealed off the ends of the tubes.

Hydrostatic   **Quick Reference:** Pressure exerted by fluid.

Advanced Reference: Hydrostatics is the branch of physics that deals with the study of fluids at rest.

Hydrous   **Quick Reference:** (hi-dros) Containing water.

Advanced Reference: The opposite of anhydrous which indicates 'no water'.

Hygiene hypothesis   **Quick Reference:** Condition related to *immunity*.

Advanced Reference: Belief is that exposure to naturally occurring infections and microbes might essentially immunise against the development of *asthma* and *allergies*.

Hygrometer   **Quick Reference:** Instrument for measuring the amount of moisture in the atmosphere.

Advanced Reference: In the context of operating theatres, the relative humidity is the amount of moisture present in the air compared to the amount which would saturate it at the same temperature. Being both too high (moist) and too low (dry) have inherent hazards with 50%–55% being regarded as safe and comfortable for most situations.

Hyoid bone   **Quick Reference:** (high-oid) Small bone to which the tongue is attached.

Advanced Reference: Small u-shaped bone in the front of the neck situated below the jaw and above the larynx to which many surrounding muscles attach.

Hyoscine **Quick Reference:** (high-o-seen) Alkaloid drug with hypnotic properties. Buscopan.

Advanced Reference: Obtained from belladonna, it is an anticholinergic agent with similar properties to atropine causing sedation and tachycardia. Used as an alternative in premedication.

Hyper **Quick Reference:** Above or too much.

Advanced Reference: A prefix indicating over or above the normal, as in hypertension (high blood pressure), hyperglycaemia (high blood sugar), hyperpyrexia (abnormally high body temperature).

Hyperalgesia **Quick Reference:** An increased response to stimulus.

Advanced Reference: Usually refers to sense of pain. Also referred to as hyperalgia.

Hyperalimentation **Quick Reference:** Administration or consumption of nutrients beyond normal requirement.

Advanced Reference: May apply to intravenous feeding with those who cannot take food via the *alimentary* tract.

Hyperbaric **Quick Reference:** A greater than normal pressure, weight or specific gravity.

Advanced Reference: In relation to theatres, hyperbaric (heavy) drugs are used in spinal analgesia. Also hyperbaric oxygen chambers are used to treat patients with impaired circulation or gangrene.

Hypercapnia **Quick Reference:** Excess concentration of carbon dioxide in the blood.

Advanced Reference: Can be due to respiratory obstruction, cessation of ventilation, or defective carbon dioxide absorber.

Hypercoagulable **Quick Reference:** An increased tendency of the blood to coagulate.

Advanced Reference: Condition in which there is an abnormally increased tendency toward blood clotting. There are numerous states and causes, i.e. medications, female hormones, contraceptive pill and aspects of undergoing surgery.

Hyperemesis gravidarum **Quick Reference:** Excessive vomiting during pregnancy. Hyper = over, emesis = vomiting, gravidarum = pregnant state.

Advanced Reference: Condition commonly seen in the first 12 weeks of pregnancy characterised by episodic vomiting which may be more pronounced in the morning. Also referred to as morning sickness.

Hypermetabolism **Quick Reference:** Abnormally increased metabolism.

Advanced Reference: The condition therefore increases the utilisation of oxygen, nutrients and other needs of the body.

Hyperpathia **Quick Reference:** A syndrome related to pain.

Advanced Reference: An abnormally exaggerated response to painful stimuli.

Hyperplasia **Quick Reference:** Increased production and growth of tissue.

Advanced Reference: The increase in amount of tissue or size of an organ due to enlargement of its cells rather than by multiplication.

Hypersensitivity   **Quick Reference:** Condition commonly associated with *allergic* reaction.

Advanced Reference: A tendency to respond abnormally to a particular *antigen*.

Hypertension   **Quick Reference:** A blood pressure reading above the recommended norm.

Advanced Reference: May be a disease in its own right or symptoms of a recognised disease. These can include renal hypertension and pulmonary hypertension. Continued and prolonged hypertension can lead to damage in other areas and organs such as stroke and kidney failure. Often termed the silent killer.

Hyperthermia   **Quick Reference:** Usually indicates a core body temperature greater than 40 °C.

Advanced Reference: Can be created accidentally, in instances such as *malignant hyperthermia* or induced therapeutically. The opposite of *hypothermia.*

Hypertonic   **Quick Reference:** A solution with a higher osmotic pressure than normal (isotonic).

Advanced Reference: Hypertonic saline has a higher osmotic pressure than normal saline. *Mannitol* is a hypertonic solution and is used to draw fluids from the tissues and treat oedema. The opposite is hypotonic, a fluid with a lower osmotic pressure than normal saline.

Hypertrophy   **Quick Reference:** Excessive or increased growth of tissue.

Advanced Reference: The increase in the size of tissue or organ due to enlargement of its cells rather than by cell multiplication.

Hyperuricaemia   **Quick Reference:** Excess *uric acid* in the blood.

Advanced Reference: A prerequisite to *gout* and may lead to renal disease.

Hyphaema   **Quick Reference:** Haemorrhage within the anterior chamber of the eye, i.e. in front of the lens.

Advanced Reference: Usually due to trauma but can also be a result of bleeding during ophthalmic surgery.

Hypnotic   **Quick Reference:** Drug used to promote sleep, narcosis.

Advanced Reference: Related in action to sedatives and narcotics, differences being in terms of potency and effect. Benzodiazepines are the most widely used as hypnotics.

Hypo   **Quick Reference:** Prefix indicating below or less.

Advanced Reference: Indicates below normal as in hypotension (low blood pressure), hypoglycaemia (low blood sugar) and hypochondrium (below the ribs).

Hypoalgesia   **Quick Reference:** Decreased sense of pain.

Advanced Reference: Diminished response to a normally painful stimulus.

Hypocapnia **Quick Reference:** Low carbon dioxide in the blood. Also referred to as acapnia.

Advanced Reference: Situation when there is a deficiency of carbon dioxide in the blood. Causes include hyperventilation or excessively deep breathing leading to **respiratory alkalosis**. First-aid treatment can involve re-breathing into a paper bag.

Hypochlorite **Quick Reference:** Related to antiseptics and disinfectants.

Advanced Reference: A salt of hypochlorous acid which has both antiseptic and disinfectant properties and when decomposed yields active chlorine. Milton® is an example of hypochlorite.

Hypochondriac **Quick Reference:** Someone with a morbid preoccupation with their health. Also referred to as health anxiety disorder (HAD).

Advanced Reference: This often extends to a belief in the existence of a physical disease although there is no evidence to support it.

Hypochondrium **Quick Reference:** Area of the abdomen below the ribs.

Advanced Reference: The upper lateral parts of the abdomen lying to the right and left of the **epigastric** region.

Hypodermic **Quick Reference:** Below or under the skin.

Advanced Reference: The term usually refers to hypodermic needles and subcutaneous injections.

Hypoglycaemia **Quick Reference:** (hypo-gli-seem-ea) Deficiency of sugar in the blood.

Advanced Reference: The usual cause is a lack of intake/fasting or an imbalance between sugar levels and available insulin. The excess of insulin uses up glucose from the blood by increased consumption. In diabetic patients, this can arise from too much insulin being administered or the wrong diet. Symptoms include perspiration, fainting, delirium and eventual coma if not treated.

Hypokalaemia **Quick Reference:** Abnormally low potassium concentration in the blood.

Advanced Reference: May result from excessive loss by renal or gastrointestinal routes, from decreased intake or because of transcellular shift.

Hypomania **Quick Reference:** Non-psychotic form of mania (a manifestation of bipolar disorder) and of lesser intensity.

Advanced Reference: Characterised by increased levels of energy, physical activity, talkativeness and inflated self-esteem.

Hyponatraemia **Quick Reference:** (hypo-nat-reem-ea) Low level of **sodium** in the blood. A blood sodium level below the norm of 135–150 mmol/l.

Advanced Reference: Can be due to excessive diarrhoea and vomiting, sweating, burns and certain renal conditions. Treatment is usually with 0.9% **sodium chloride** but in severe cases **hypertonic** saline may be used. In the theatre setting it is seen as ***TUR syndrome*** (water intoxication) caused when bladder irrigation fluid (usually 1.5% ***Glycine***) enters the circulation via the blood vessels of the prostatic bed during ***trans urethral resection of the prostate*** (TURP). Symptoms include perspiration, excitement, delirium and, if not treated in time, coma.

Hypoperfusion   **Quick Reference:** Decreased ***perfusion*** through an organ.

Advanced Reference: If prolonged may result in permanent cellular dysfunction, e.g. (***acute***) renal failure following ***shock.***

Hypoplasia   **Quick Reference:** Hypo = low, plasia = development or formation.

Advanced Reference: Incomplete or underdevelopment of an organ or tissue. Less severe than ***aplasia***.

Hypospadias   **Quick Reference:** Congenital malformation of the penis.

Advanced Reference: The genital folds fail to unite in the midline and the opening of the urethra may be found elsewhere on the under-surface of the penis or even in the ***perineum.***

Hypotensive anaesthesia   **Quick Reference:** Refers to techniques used to lower blood pressure (BP) during general anaesthesia (GA).

Advanced Reference: The aim is to lower BP and so improve operating conditions for the surgeon as well as reduce blood loss. Commonly used in ENT (ear, nose and throat) surgery. May involve a number and range of drugs which directly lower BP or combinations of anaesthetic agents and drugs. Patient positioning (head-up/foot-down) is also used as a method or in combination with drugs. For certain procedures, epidural and spinal analgesia techniques are utilised for the same purpose.

Hypothalamus   **Quick Reference:** Part of the brain that lies below the third ventricle and below the thalamus.

Advanced Reference: It controls the vegetative functions, such as body temperature, appetite, BP, fluid balance and sleep.

Hypothermia   **Quick Reference:** A lowering of body temperature.

Advanced Reference: Body temperature below the normal range. Can be accidental, which occurs if normal homeostasis fails and heat loss exceeds heat production, or deliberately induced as for surgery in order to slow metabolism and therefore oxygen need. Measured sometimes as mild, moderate and severe. Said to become a clinical problem when the core temperature falls below 36 °C. Warming from hypothermia is usually carried slowly as rapid heating could cause vasodilatation and hypotension.

Hypothyroidism   **Quick Reference:** Deficient activity of the ***thyroid*** gland resulting in lower metabolic rate.

Advanced Reference: Due to failure of the ***pituitary*** gland to secrete a ***hormone*** that stimulates the thyroid. May also be due to inflammatory conditions, surgical removal, irradiation or a ***congenital*** defect.

Hypovolaemia   **Quick Reference:** Reduced quantity of blood or decreases in circulating volume.

Advanced Reference: Indicates a reduction in circulating blood volume usually due to bleeding, leading to a drop in BP and tissue perfusion and eventual hypovolaemic shock. As bleeding continues, cardiac output cannot compensate for anaemia as the Hb falls below 7–8g d/l.

Hypoxia   **Quick Reference:** Deficiency of oxygen in the tissues.

Advanced Reference: Related to *anoxia* in which tissues receive inadequate or literally no oxygen. Also *hypoxia*. All recognised clinically by the presence of *cyanosis.*

Hysterectomy   **Quick Reference:** Surgical removal of the uterus.

Advanced Reference: Removal of the uterus, either via the abdomen or vagina. Performed for a variety of reasons including cancer and excessive bleeding. The abdominal approach can involve various degrees of organ/tissue removal including, sub-total, total, *Pan* and *Wertheims,* which is the removal of uterus, Fallopian tubes, ovaries, upper part of vagina plus pelvic lymph glands.

Hysterogram   **Quick Reference:** X-ray examination of the uterus and Fallopian tubes.

Advanced Reference: Also termed hysterosalpingogram and hysterosalpingography. Involves injection of a contrast medium via the vagina/cervix through the uterus and Fallopian tubes to determine patency.

Hysteroscopy   **Quick Reference:** Inspection/examination of the uterus through a rigid telescope.

Advanced Reference: A gynaecological procedure that is used as a diagnostic tool to inspect the endometrial lining of the uterus. Great care must be taken to initially establish the depth of the uterus by using a uterine sound because of potential risk of puncture, mainly of the fundus, by the telescope.

Hysterotomy   **Quick Reference:** Opening into the uterus.

Advanced Reference: Usually involves surgical opening into the uterus in order to remove a fetus.

Iatrogenic   **Quick Reference:** Caused by treatment or disease.

Advanced Reference: A disorder or condition actually caused by a physician or practitioner during the course of treatment and within a health-care facility.

Icilin   **Quick Reference:** Compound related to *Menthol* but has more potent cooling effect. (Chemical formula – $C_{16}H_{13}N_3O_4$.)

Advanced Reference: Its cooling effects are being investigated as a suitable analgesic.

Idiopathic   **Quick Reference:** Of unknown causation.

Advanced Reference: A term applied to diseases when their cause is unknown or of spontaneous origin.

I:E ratio   **Quick Reference:** Inspiratory:expiratory ratio.

Advanced Reference: Refers to the ratio between inspiration and expiration, usually when a patient is being mechanically ventilated. The ratio is normally 1:2.

i-gel™   **Quick Reference:** Supraglottic airway device (SAD) made of a non-latex gel material.

Advanced Reference: A single-use airway device that sits over the larynx once inserted and has a non-inflatable cuff. It is inserted without the use of a laryngoscope or introducer and incorporates a gastric channel designed for suctioning and insertion of a nasogastric tube as well as an integral bite-block. Intended to be used for securing the airway for spontaneous breathing and intermittent positive pressure ventilation (IPPV) in both routine and emergency anaesthetics where the patient has been fasted.

Ileo-anal pull through   **Quick Reference:** Also referred to as pelvic pouch and J-pouch. Alternative *colostomy* or *ileostomy* technique following various methods of bowel resection.

Advanced Reference: In this procedure an internal pouch is constructed from the *rectum*, allowing waste to gather there before being expelled at intervals in the normal way.

Ileostomy   **Quick Reference:** An artificial opening between the ileum and the exterior (abdominal wall).

Advanced Reference: Created surgically in the right lower abdominal wall when the colon (large bowel) has been removed. Due to such causes as *ulcerative colitis*.

Ileum   **Quick Reference:** A section of the small intestine.

Advanced Reference: Involves the last three-fifths of the small intestine between the jejunum and caecum below.

Ileus   Quick Reference: An obstruction of the intestine.

Advanced Reference: Intestinal obstruction due to a number of causes including obliteration of the lumen by a tumour, strangulation, twisting or paralysis. Signs include abdominal distension and vomiting.

Iliac crest   Quick Reference: Iliac is a suffix indicating the ilium. Crest is a ridge or protuberance, usually of a bone.

Advanced Reference: Refers to the external bony prominence of the outer pelvis felt under the skin at waist level and used regularly as a landmark for surgery and for identifying *vertebrae* level during *epidural* and *spinal* analgesia as it is level with lumbar spine space L4–5. Also termed superior iliac spine.

Image intensifier   Quick Reference: A mobile X-ray machine also referred to as the C-Arm because of its shape.

Advanced Reference: Used in theatres for situations other than straight X-ray films. Most commonly used in orthopaedics. It amplifies the fluoroscopic optical image and projects it on to a viewing screen. The C-shape enables access to difficult areas and positions used during surgery and can facilitate screening from anterior to lateral positions as well as being capable of producing standard X-ray films.

Immobilisation   Quick Reference: Fixation of a body part.

Advanced Reference: Indicates the fixation of a body part so that it cannot move during or after surgery or treatment, as with the setting of a fracture.

Immune system   Quick Reference: Indicates the cells and organs of the body concerned with *immunity*.

Advanced Reference: These include the *spleen*, bone *marrow, thymus* gland, *tonsils, antibodies* and white blood cells (*lymphocytes*).

Immunity   Quick Reference: The process in the body of identifying and eradicating invading organisms and foreign matter.

Advanced Reference: The word indicates the resistance to subsequent attacks conferred by one attack of an infectious disease or by a simulated attack such as vaccination (immunisation). Immunology is the study of immunity and the body's defence system.

Immunogenic   Quick Reference: Producing *immunity*.

Advanced Reference: Evoking an immune response. An immunogen is any substance that provokes the immune response when introduced into the body.

Immunoglobulin   Quick Reference: Any of the glycoproteins that function as antibodies.

Advanced Reference: Includes antibodies that are important in allergic responses.

Immunosuppressants **Quick Reference:** Class of drugs used to inhibit the body's resistance to the presence of foreign tissue. *Ciclosporin* is an example.

Advanced Reference: Such drugs are used to suppress tissue rejection following transplantation or donor grafting but in turn their use creates the risk of unopposed infection.

Immunotherapy **Quick Reference:** To use the body's own natural defence system as treatment.

Advanced Reference: It was once thought that the *immune system* was only effective against diseases caused by bacteria and viruses but it is now known that it plays a role in protection against additional conditions such as *cancer*.

Impaction **Quick Reference:** The wedging together of two objects making separation difficult.

Advanced Reference: Can relate to: teeth, when two can be impacted together or when one is locked into a socket; fracture, where the broken bone ends are pushed into each other; faeces, which occurs in chronic constipation and the faeces cannot be passed naturally out of the rectum.

Impactor **Quick Reference:** Orthopaedic instrument. Also referred to as a driver.

Advanced Reference: Used to drive an implant into the bone.

Impedance **Quick Reference:** It is the resistance to alternating current (AC) flow in an electrical circuit.

Advanced Reference: The unit of impedance is the *ohm*. Involves resistors and *capacitors*. *Conductors* are substances with low impedance and those with high impedance are known as *insulators*.

Implant **Quick Reference:** To set into.

Advanced Reference: Term used to indicate setting or fixing a device into the body. Examples are implantation of a prosthesis, embryo implant or radiological implant.

Implantable gastric stimulator **Quick Reference:** Device designed as an appetite depressant.

Advanced Reference: It sends out electronic signals to the vagus nerve then relays messages of satiety to the brain which reduces the desire to eat.

Implantable injection port **Quick Reference:** Refers to injection ports that are an integral part of central lines and implanted under the skin. Available as brand names such as Port-a-Cath™ and Medi-Port™.

Advanced Reference: They facilitate the injection of medications via the skin instead of an external port as they have a lower risk of infection. Used for patients on long-term treatment.

Impotence **Quick Reference:** Inability in the male to achieve or maintain an erection.

Advanced Reference: Can be due to disease (i.e. diabetes), endocrine disorders, current medications, trauma or be psychological in origin.

Imuran® **Quick Reference:** Proprietary preparation of the cytotoxic drug azathioprine.

Advanced Reference: Used to suppress tissue reaction and rejection following donor grafting or transplant.

Inadvertent hypothermia (IH) **Quick Reference:** Unexpected drop in body temperature.

Advanced Reference: Usually refers to postoperative situations when potential heat loss and temperature drop have not been anticipated. Commonly due to unplanned extended operative duration or a physiological response to anaesthetic agents.

Incidence **Quick Reference:** Number of times an event occurs.

Advanced Reference: In epidemiology, the number of new cases of an event (e.g. disease) in a particular period.

Incident reporting **Quick Reference:** Written or verbal reporting of an incident/event or series of occurrences that are considered untoward, unwanted, abnormal, or needing correction.

Advanced Reference: Refers to any event that is inconsistent with desired outcomes or routines within a health-care setting. Primarily refers to patient situations but can indirectly involve staff behaviour.

Incision **Quick Reference:** A surgical cut into the body tissues using a scalpel and blade.

Advanced Reference: To gain access to underlying structures and organs. There are various named to suit the operation or site, i.e. midline, lower midline, paramedian (*laparotomy*), **grid iron** (appendicectomy), sub-costal (gallbladder*)*, **Pfannenstiel** (hysterectomy, Caesarean section, prosta-tectomy).

Incisor **Quick Reference:** The front teeth in each jaw.

Advanced Reference: Two on each side of the midline, totalling four in each jaw.

Incompatibility **Quick Reference:** Unable to coexist.

Advanced Reference: In relation to tissue transplantation, there may be rejection because donor and recipient antibodies are incompatible.

Compatibility indicates the opposite, i.e. capable of harmonious coexistence and with reference to bodily tissues and blood, able to tolerate the presence of foreign material.

Incontinence **Quick Reference:** Inability to control bladder or bowel.

Advanced Reference: Due often to degeneration and diseases of the nervous system and, particularly in women, weakness of the pelvic muscles (stress incontinence) after childbirth, but it can also happen following surgery (*TURP*).

Increment **Quick Reference:** To deliver/administer small amounts of a total dose.

Surgical incisions

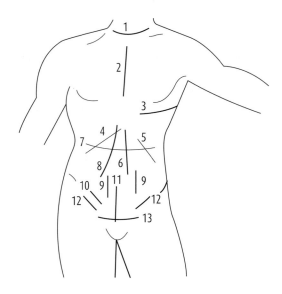

Incision	Used For
1. Collar	Thyroid
2. Sternal split	Cardiac procedures
3. Lateral thoracotomy	Thoracic, cardiac procedures
4. Right subcosta (Kocher)	Gallbladder, biliary procedures
5. Left subcostal	Splenectomy, high gastric procedures
6. Upper midline or median upper abdominal	Stomach, duodenum, pancreas
7. Upper transverse	Abdominal exploration, hiatal hernia repair
8. Right upper paramedian	Stomach, duodenum, pancreas
9. Right or left lower paramedian	Pelvic structure, colon
10. McBurney	Appendectomy
11. Lower midline or median lower abdominal	Uterus, urinary bladder
12. Right or left oblique	Hernia repair, groin exploration
13. Pfannenstiel or transverse	Uterus, tubes, ovaries

Fig. 10. Common surgical incisions.

Advanced Reference: Describes the intermittent injection of drugs by small amounts when a bolus could be contraindicated.

Incubator **Quick Reference:** Apparatus used to provide a controlled environment.

Advanced Reference: In hospitals they are found in Special Care Baby Units (SCBU), and in laboratories for the cultivation of micro-organisms. Involves the control of light, heat, moisture and oxygen.

Indicator tape **Quick Reference:** Refers to a number of colour-change tapes used in various sterilisation processes.

Advanced Reference: The most common are those in steam and ethylene oxide sterilisers. They indicate exposure to the process rather than being a guarantee of sterility.

Indigo-carmine **Quick Reference:** A dye used usually in a 0.4% solution.

Advanced Reference: Given intravenously when testing renal function and for identifying vessels such as ureters and thyroid during surgery. Also used for confirming patency of Fallopian tubes during *hysterogram*.

Induce **Quick Reference:** To initiate or stimulate the start of an activity.

Advanced Reference: To induce labour, to induce an abortion, induction of anaesthesia. An enzyme induces a metabolic activity.

Induction **Quick Reference:** To begin or set in motion. To *induce*.

Advanced Reference: Used commonly with reference to anaesthesia or labour.

Inert **Quick Reference:** Not causing or instigating any reaction. Inert gases are present in air but play no part in respiration, i.e. nitrogen.

Advanced Reference: Used in relation to implants and prostheses made of inert materials, which indicates they will cause little or no tissue or biological reaction, e.g. titanium joints, silicone catheters.

Infarct (ion) **Quick Reference:** Area of dead tissue following an interruption in blood supply.

Advanced Reference: Caused by a starvation in blood supply usually due to a blockage, e.g. thrombosis, which leads to scarring and death of tissue. The segment of tissue lost is called an infarct. Common sites affected are the heart (coronary thrombosis) and mesentery (mesenteric infarct).

Infiltration **Quick Reference:** Indicates the injection of local anaesthetic into the subcutaneous and intradermal tissue.

Advanced Reference: Technique used for minor surgical procedures, primarily for pain relief but also carried out with local anaesthetic containing adrenaline as a way of reducing bleeding in an operative area. Infiltration of an incision following surgery is a common method of providing immediate pain relief, sometimes leaving a small catheter in place for continuing top-up into the postoperative period.

Inflammation **Quick Reference:** The local reaction of the body to damage caused by injury and/or infection.

Advanced Reference: Inflammation is the natural response to injury of almost any kind and is the first stage of healing. The classic signs are redness and swelling combined with heat and pain.

Influenza **Quick Reference:** Acute infection with the respiratory virus A, B, or C.

Advanced Reference: Mostly seasonal and spread by droplets in the breath of infected people. Incubation period is between one and four days and symptoms include high temperature, shivering, headache, aching pain in the bones and muscles, cough, loss of appetite and severe *malaise*.

Infraclavicular **Quick Reference:** Below the clavicle.

Advanced Reference: Term donating anatomical approach such as for nerve block (shoulder) when targeting the *brachial plexus*. The alternative is subclavian, which is more commonly used when referring to the vein for *CVP* monitoring.

Infraorbital **Quick Reference:** Infra = below, beneath, inferior; orbital = orbit.

Advanced Reference: Normally indicates the area including nerves and arteries involved in the eye.

Infrared **Quick Reference:** Electromagnetic radiation beyond the red end of the spectrum.

Advanced Reference: Infrared comprises long invisible rays which are therapeutically in numerous forms, mainly to produce heat in tissues when treating injury. Classified as non-ionising radiation.

Infusion **Quick Reference:** The slow injection of fluids and/or medication.

Advanced Reference: The IV administration of fluids, often with added drugs, being infused slowly usually controlled by either mechanical or electronic devices, as opposed to direct bolus injection.

Inguinal **Quick Reference:** (in-gwine-al or in-gwi-nal) The groin.

Advanced Reference: The inguinal region comprises the fold in front of the hip joint where the muscles of the abdomen and thigh meet. The part where the abdomen surrounds the inguinal canal is a common site for *hernia*.

Inhalation **Quick Reference:** To breathe in.

Advanced Reference: The inhalation(al) method is a way of delivering medication into the body using aerosol, spacer, nebuliser, or a vaporiser, as is common in anaesthesia.

Inherent **Quick Reference:** Refers to the natural characteristics.

Advanced Reference: Those that are innate and part of a person. To possess by *genetic* transmission.

Injection **Quick Reference:** The act of administering medications (in liquid form) into the body.

Advanced Reference: Carried out usually with a syringe and/or needle via many routes, i.e. intravenous (IV), intramuscular (IM), subcutaneous, intra-dermal, intraosseous, intrathecal.

Inoculation **Quick Reference:** Introduction of foreign matter into a living organism.

Advanced Reference: In humans it indicates injecting vaccines to prevent disease. With a culture medium in the laboratory setting it usually means introducing a micro-organism for propagation.

Inoperable **Quick Reference:** Term used with reference to surgery when a condition has progressed too far to benefit from surgical intervention.

Advanced Reference: This can be applied at an early stage when a surgeon indicates the surgery would be of no benefit but can also be decided when a patient is actually undergoing an intended or exploratory procedure.

Inotropic **Quick Reference:** Anything that affects the force of muscle contraction.

Advanced Reference: Usually applied to mean cardiac drugs which may have a positive or negative effect, i.e. beta-blockers which are intended to calm the heart muscle as well as those with a stimulating action, i.e. adrenaline. All are said to have an inotropic effect.

Instrument count **Quick Reference:** Refers to counting all surgical instruments prior to surgery.

Advanced Reference: It is the role and responsibility of the scrub practitioner to keep a check of all instruments used, before, during and after surgery and inform the operating surgeon of any discrepancies prior to closure. In spite of rigorous policies and procedures, there continue to be incidents involving all manner and size of instruments left inside patients.

Insufflation **Quick Reference:** To blow air, gas, or powder down a tube.

Advanced Reference: Indicates the blowing of air/gas into a body cavity, e.g. insufflation of carbon dioxide into the peritoneal cavity for creating better viewing conditions during laparoscopy, or blowing gas through a Fallopian tube to establish patency. Carried out with various forms of insufflator to suit the procedure.

Insulation **Quick Reference:** Means of preventing the passage of heat by conduction, convection or radiation, as well as the flow of electricity.

Advanced Reference: A vacuum is often utilised as an insulator by preventing conduction and convection.

Insulin **Quick Reference:** A hormone produced in the pancreas.

Advanced Reference: Insulin is released into the blood stream where it promotes the uptake of glucose for use by the body cells. Without it glucose is neither consumed as a fuel nor adequately stored, which leads to the dangerous situation of accumulation.

Insulinoma **Quick Reference:** Tumour occurring in the *pancreas*.

Advanced Reference: More precisely, a tumour of the beta cells in the *Islets of Langerhans* which leads to overproduction of *insulin*.

Insulin shock Quick Reference: *Hypoglycaemia*.

Advanced Reference: Alternative term for low blood sugar.

Intensive care Quick Reference: Shortened term which indicates an Intensive Care Unit (ICU).

Advanced Reference: Also termed Intensive Therapy Unit (ITU) but both indicate a specialised ward/unit for patients requiring intensive treatment following surgery, trauma or a debilitating disease. Usually indicates the severity of a condition if a general ward and/or High Dependency Unit (HDU) cannot cope with or provide the treatment needed.

Intercostal Quick Reference: Indicates the area between the ribs.

Advanced Reference: Used to describe the space housing the blood vessels, nerves and muscles lying between the ribs.

Intercurrent Quick Reference: Occurring during the progress of another event or activity.

Advanced Reference: Illness or condition arising during the course of another established illness or condition. Intercurrent disease.

Interferon Quick Reference: Group of glycoproteins that exert antiviral activity and strengthen the immune system and its ability to find and destroy cancer cells.

Advanced Reference: Almost all human cells produce interferon naturally but they are also prepared artificially.

Intermittent Quick Reference: At intervals, rather than all at one time.

Advanced Reference: Used in relation to injection, to pain and to ventilation: intermittent injection, i.e. delivering increments of a drug rather than a single dose; intermittent pain, i.e. a pain that is not constant; and intermittent positive pressure ventilation (*IPPV*) of the lungs.

Intermittent claudication Quick Reference: Pain that is instigated by and aggravated after exercise.

Advanced Reference: Due to arterial disease where there is a poor supply of oxygen to an area and muscle. Often affects the calf in those with an interrupted blood supply to the legs, who are sometimes referred to as an arteriopath. Besides the reduced oxygen supply, the pain is also due to the muscle's inability to get rid of waste products such as lactic acid.

International unit Quick Reference: (i.u.) Unit of measurement. Used with insulin, heparin, hormones and vitamins.

Advanced Reference: Not part of the Système International d'Unités (Metric system). It is the unit of measurement for the amount of a substance and does not translate or equate to SI units; it differs from substance to substance although it is a unit of potency for similarly active substances.

Interpolated (beat) Quick Reference: A cardiac contraction occurring exactly between two normal beats.

Advanced Reference: Happens without altering *sinus* rhythm.

Interscalene Quick Reference: Between the muscles (*scalene*) of the neck.

Advanced Reference: Term donating approach or reference point used commonly during shoulder nerve block insertion.

Interstitial Quick Reference: Indicates between the tissues, the tissue spaces. Outside of the cells.

Advanced Reference: As opposed to intercellular, i.e. within the cells. The fluid in which the cells are bathed. Sometimes termed background tissue.

Intertrochanteric Quick Reference: Pertaining to the space between the greater and lesser trochanters.

Advanced Reference: A hip fracture through the trochanters is termed an intertrochanteric fracture.

Intestinal bag Quick Reference: A surgical sundry used to hold the intestines during abdominal surgery.

Advanced Reference: A clear plastic bag which houses the intestines temporarily during such procedures as resection of abdominal aneurysm. The objective is to limit evaporation (heat and fluid loss) while other areas are being operated on. The clear nature of the container also allows for continual monitoring.

Intestine Quick Reference: The *alimentary* canal after it leaves the stomach.

Advanced Reference: Comprised of the small intestine, duodenum, pylorus, jejunum, ileum, and large intestine and terminates at the anus.

Intima Quick Reference: The inner layer of the wall of an artery or vein.

Advanced Reference: Composed of a lining of endothelial cells and an elastic membrane.

Intracranial pressure monitoring Quick Reference: (ICPM) Used most commonly in ITU for patients with raised intracranial pressure.

Advanced Reference: Often used when there are head injuries, or viral *encephalitis*-related cerebral *oedema* and when treatments such as sedation and muscle relaxants may obscure neurological status.

Intralipid Quick Reference: Intravenous nutritional supplement.

Advanced Reference: Seen mostly as part of a *TPN* regime with ITU or postoperative patients. It is an emulsion of fats, importantly essential *fatty acids*, given primarily as an energy source. The two induction agents propofol and etomidate are supplied in an emulsion of intralipid.

Intramuscular Quick Reference: Indicates into a muscle.

Advanced Reference: As with an intramuscular injection.

Intraocular Quick Reference: Within the eyeball.

Advanced Reference: Used to describe the pressure inside the eye, as in *glaucoma*.

Intraosseus **Quick Reference:** Indicates entering a bone.

Advanced Reference: An intraosseus infusion is to administer fluids into the bone (marrow). Used in emergency situations when an intravenous line cannot be established and with children.

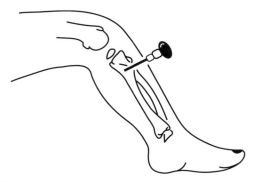

Fig. 11. Insertion of intraosseous needle in the right tibia.

Intrathecal **Quick Reference:** Within a sheath.

Advanced Reference: As with intrathecal injection, i.e. the injection of local anaesthetics into the spinal column.

Intra-vas device **Quick Reference:** (IVD) Male contraceptive device.

Advanced Reference: Inserted surgically via the *scrotum* into the *vas deferens* and works by blocking the vas and obstructing the flow of *sperm*.

Intravenous **Quick Reference:** Indicates into the vein.

Advanced Reference: Can be used to indicate an injection or an infusion.

Intubating axis **Quick Reference:** To orally intubate, the path from the incisor teeth to the larynx should be a straight line.

Advanced Reference: The path has three axes: oral axis, pharyngeal axis and laryngeal axis.

Intubation **Quick Reference:** To introduce a tube (into the body).

Advanced Reference: The term most commonly refers to intubation of the trachea with an endotracheal tube.

Intussusception **Quick Reference:** Condition in which part of the intestine telescopes into the next segment.

Advanced Reference: Most cases occur in infants but can be seen in adults. Examples are the large intestine invaginating into itself or the last portion of the ileum prolapsing into the caecum. Can lead to obstruction which requires surgical intervention.

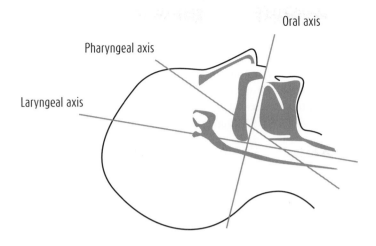

The three axes with the head in neutral position.

Intubating axis

Fig. 12. Used with permission from Update in Anaesthesia (www.world-anaesthesia.org)

Invaginate   **Quick Reference:** To fold inwards.

Advanced Reference: This folding inwards can lead to the formation of a pouch, as with intussusception of the intestine.

Inverse square law   **Quick Reference:** Equation in relation to the travel and spread of *X-ray radiation*.

Advanced Reference: The intensity of radiation is inversely proportional to the square of the distance between a point source and the irradiated surface. For related safety reasons this equates approximately as: double your distance, quarter the dose.

Involution   **Quick Reference:** Indicates the return to normal size of the uterus after childbirth.

Advanced Reference: Also used to indicate the shrinking of tissues and organs which may occur in old age.

Iodine   **Quick Reference:** A naturally occurring element.

Advanced Reference: In medicine, it is essential for the correct functioning of the thyroid gland and also used in solution as an effective antiseptic.

Ion   **Quick Reference:** A charged subatomic particle.

Advanced Reference: An atom or group of atoms that carry a positive or negative charge as a result of having lost or gained one or more electrons.

Ionisation   **Quick Reference:**   Term used with reference to high-energy electromagnetic waves, such as X-rays and gamma rays.

Advanced Reference: Ionising radiation is so-called because when the waves pass through matter they cause ionisation (change), whereby neutral atoms acquire a temporary electric charge. Ionising radiation has penetrative powers whereas non-ionising does not. ***Ultraviolet*** and ***infrared*** are examples of non-ionising radiation.

Iris **Quick Reference:** The coloured part of the eye.

Advanced Reference: Situated behind the cornea and comprises two muscle layers which alter the size of the pupil and so control the amount of light entering the eye. Iritis is inflammation of the iris and iridectomy is the removal of part of the iris, usually due to glaucoma.

Iron **Quick Reference:** Naturally occurring metallic element. Ferrous.

Advanced Reference: Haemoglobin (Hb) is made up of an iron compound (haem). Iron deficiency ***anaemia*** is a common type of this condition.

Irradiation **Quick Reference:** Exposure to radiation.

Advanced Reference: May also be for therapeutic purposes, as in the treatment of cancers.

Irrigation **Quick Reference:** To supply a stream of water or alternative fluid.

Advanced Reference: There are many examples: the washing out of a cavity or wound by a stream of continuous flow, eye irrigation following injury, irrigation of the bladder during and following ***TURP Lavage***.

Ischaemia **Quick Reference:** (is-keem-ea) Inadequate blood supply to a body part.

Advanced Reference: Can be due to many causes; a disease of the blood vessels and spasm and if prolonged can bring about the death of tissue. A common example is myocardial ischaemia, which occurs when the heart muscle receives inadequate blood supply due to thrombosis/spasm.

Ischial **Quick Reference:** Pertaining to the ischium.

Advanced Reference: The lower ***posterior*** part of the ***pelvis*** upon which one sits. The actual part that bears the weight of the sitting body is the ***tuberosity*** of the ischium.

Ischiorectal abscess **Quick Reference:** An abscess occurring between the rectum and the ***ischium***.

Advanced Reference: This type of abscess is often associated with a fistula in ano (a communication between the rectum and the skin at the anus).

Islets of Langerhans **Quick Reference:** Specialised cells within the pancreas.

Advanced Reference: A cluster of cells in the pancreas which produce ***insulin*** and ***glucagon***, which are released directly into the circulation where they play a part in glucose metabolism.

Isobaric **Quick Reference:** Having equal or constant pressure and weight.

Advanced Reference: Relates to solutions having the same density.

Isoelectric line **Quick Reference:** Baseline of an ECG reading. The resting potential.

Advanced Reference: Period between the S wave and the beginning of the T wave. Displaying no variation in electrical potential.

Isoflavones **Quick Reference:** Plant-based substances used in the treatment of menopausal symptoms.

Advanced Reference: They mimic the actions of oestrogens. Soy-based products are a rich source of isoflavones.

Isoflurane **Quick Reference:** A volatile anaesthetic agent.

Advanced Reference: A colourless agent that allows rapid induction and recovery from anaesthesia.

Isograft **Quick Reference:** Type of tissue graft.

Advanced Reference: A graft carried out between identical individuals.

Isolated forearm technique **Quick Reference:** Technique used in the prevention of awareness during general anaesthesia.

Advanced Reference: Involves placement of a *tourniquet* on the upper arm that is inflated to above systolic blood pressure prior to administration of a *muscle relaxant* with the intention of excluding the lower portion of the arm and hand from paralysis and so allowing the patient to display awareness by movement during surgery either spontaneously or following auditory command.

Isolation **Quick Reference:** Separation of an infected patient from others.

Advanced Reference: Usually involves an isolation ward or area with the intention of preventing the spread of infective organisms. Also used for patients with a deficient immune system when recovering from a related condition. Likened to the term barrier nursing.

Isomers **Quick Reference:** Molecules with the same chemical formula.

Advanced Reference: They have the same number and types of atoms but in a different structure and also have the same kind of bonds between atoms.

Isoprenaline **Quick Reference:** Cardiac stimulant closely related to adrenaline. Saventrine®.

Advanced Reference: Increases both the heart rate and force of contraction and often used to treat extremely slow heart rate. May also be used in treating bronchospasm. Sometimes referred to as a chemical pacemaker.

Isopropyl **Quick Reference:** Clear, colourless alcohol. C_3H_8O.

Advanced Reference: Used as a 70% solution for skin prepping and general cleaning of clinical surfaces.

Isotonic **Quick Reference:** Refers to solutions which have the same osmotic pressure as plasma.

Advanced Reference: Intravenous normal saline (0.9% sodium chloride) is isotonic with plasma, which means that it will not draw fluid from surrounding tissues or be absorbed into them. *Hypertonic* solutions will withdraw fluid from the tissues into the adjacent veins.

Isotope **Quick Reference:** A chemical element having the same atomic number as another.

Advanced Reference: However, it has different physical properties and atomic mass, i.e. a different number of nuclear neutrons.

Isthmus   **Quick Reference:**   Narrowed connection between two larger structures.

Advanced Reference: Constriction or narrow passage connecting two larger parts of an organ or anatomical structure. Band of tissue joining the two lobes of the **thyroid** gland. The isthmus of the **eustachian** tube, isthmus of the uterus.

IUCD   **Quick Reference:**   Intra-uterine contraceptive device. Female contraceptive method.

Advanced Reference: Usually made from plastic or metal and inserted into the uterine cavity and interrupts the normal environment for the egg.

Ivor Lewis   **Quick Reference:**   Oesophagectomy. Surgical procedure for tumours of the oesophagus.

Advanced Reference: Procedure carried out for the treatment of growths in the upper third of the oesophagus.

IVP   **Quick Reference:**   Intravenous **pyelogram**. Radiological technique for demonstrating the outline and function of the kidneys, ureters and bladder.

Advanced Reference: Involves the intravenous injection of a radio-opaque dye and as this is excreted by the kidneys, X-rays are taken to ascertain outline, function and general performance and any obstruction to flow.

J

Jaboulay amputation Quick Reference: Also known as hind-quarter amputation.

Advanced Reference: Involves amputation of the whole lower limb with corresponding iliac bone, through the sacro-iliac joint. This is regarded as a mutilating operation and is usually performed because of a chondro-sarcoma of the pelvis or upper femur.

Jaboulay pyloroplasty Quick Reference: A side-to-side gastroduo-denostomy.

Advanced Reference: It is carried out when the pylorus and proximal duodenum are extensively scarred by peptic *ulcer* disease.

Jack-Knife Quick Reference: Patient operating position.

Advanced Reference: Involves the patient lying on their stomach (*prone*) with the hips flexed and knees bent at 90° and arms outstretched towards the front. Used for various spinal and rectal procedures.

Jackscrew Quick Reference: A threaded screw.

Advanced Reference: Device used in orthopaedic appliances for the separation or approximation of teeth or jaw segments.

Jackson-Rees T-Piece Quick Reference: A modification of the *Ayer's T-Piece*.

Advanced Reference: The Jackson-Rees version is a modification to the Ayer's paediatric circuit and ensures that fresh gas flow (FGF) remains separate from the expired gas. The modifications followed on from the *Jackson-Rees T-tube*.

Jackson-Rees T-tube Quick Reference: Paediatric endotracheal tube that incorporates a suction arm.

Advanced Reference: The T-shape allowed for FGF with flow across the intersection of the T. There was a removable bung at the top end of the tube used for suction. The remaining end of the T-shape was open-ended, usually with a connected piece of anaesthetic tubing which allowed expired gas to escape under positive pressure exerted by the patient.

Jacob's chuck Quick Reference: The holding jaws on a power drill used in orthopaedic surgery.

Advanced Reference: The Jacob's chuck has three equal jaws that move in and out on an axis so as to allow the insertion of drills or guide wires of all different sizes.

Jacque's catheter Quick Reference: (jakes) Red-rubber catheter/tubing.

Advanced Reference: Often used as a tourniquet for fingers and toes.

Jarvik   **Quick Reference:** Name associated with an artificial heart.

Advanced Reference: Named after its inventor, Robert Jarvik. The heart was intended as a bridge to transplantation rather than a permanent device or pump to aid/rest the ventricles.

Jaundice   **Quick Reference:** A yellowish discoloration of the skin, whites of the eyes (conjunctiva) and mucous membranes.

Advanced Reference: Due to the presence of bilirubin (bile pigment) in the blood and tissues. The pigment accumulates in the blood if: (1) too much is produced, (2) the liver does not dispose of it, (3) the bile ducts are obstructed. A trace of jaundice is common in the first few days of life but is not usually an on-going problem.

Javid shunt   **Quick Reference:** Bypass device used when operating on the carotid artery.

Advanced Reference: Consists of a length of tubing and works as a temporary measure to bypass the artery during *endarterectomy*.

Jaw thrust   **Quick Reference:** Procedure used to establish a clear airway.

Advanced Reference: Involves lifting the patient's jaw forward from its normal anatomical position, therefore raising the tongue and preventing obstruction of the airway. Utilised with patients who have cervical neck injury.

Jejunostomy   **Quick Reference:** An artificial opening into the *jejunum*.

Advanced Reference: The insertion of a feeding catheter into the jejunum. It is performed when there is obstruction of the gastric tract superior to the jejunum, or when a partial gastrectomy has been carried out. The feeding tube gives a direct route for liquid nutrients to be inserted into the *jejunum*.

Jejunum   **Quick Reference:** A section of small bowel directly following the duodenum.

Advanced Reference: The jejunum is approximately 2–4 cm in length in the normal adult and supports absorption from the breakdown of food by gastric enzymes. Absorption takes place through the villi which line the jejunum as well as the continual motion of contents by *peristalsis*.

Jelly   **Quick Reference:** A term used to indicate lubricating jelly.

Advanced Reference: Used regularly for lubrication in urology and gynaecology, and also used in anaesthesia for lubricating ET tubes, *stylettes* and *bougies*. Usually involves a water-based solution such as KY jelly® but other products containing lignocaine (2%) are often used mistakenly in the same manner. The latter form has its place as a lubricant but also to prevent discomfort when inserting scopes into sensitive areas, e.g. cystoscopes into the urethra, with a conscious patient.

Jelonet®   **Quick Reference:** Brand name for paraffin gauze.

Advanced Reference: A wound dressing impregnated with paraffin jelly used for burns and wounds.

Jet ventilator   **Quick Reference:** Type of high-frequency patient ventilator.

Advanced Reference: The jet ventilator was designed to deliver very high respiratory rates (200/300 p.m.) combined with small tidal volumes. Intended for use in ITU with chest injury patients.

Jeweller's forceps   **Quick Reference:** Fine non-toothed dissecting forceps.

Advanced Reference: Jeweller's forceps are used during microvascular surgery to dissect tissues or to hold the ends of vessels and delicate tissue, often using a surgical microscope.

Jewellery   **Quick Reference:** With reference to theatre, argument continues over the wearing of jewellery by staff, but in relation to patients the universal policy is still to either remove where possible or secure and cover.

Advanced Reference: With regard to staff, in general it is accepted that jewellery should not be worn in theatre as it can harbour bacteria as well as there being the potential for it to fall into wounds or even scratch patients. However, the removal of wedding rings is optional, as being ordered to remove it can contravene a person's human rights.

Jobson Horn probe   **Quick Reference:** Non-traumatic curette.

Advanced Reference: The probe has a small circular shape at the end of a fine shaft, with the purpose being to scoop out any ear cavity content such as wax and foreign objects.

Joint   **Quick Reference:** The point where two or more bones meet.

Advanced Reference: An articulation.

Jols retractor   **Quick Reference:** A retractor used during thyroid surgery.

Advanced Reference: Half-moon in shape with a spring-loaded towel clip on either end. The clamp is placed at each side of the surgical incision at approximately right angles, with each towel clip holding the skin edge. The middle knurled adjuster is used to expand the two ends of the clamp outwards creating maximum exposure of the surgical area.

Joule   **Quick Reference:** (jule) SI unit of energy.

Advanced Reference: Joule refers to energy or amount of work done. Sometimes equated to watts times second. Most commonly encountered as the usable power on defibrillators.

J-pouch   **Quick Reference:** Faecal reservoir.

Advanced Reference: Formed surgically by folding over the lower end of the ileum in an ileo-anal anastomosis.

J-suture   **Quick Reference:** J-shaped multi-use surgical suture needle.

Advanced Reference: The unique shape enables the surgeon to close deep layers of the wound without perforation of the underlying organs. Also used to close laparoscopic trocar incisions. Available in eyed and eyeless design allowing for choice of suture material.

Judd Allis tissue forceps   **Quick Reference:** Atraumatic tissue forceps.

Advanced Reference: Judd Allis forceps have slightly bevelled jaws that can be used to grip or hold delicate tissue without causing unnecessary damage.

Jugular   **Quick Reference:** Indicates the jugular vein, situated on both (lateral) aspects of the neck.

Advanced Reference: There is an external and internal jugular vein commonly feeding into the superior vena cava returning deoxygenated blood to the right atrium. The external is more visible because of its more superficial position just under the skin surface. It is regularly used for insertion of a CVP line and can be identified by using adjacent landmarks.

Juxtaposition   **Quick Reference:** To position side by side.

Advanced Reference: The act of placing two or more things side by side or adjacent to one another.

J-wire   **Quick Reference:** Flexible wire with curved J-tip.

Advanced Reference: A variation on the *Seldinger* wire, the J-wire is used as an introduction aid for venous and arterial cannulation but has the advantage of causing less trauma to the vessel walls and tends to better negotiate tortuous routes through the vessels.

Kaltostat® **Quick Reference:** Type of wound dressing.

Advanced Reference: These dressings absorb exudate from wounds and turn to a gel which is then easily removed by syringing with saline. The gel also provides a moist covering for wound surfaces which enhances normal healing.

Kaolin **Quick Reference:** Compound used in the treatment of diarrhoea.

Advanced Reference: Sometimes mixed with morphine (Kaolin-morph). Its original source is China clay.

Kefzol® **Quick Reference:** Proprietary antibiotic.

Advanced Reference: A preparation of the cephalosporin cephazolin.

Keller's **Quick Reference:** An operation to correct deformity of the big toe.

Advanced Reference: Also referred to as *hallux valgus* procedure. Commonly identified as a bunion.

Keloid **Quick Reference:** An overgrowth of scar tissue at the site of a wound.

Advanced Reference: Associated with scar tissue; instead of a gradual shrinking and disappearing, the affected area spreads and causes puckering of the surrounding tissue.

Kelvin **Quick Reference:** SI unit of temperature.

Advanced Reference: Based on an absolute temperature scale where zero Kelvin is the temperature at which molecular motion ceases.

Keratin **Quick Reference:** Fibrous protein found in skin and hair.

Advanced Reference: Fingernails and the outer layer of the skin are also composed of this protein and it is part of the structure of tooth enamel.

As it is insoluble in gastric juice, keratin is used as a coating for pills designed to dissolve in the *intestine*.

Keratoma **Quick Reference:** Horny growth of the skin.

Advanced Reference: Involves excessive growth of the *epidermis*.

Keratome **Quick Reference:** A surgical knife used in ophthalmic surgery.

Advanced Reference: A trowel-shaped blade for incising the cornea.

Kerrison Rongeur **Quick Reference:** Bone nibbler.

Advanced Reference: Used in orthopaedics and neurosurgery, e.g. laminectomy. Available with an upward or downward bite.

Ketamine **Quick Reference:** Anaesthetic agent. Alternative name is ketelar.

Advanced Reference: Termed a dissociative anaesthetic agent. May be given intravenously (IV) or intramuscularly (IM). Known to produce hallucinations and nightmares.

Ketones Quick Reference: Products of incomplete fat metabolism.

Advanced Reference: Ketones are compounds containing the carboxyl group. Seen in relation to diabetic patients and acknowledged as being present when the breath has a smell resembling 'pear drops'. Poisoning by ketones is termed ketosis.

Ketonuria Quick Reference: (key-tone-your-ea) Excessive concentration of *ketone* bodies in the urine.

Advanced Reference: Commonly occurs in *diabetes* mellitus. Also called acetonuria and hyperketonuria.

Ketorolac Quick Reference: A non-steroidal anti-inflammatory drug (NSAID).

Advanced Reference: Has moderate analgesic properties with anti-inflammatory action.

Key-ed filling system Quick Reference: System for filling anaesthetic vaporisers.

Advanced Reference: Designed to prevent filling with an incorrect agent as well as preventing spillage and consequent pollution.

Khat Quick Reference: (cat) Plant whose leaves are chewed and bring on mild cocaine and amphetamine-like effects, producing euphoria and hallucinations while also causing depression, constipation and loss of apetite. Also referred to as kat or gat.

Advanced Reference: It is used traditionally by those from countries such as Somalia, Ethiopia, Yemen and the Arabian Peninsula. Has *amphetamine*-like effects that can cause cardiac irregularities, especially in those with existing heart problems. Also suspected of causing liver damage and oesophageal cancer. It is not a classified drug or illegal in the UK but is banned in such countries as USA, Canada, Sweden, Norway and Ireland.

kHz Quick Reference: kilohertz.

Advanced Reference: The unit of frequency.

Kidney Quick Reference: Organs of the urinary system sited in the *lumbar* region.

Advanced Reference: Chief component of the urinary system, responsible for producing *urine*. Additional functions include filtration of the blood, maintenance of pH, re-absorption and secretion of salts and sugars, and involvement in the adjustment of blood pressure.

Kidney bridge Quick Reference: Elevation facility incorporated into many operating tables or fitted as an attachment.

Advanced Reference: The bridge may be integral to the table design or come as an attachment and is elevated during kidney surgery with the patient in the lateral position. Intended to provide improved access and visualisation to the kidney area during surgery. Sometimes used in combination with Jack-knifing of the table but improper use can lead to injury and reports of vena-caval occlusion have been reported.

Kidney sling   Quick Reference: A surgical sundry used to position and lower the kidney during transplantation.

Advanced Reference: Use of the sling can prevent unnecessary handling of the kidney during surgery as it is used to lower the kidney into the correct anatomical position prior to connecting of the vein, artery and ureter.

Kilogram   Quick Reference: SI unit of mass.

Advanced Reference: Equal to 1000 g. Kilo denotes a factor of 1000.

Kinetics   Quick Reference: Pertaining to or indicating motion.

Advanced Reference: The science of the relationship between the motion of bodies and the forces acting upon them. Kinematics is the branch of *biomechanics* concerned with the study of movement, particularly the time taken to carry out an activity.

Kinins   Quick Reference: Substances present in the body that are powerful vasodilators.

Advanced Reference: Also thought to be involved in inducing pain while also playing a part in the triggering of allergy and anaphylaxis.

Kiss of life   Quick Reference: A lay term for mouth-to-mouth resuscitation.

Advanced Reference: Relates to the expired air method of artificial respiration as used in cardiopulmonary resuscitation (*CPR*).

May also indicate the mouth-to-nose alternative used in small babies and those with mouth trauma.

Klebsiella   Quick Reference: A type of bacteria.

Advanced Reference: Short rod-shaped bacilli, Gram-negative and non-spore-forming bacteria which can cause infections in the lungs, intestines and urinary tract. The various strains are *K. pneumoniae* (pneumonia and respiratory infections), *K. rhinoscleromatis* (infections of the nose and pharynx), *K. oxytoca* (urinary tract infections).

Knee   Quick Reference: The joint between the *femur* and *tibia*.

Advanced Reference: A hinge joint formed between the lower end of the femur and upper aspect of the knee.

Knee-elbow   Quick Reference: Surgical operating position.

Advanced Reference: There are a number of variations to this position which is used mainly for spinal surgery. Involves the patient being placed in a crouched position, sometimes over a frame, resting on their knees and elbows. Due to the precarious nature of this position, there are many inherent and potential hazards. Also referred to as knee-chest position.

Knife   Quick Reference: Surgical scalpel.

Advanced Reference: Indicates both the handle and interchangeable blade used during surgery.

Koch pouch   Quick Reference: Form of *ileostomy*.

Advanced Reference: An internal pouch constructed from small intestine which stores waste products until they are ready to be irrigated by inserting a tube into the *stoma*, which is closed over by a one-way nipple valve. This method negates the use of an external ostomy bag.

Kocher's forceps   Quick Reference: (cock-ers) Toothed surgical forceps.

Advanced Reference: A toothed self-retaining forceps used to hold tissue that requires extra grip.

Koilonychia   Quick Reference: Spoon-shaped finger nails.

Advanced Reference: Often found in chronic *anaemia* and may also be brittle.

Konakion®   Quick Reference: Neonatal vitamin K.

Advanced Reference: Used to protect babies from vitamin K deficiency at birth. Since 2006 has been replaced by Konakion MM® paediatric version, which can also be used to reverse the effects of anticoagulant therapy in babies and infants.

Korotkoff sounds   Quick Reference: Sounds heard with a stethoscope when placed over the *brachial* artery during non-invasive blood pressure reading.

Advanced Reference: The sounds are thought to be due to vibration caused by blood turbulence within the artery. These are different from the lubb-dupp sounds associated with listening to the heart over the chest and are due to closing of the heart valves.

Kraske's position   Quick Reference: (kras-keys) Modification of the *prone* position.

Advanced Reference: Useful for surgical access during proctological procedures on the anus and rectal region. A variation of the *Jack-Knife* position.

KUB   Quick Reference: Abbreviation for kidney, ureter and bladder.

Advanced Reference: Term used in relation to radiograhic examination when determining location, size, shape and malformation of the above organs.

Kuntscher nail   Quick Reference: An orthopaedic device used in fracture correction.

Advanced Reference: An *intramedullary* nail used to stabilise long-bone fractures of such areas as the *femur*.

K (vitamin)   Quick Reference: Fat-soluble vitamin involved in the clotting of blood.

Advanced Reference: Vitamin K is needed for the formation of the enzyme thrombin, without which blood cannot clot. Formed in the body by intestinal bacteria, vitamin K is found in green vegetables; there are synthetic versions as well. Can only be absorbed in the presence of bile, therefore if the flow of bile is obstructed vitamin K is poorly taken up. Newborn babies are sometimes short of this vitamin and so, to prevent undue bleeding, they are given it in the diet until bacteria in the intestine take over.

Kyphosis   Quick Reference: (kie-fosis) Curvature of the spine.

Advanced Reference: The curvature is directed forward in a concave manner giving a hunchback appearance.

L

Labetalol **Quick Reference:** Drug used to treat hypertension and lower blood pressure (BP) for surgical purposes.

Advanced Reference: It is a combined alpha- and beta-blocking agent used for treating hypertension. In theatres, often used as an infusion for lowering BP in order to limit blood loss. Available as Trandate®.

Labia **Quick Reference:** Lip.

Advanced Reference: There are two pairs of labia at the entrance to the vagina, i.e. the labia majora and the labia minora, which together form part of the female external genitalia known as the *vulva*.

Labile **Quick Reference:** Indicates being prone to frequent swings and changes, unstable.

Advanced Reference: Term frequently applied to a patient's blood pressure when it is fluctuating regularly.

Labour **Quick Reference:** The process of giving birth (*parturition*).

Advanced Reference: Labour consists of three stages: the first stage starts with the onset of labour pains until there is full dilatation of the cervical *os*; the second stage lasts until the baby is delivered; and the third stage continues until the placenta is expelled.

Labyrinth **Quick Reference:** (lab-rinth) Any intricate or convoluted closure.

Advanced Reference: The labyrinth of the ear consists of the cochlea and semicircular canals which form the inner ear and are the organs of balance and hearing. The bony labyrinth indicates the bony canals of the inner ear and the membranous labyrinth is the soft structure inside the bony canals. Labyrinthectomy is the excision of the labyrinth, and labyrinthitis (which causes vertigo) is inflammation of the labyrinth.

Laceration **Quick Reference:** (las-air-a-shun) The act of tearing.

Advanced Reference: A laceration is a wound with torn and ragged edges, as opposed to an incision or cut which may not have neat and symmetrical edging.

Lacri-lube **Quick Reference:** Form of liquid paraffin used as an eye lubricant.

Advanced Reference: Used to hold down, protect and lubricate the eyes during anaesthesia.

Lacrimal **Quick Reference:** Pertaining to tears. To lacrimate = to cry.

Advanced Reference: Refers to the parts or structures concerned with the secretion and drainage of tears. Lacrimation is the act of shedding tears or eye watering.

Lactase   Quick Reference: An enzyme of the intestinal juices.

Advanced Reference: Lactase is involved in the breakdown of lactose into dextrose and galactose.

Lactation   Quick Reference: Formation of milk.

Advanced Reference: Commonly refers to breast milk and the period during which the child is nourished from the breast.

Lacteals   Quick Reference: Lymphatic capillary or duct.

Advanced Reference: Lymphatic ducts in the small intestine which absorb digested fats.

Lactic acid   Quick Reference: It is an end-product of glucose metabolism.

Advanced Reference: Produced in muscles by the breakdown of glucose in the absence of oxygen. Formed when there is an oxygen debt in exercise, and it is the cause of cramp.

Lactobacillus   Quick Reference: Group of *aerobic Gram-positive* rod- and *coccus*-shaped bacteria that produce lactic acid as an end-product.

Advanced Reference: Normally resident in the *vagina* maintaining an acid environment which prevents the growth of bacteria or *yeasts* that cause infection.

Lactose   Quick Reference: Milk sugar.

Advanced Reference: A compound of the simple sugars galactose and glucose. In the intestine the galactose is broken down to form glucose.

Lahey swab   Quick Reference: (lay-he) Small swab used for blunt dissection. Also known as a pledglet or peanut.

Advanced Reference: Used in many surgical specialities especially vascular, they are always mounted on an instrument such as an artery forceps. Although referred to as swabs, their main intention is for blunt dissection rather than absorption of blood.

Laminar   Quick Reference: In layers, horizontal. Laminar flow refers to a type of air flow system utilised in operating theatres.

Advanced Reference: An air flow system used mainly in orthopaedics to remove particulate matter from the air and so aiding the prevention of airborne infections during surgery. The flow is in one constant direction and at a high velocity.

Laminates   Quick Reference: Materials produced by bonding together two or more different materials.

Advanced Reference: This can involve glass, plastics, or wood, making the laminate much stronger than the individual components alone.

Laminectomy   Quick Reference: General termed applied to surgical procedures involving the spinal cord or intervertebral discs.

Advanced Reference: The name indicates removal of the lamina or overlying vertebral arches, and it is a basic procedure for treating a number of spinal-related problems, e.g. prolapsed disc, nerve and pressure release and excision of tumours.

Lancet   **Quick Reference:** Surgical knife.

Advanced Reference: It is of a double-edged design and originally used for opening abscesses and blood letting.

Landmarks   **Quick Reference:** Refers to anatomical landmarks in relation to treatment.

Advanced Reference: A number are commonly used, e.g. iliac crest, umbilicus, quadrants of the abdomen, xiphoid process, sternal notch.

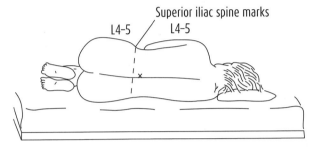

Fig. 13. Superior iliac spine.

Langenbeck   **Quick Reference:** Name of a number of different surgical instruments.

Advanced Reference: More usually a retractor but there is also a Langenbeck periosteal elevator.

Langer's lines   **Quick Reference:** Anatomical lines along which most of the supporting fibres of the skin are arranged.

Advanced Reference: They determine the direction in which the skin folds or creases if pinched. Are of interest during surgery in that incisions along them are less likely to stretch than those at a diagonal to them, therefore affecting the cosmetic outcome.

Lanolin   **Quick Reference:** Fat obtained from sheep wool.

Advanced Reference: Used as a base for ointments, one reason being that it can penetrate the skin. It is capable of absorbing and mixing with water but can cause sensitisation and provoke a reaction.

Laparoscopic surgery   **Quick Reference:** Indicates the use of telescopes (flexible and rigid) as an alternative to open surgery.

Advanced Reference: Alternative terms are: key-hole surgery, minimally invasive surgery and even incision-less surgery. In the pure sense, laparoscopic refers to entering the abdominal cavity but the term is used loosely with regard to the use of endoscopes although each surgical speciality has its own unique versions, e.g. arthroscopes in orthopaedics, hysteroscopes in gynaecology and cystoscopes in urology. The effect has been to both replace and complement open techniques and this combined approach is now common practice in all specialities. The benefits of laparoscopic surgery include: shorter hospital stay, reduced and limited anaesthetic input, reduced recovery time, lower post-operative infection rates, less pain and therefore reduced medication needs, improved cosmetic outcomes and it is reported to have overall financial savings. Tele-robotic and remote surgery where cameras and robotic instruments are at the operating site and the operator at a remote consul, sometimes in another country, are also undergoing rapid development.

Laparoscopy   **Quick Reference:** Endoscopic examination of a body (abdominal) cavity using a laparoscope.

Advanced Reference: The endoscope is introduced through the abdomen wall into the peritoneal space following insufflation with carbon dioxide which creates a pneumoperitoneum that provides enhanced working conditions.

Laparotomy   **Quick Reference:** Surgical opening of the abdominal cavity.

Advanced Reference: Used commonly to indicate a surgical exploration of the abdomen.

Largactil®   **Quick Reference:** Drug used primarily as a tranquilliser.

Advanced Reference: A preparation of chlorpromazine hydrochloride. Also used as an antipsychotic agent.

Large intestine   **Quick Reference:** The bowel.

Advanced Reference: It is approximately 1.5 metres long, sits draped around the *small intestine* and consists of the caecum, rectum and anal canal.

Laryngeal mask airway   **Quick Reference:** LMA. Airway device.

Advanced Reference: Invented and immediately became popular in the 1980s. Often described as an option between an oropharyngeal airway and an endotracheal tube. Provides a hands-free airway access without the need for laryngoscopy and intubation or the need for muscles relaxants as it sits above the vocal cords and larynx. Estimates are that it has replaced approximately 80% of intubations in the theatre setting. Hopes for it to be used by non-medical staff such as paramedics have not become a reality mainly due to the nature of their need being emergency work and the LMA in situ not protecting the airway in the event of aspiration. A number of variations, e.g. flexible, intubating and paediatric sizes, are also available.

Laryngeal tube   **Quick Reference:** (LT) Airway device, S-shaped with two cuffs, inserted blindly and used as an alternative to ventilation with a face mask or LMA.

Advanced Reference: A small oesophageal cuff at the distal end intended to block entry into the oesophagus while also reducing gastric inflation, and a larger pharyngeal cuff which stabilises the tube and blocks the oro and nasopharynx. Ventilation is via a hole positioned between the two cuffs which aligns with the larynx.

Laryngectomy   **Quick Reference:** (larin-gec-tommy) Surgical removal of the *larynx*.

Advanced Reference: Removal of the entire or a portion of the larynx usually as a measure in the treatment of cancer.

Laryngoscope   **Quick Reference:** An instrument for looking into and examining the pharynx and larynx.

Advanced Reference: An illuminated device most commonly associated with intubation in anaesthetics, although also used in ENT surgery on a regular basis. Numerous variations in both re-usable and disposable varieties are available to suit the needs of a range of scenarios.

Laryngospasm   **Quick Reference:** Spasmodic closure of the larynx and vocal cords.

Advanced Reference. Involves closure or partial closure of the vocal cords and so obscures the entrance into the larynx and threatens oxygen supply. Prime times for it to happen are at both induction and arousal from anaesthesia due to irritation from secretions, laryngoscope/airway insertion and suctioning. Treatment can involve administration of a short-acting muscle relaxant to facilitate intubation, or, if possible, sedation and relaxation with gases, volatiles and/or drugs.

Larynx   **Quick Reference:** (lar-rinx) Voice box.

Advanced Reference: The major function of the larynx is the production of the voice as it contains the vocal cords. It is lined with mucous membrane, is continuous with the throat above and the trachea below.

Laser   **Quick Reference:** Acronym for light amplification by stimulated emission of radiation.

Advanced Reference: Laser is the application of the fact that light is a form of energy. With ordinary light, the energy is diffuse but with a laser the beam is organised and concentrated. Utilised in hospitals as a cutting and coagulating tool in numerous types of surgery.

LASIK   **Quick Reference:** Acronym for laser-assisted in-situ keratomileusis. An ophthalmic procedure to correct refractive disorders.

Advanced Reference: It involves reshaping of the *cornea*.

Lasix®   **Quick Reference:** Proprietary diuretic. Frusemide.

Advanced Reference: A loop diuretic that is useful for reducing fluid levels when required in heart failure, kidney malfunction and general oedema. Works by inhibiting reabsorption in the Loop of Henle.

Late stent thrombosis   **Quick Reference:** Refers to clots that form on metal arterial stents.

Advanced Reference: Clots form on the uneven surfaces months or years after insertion and can break free and move to other parts of the body.

Latent heat   **Quick Reference:** Heat which is used to bring about a change in state, not in temperature.

Advanced Reference: Refers to the amount of heat energy needed to change the state of any substance without a change in temperature, as in solid to liquid, or liquid to gas.

Lateral **Quick Reference:** Indicates to the side. Away from the midline.

Advanced Reference: A surgical operating position. Left lateral indicates the patient lying on their left side.

Latex **Quick Reference:** Latex rubber. Basically a milky fluid of the rubber plant made up of various gums, resins, fats and waxes.

Advanced Reference: It is the source of rubber and is used in numerous hospital-based products with surgical gloves being one of the more familiar. The incidence of *latex allergy* has increased dramatically and its prevention is foremost amongst policies in all operating theatres.

Latex agglutination test **Quick Reference:** Carried out to detect the presence of the rheumatoid factor.

Advanced Reference: A test that has become standard in the diagnosis of rheumatoid arthritis.

Latex allergy **Quick Reference:** Hypersensitivity to latex.

Advanced Reference: Allergic reaction most commonly connected with the wearing of latex gloves, correctly called contact dermatitis. Reactions can range from minor redness and irritation to full *anaphylactic* reaction. Thought to be due mainly to the proteins in the latex whereas originally there was indecision over the primary source, with glove powder highly suspected, along with starches and other chemicals used in glove production. There are many alternatives available for both scrub and other staff, many manufactured from derivations of *PVC*.

Latissimus dorsi **Quick Reference:** A back muscle.

Advanced Reference: It is the flat muscle which covers the central and lower back. Said to be one of the largest muscles in the body.

Laughing gas **Quick Reference:** Nitrous oxide.

Advanced Reference: Anecdotally said to produce euphoria and a feeling of happiness. Nitrous oxide has both anaesthetic and analgesic properties.

Lavage **Quick Reference:** To wash.

Advanced Reference: In relation to the heath-care setting, it indicates to wash out a body cavity, e.g. peritoneal lavage, pulmonary lavage.

Lead apron **Quick Reference:** Radiation protection apron.

Advanced Reference: In relation to theatres, worn during surgical procedures when X-rays are to be used. Fits over the shoulders and should be of adequate length to cover the reproductive organs. Comprised of a thin lead sheet covered with plastic or leather. Great care is needed with their handling and storage as the lead is naturally prone to cracking if creased and will therefore lose its intended protective qualities.

Lean tissue **Quick Reference:** Anaesthetic term relating to body weight.

Advanced Reference: Used in relation to assessing drug dosage and distribution throughout the body but referring to real body weight and not weight due to excess fat.

LeFort **Quick Reference:** A classification of facial fractures.

Advanced Reference: The LeFort classification is a useful guide to determine the appropriate method of reduction and stabilisation. LeFort 1 involves a *transverse* fracture of the maxilla, while LeFort 2 is a pyramidal fracture of the frontal process of the maxilla, nasal bones and orbital floor. LeFort 3 includes both *zygomas*, namely both maxilla and nasal bones, as well as the *ethmoid, sphenoid* and outer orbital bones.

Left ventricular assist device **Quick Reference:** (LVAD) Device used to support patients with certain forms of heart failure, usually while they await heart transplant.

Advanced Reference: It takes over the work of the left ventricle, in effect resting the biological heart, but in some patients it has been seen that their heart actually undergoes a degree of recovery and regeneration.

Legionnaire's disease **Quick Reference:** Disease spread via airborne water droplets.

Advanced Reference: The name stems from an outbreak of a pneumonia-like condition which occurred in Philadelphia (USA) in 1976 at a convention of the American Legion in which 29 people died. As a result, a new organism was identified and named *Legionella pneumophilia*. It was discovered that the infection came from the water-cooled air-conditioning system, which if not maintained regularly harbours and becomes a source of spread. Simply adding chlorine to the water reservoir is an adequate precaution. Cannot be spread direct from person to person.

Lens **Quick Reference:** A device that makes beams of rays passing through it either converge or diverge.

Advanced Reference: In the eye the lens is the transparent structure situated behind the pupil that helps to *refract* incoming light and focus it onto the *retina*.

Leptin **Quick Reference:** A protein hormone. From the Greek – leptos, meaning thin.

Advanced Reference: Plays a key role in regulating energy intake and expenditure, including appetite and metabolism.

Lesion **Quick Reference:** Non-specific term referring to the damage done to tissues.

Advanced Reference: Involves a pathological change in a body tissue which can be due to injury or a disease process.

Lesser curvature **Quick Reference:** Concave curve of the stomach.

Advanced Reference: It is the boundary of the stomach that forms a short concave curvature on the right side between the oesophagus and duodenum.

Lethidrone **Quick Reference:** Alternative name is nalorphine, a narcotic antagonist.

Advanced Reference: Nalorphine neutralises the pain-relieving action of morphine, pethidine and similar narcotics.

Leuc(o) **Quick Reference:** Prefix indicating white.

Advanced Reference: Used in relation to both white cells and the white matter in the brain.

Leucocyte **Quick Reference:** The white cells in the blood.

Advanced Reference: The total number is raised during infection while being abnormally low in other conditions. Leucocytosis indicates an increase in white cell count and leucopaenia a decrease.

Leucotomy **Quick Reference:** Neurosurgical procedure.

Advanced Reference: Involves cutting of certain fibres (frontothalmic) in the brain as a treatment of some insanity disorders. The original operation involved the injection of alcohol to destroy the fibres rather than physically severing them.

Leukaemia **Quick Reference:** Malignant disease involving overproduction of white blood cells.

Advanced Reference: May be acute or chronic and, according to the type involved, can be divided into myeloid or lymphatic.

Levobupivacaine **Quick Reference:** Local anaesthetic agent.

Advanced Reference: Has less cardiovascular and *central nervous system* (CNS) toxicity than *bupivacaine*. Very potent with a trend towards a longer sensory block and when used for *epidural* produces less pronounced motor block.

Levophed® **Quick Reference:** A vasoconstrictor agent.

Advanced Reference: It is in fact noradrenaline and is used to raise the blood pressure in severe hypotension.

LFA **Quick Reference:** Low friction arthroplasty.

Advanced Reference: Referred originally to the Charnley (Sir John) total hip replacement. Made of stainless steel with a small femoral head, high-density *polyethylene* cup and secured with acrylic *cement*.

Lice (louse) **Quick Reference:** A parasitic insect.

Advanced Reference: There are many varieties but only two that directly affect humans, e.g. head and body lice, which are spread by direct contact.

Ligaclip **Quick Reference:** A metal surgical clip used for haemostasis of bleeding points.

Advanced Reference: Supplied on an applicator, they are placed on vessels and pinched shut, which then occludes the lumen and stops the flow of blood.

Lightening **Quick Reference:** A stage of the pregnancy cycle when after the 36th week the head of the fetus engages in the brim of the pelvis.

Advanced Reference: The uterus and its contents descend a little in the abdomen and relieve the feeling of distension.

Lignocaine **Quick Reference:** A local anaesthetic agent.

Advanced Reference: Also termed lidocaine. Used in various percentage strengths and also with an added vasoconstrictor (adrenaline). Also used as an antiarrhythmic in the management of ventricular tachycardia and ventricular ectopic beats. Ointment and gel versions (usually 2%) are available for use when inserting scopes. Also available as a 4% throat spray as well as syrup for gastroscopy.

Limbic (system) **Quick Reference:** System of brain structures.

Advanced Reference: Region that governs emotions and behaviour.

Limbus **Quick Reference:** A border or edge of certain structures.

Advanced Reference: The limbus of the eye is where the cornea joins the conjunctiva.

Linctus **Quick Reference:** A syrup.

Advanced Reference: Medium used to carry medicines, e.g. cough mixtures.

Linea alba **Quick Reference:** A fibrous band.

Advanced Reference: A fibrous band running vertically along the middle of the anterior abdominal wall, formed by the junction of the flat tendons of the external oblique, internal oblique and transverse muscles after they have split to enclose the two longitudinal rectus muscles.

Linear **Quick Reference:** Of length. Indicating one dimension.

Advanced Reference: A straight path. When particles travel in a straight line only. X-rays travel in straight lines prior to being prone to scatter. In laminar flow systems, the air travels in a linear manner, i.e. straight line.

Linen **Quick Reference:** Termed used generally to indicate theatre clothing and drapes.

Advanced Reference: All theatre-related clothing, drapes (where applicable) and instrument wrappings are included within the term even though most of these items are now made from synthetic materials.

Lingual **Quick Reference:** Of the tongue. Linguistic, to talk.

Advanced Reference: Term used to indicate the tongue. Teeth have a lingual surface which is the surface adjacent to the tongue. Something said to be linguiform is tongue-shaped. Sublingual and hypoglossal indicate the area of the mouth beneath the tongue.

Lipaemia **Quick Reference:** Excess fat in the blood.

Advanced Reference: Often associated with diabetes. Can also include cholesterol.

Lipase **Quick Reference:** An enzyme.

Advanced Reference: Lipase is involved in the breakdown of fats and is present in pancreatic juice and assists in converting them to fatty acids and glycerol.

Lipid   Quick Reference: Fatty substance.

Advanced Reference: A group of fatty substances that are insoluble in water but soluble in alcohol and form an important part of the diet.

Lip(o)   Quick Reference: Prefix for fat.

Advanced Reference: Lipid and lipoid refer to fat-like substances such as cholesterol.

Lipoma   Quick Reference: Benign tumour often occurring just below the skin.

Advanced Reference: Lipomas are relatively harmless and composed of fat cells.

Liposuction   Quick Reference: Surgical removal of fat, utilising suction. Also referred to as lipoplasty and lipectomy.

Advanced Reference: The removal of fat deposits, especially for cosmetic reasons, often carried out endoscopically. Ultrasonic-assisted lipoplasty (UAL) uses high-frequency sound waves to liquefy fat beneath the skin which is then removed with suction.

Listers   Quick Reference: Scissors used for cutting Plaster of Paris bandages.

Advanced Reference: Of an offset (handle upward) angle design and have no sharp edges on the lower blade so as to avoid skin injury.

Lithium   Quick Reference: Metallic element, symbol Li.

Advanced Reference: Used in the treatment of manic depression and more recently an ointment in the treatment of dermatitis.

Lithopaxy   Quick Reference: Crushing of a bladder stone.

Advanced Reference: Carried out with a lithotrite, followed by irrigation to flush out the fragments.

Lithotomy   Quick Reference: Originally indicated cutting into the bladder to remove a stone. Litho = stone.

Advanced Reference: The patient for this procedure was positioned with legs elevated into stirrups, i.e. legs raised and slightly head down tilt; hence, the position became known as lithotomy. Now the term indicates when the patient is supine with their legs in stirrups. Often used for gynaecology, urology and anal/rectal access. Placing the legs into position must be done in a synchronous movement in order to avoid spinal injury and hernia.

Lithotomy tray   Quick Reference: Instrument tray used when the patient is in the *lithotomy* position.

Advanced Reference: Attaches to the bottom end of the table when the end section has been removed or dropped. Used for holding instruments when operating on the vaginal, anal and perineal region.

Lithotripsy   Quick Reference: The crushing of a stone.

Advanced Reference: Procedure for breaking down renal stones, either directly or using shock wave (extracorporeal shock wave lithotripsy – ESWL).

Litmus   Quick Reference: Naturally occurring blue colouring matter.

Advanced Reference: Litmus is turned red by acids. Alkalis turn red litmus blue.

Liver   **Quick Reference:** Literal meaning is gland. Hepatic indicates the liver.

Advanced Reference: The largest gland in the body situated in the right upper area of the abdominal cavity, just below the diaphragm. Performs numerous functions: secretes bile; removes toxins from the blood; breaks down drugs; removes nitrogen from amino acids; stores and is involved in the production of vitamins, iron and glycogen; generates heat and converts stored fat into other usable fatty products, i.e. cholesterol, glycogen to glucose when needed; and metabolises proteins.

Live-related donor   **Quick Reference:** Term used with reference to trans-plantation.

Advanced Reference: The term is used mainly in renal transplantation and refers to a donor kidney being from a live relative as opposed to an alternative method, i.e. *cadaver*.

Lloyd-Davies stirrups   **Quick Reference:** Design of lithotomy poles.

Advanced Reference: A more versatile design of stirrup that has a number of adjustable joints and anatomically shaped leg rests into which the calves can be secured. They allow for variations in positioning and are intended for use with longer operations.

Lobe   **Quick Reference:** A well-defined part of an organ.

Advanced Reference: Partition of an organ as found in the lungs, thyroid and liver. Lobectomy is the removal of only the lobe and not the entire organ.

Lobotomy   **Quick Reference:** Neurosurgical procedure.

Advanced Reference. An operation performed on the prefrontal area of the brain, intended to bring about behavioural change through severing nerve fibres.

Local anaesthetic   **Quick Reference:** LA. Involves anaesthetising (localising) one specific area of the body.

Advanced Reference: Also termed regional anaesthesia, which can involve infiltration, surface creams as well as epidural and spinal techniques using various forms of local anaesthetic agents. Also referred to as conduction anaesthesia. Various techniques come under the heading of local anaesthesia. **Surface anaesthesia** involves local anaesthetic sprays, lotions, creams applied to skin and mucous membranes. **Infiltration anaesthesia** is the injection of local anaesthetic into the tissues to be anaesthetised. Both surface and infiltration anaesthesia can also be classified as topical anaesthesia. **Field blocks** involve the injection of local anaesthetic into an area bordering on the field to be anaesthetised. **Peripheral nerve block** is the injection of local anaesthetic into the vicinity of a peripheral nerve so as to anaesthetise the area served by that particular nerve. **Nerve plexus** anaesthesia indicates injecting local anaesthetic into the vicinity of a nerve plexus so as to anaesthetise several nerves spreading out from the plexus. Intravenous local techniques include such techniques as *Bier's block*. Also included is the injection of local anaesthetic into a cavity, e.g. intrapleural and intra-articular anaesthesia. In the broad sense of the term *epidural* and *spinal* techniques are also included.

Locomotor **Quick Reference:** Relating to movement.

Advanced Reference: Usually refers to human movement involving nerves and muscles as well as bones and joints.

Log-roll **Quick Reference:** System used for turning injured casualties.

Advanced Reference: Used when a patient has suspected or confirmed spinal injury. Involves rolling the patient as a unit, with no twisting of the spine and trunk and pelvis if possible. To be performed correctly should involve a minimum of four to six people. Some variations (mainly in first-aid settings) involve tying the patient's legs in a figure of eight and arms fixed to their side for further stabilisation.

Loin **Quick Reference:** Area of the back immediately above the buttocks.

Advanced Reference: The area that extends between the thorax (lower ribs) and the pelvis (iliac crest).

Lomodex® **Quick Reference:** Proprietary form of *Dextran*.

Advanced Reference: A plasma substitute used as an infusion to increase circulating volume. Available with either saline or dextrose. Also used in the prevention of thrombosis following surgery. Available in two strengths, 40 and 70, these figures relating to the molecular weight of the dextran chains, i.e. 40 000 and 70 000 Da respectively.

Lomotil® **Quick Reference:** Medicinal preparation used in the treatment of diarrhoea.

Advanced Reference: It is a mixture of diphenoxylate hydrochloride and atropine. It reduces gut motility and allows for water absorption from the faeces.

Long QT syndrome **Quick Reference:** A disorder of the electrical rhythm of the heart. An extended repolarisation time. Often the cause of unexplained sudden death in the young.

Advanced Reference: Leads to a very fast abnormal heart rhythm known as *Torsade de Pointes*. Long QT reduces blood pumping from the heart, leading to an insufficiency of oxygen throughout the body, especially the brain, which goes on to cause unconsciousness and possible death.

Lorazepam **Quick Reference:** Antidepressant and anxiolytic.

Advanced Reference: Member of the benzodiazepine group and is used to treat anxiety, insomnia and as a premedication. Available as Ativan®.

Lordosis **Quick Reference:** Curvature of the spine.

Advanced Reference: Indicates towards the front. As with the natural curvature in the lumbar region which produces the hollow of the back.

Loss of resistance technique **Quick Reference:** (LOR) Confirmation process used in *epidural* needle insertion.

Advanced Reference: Method of ensuring that the epidural needle is entering the epidural space rather than the fluid-filled canal required for *spinal* analgesia or the surrounding tissues and structures. The anaesthetist does this with an air- or saline-filled low-resistance syringe, ensuring no resistance to injection, which is felt as the space is entered after passing through the dense ligamentum flavum.

Lotion   Quick Reference: Solutions or suspensions in water.

Advanced Reference: Lotions are used to carry medications and usually involve the active drug being left behind after evaporation of the carrier. Alcohol is often added to assist this action. Common term for many skin preparations containing Hibitane™.

Lubricant   Quick Reference: Generally refers to substances used to make entrance to body cavities easier and less uncomfortable.

Advanced Reference: KY jelly is a very common lubricant and water soluble. There are also lubricants containing local anaesthetics such as lignocaine, usually in a 2% solution, and Hibitane® cream is used mainly in obstetrics to lubricate the vulva during labour and childbirth. Usually coated on fingers and/or instruments to facilitate easier passage.

Lucid   Quick Reference: Relates to a clear state of the mind.

Advanced Reference: Indicates clear logical thinking. A lucid interval is a period of clear thinking that can occur with head injury in between periods of unconsciousness.

Luer   Quick Reference: Connecting and locking system for cannulas and tubing.

Advanced Reference: Originally just one of a number of connecting systems for intravenous catheters, sets and cannulae. Now universally used and adapted to a Luer-lock system.

Lumbar   Quick Reference: The part of the back between the lower pair of ribs and the top of the *pelvis*.

Advanced Reference: The lumbar region is supported by the five lumbar vertebrae. The lumbar plexus is a group of nerves that supply the skin and muscles of the lower abdomen, thighs and groin.

Lumbar puncture   Quick Reference: To gain access into the spinal canal to extract cerebrospinal fluid (CSF). Also referred to as spinal tap.

Advanced Reference: Involves the introduction of a needle into the spinal canal (subarachnoid space) in order to draw off a sample of CSF for examination.

Lumen   Quick Reference: Space inside a tube.

Advanced Reference: Indicates the cavity or space inside a tubular structure, as with the lumen of a blood vessel.

Lund and Browder charts   Quick Reference: Assessment tool for burns in children.

Advanced Reference: They are utilised as an alternative to or to adjust the adult-based *Rule of 9s* system according to the age of the child. However, this system is said to be more suitable for burns assessment than the Rule of 9s as it compensates for the variation in body shape with age and therefore can more accurately assess burns in children.

Lungs   **Quick Reference:** Main organs of respiration.

Advanced Reference: The lungs allow the exchange of gases into and out of the blood. Positioned either side of the heart/mediastinum with the left lung having two lobes and the right three. The lungs themselves are made up of alveoli, bronchioles, blood vessels, nerves, connective and elastic tissue.

Lupus   **Quick Reference:** Chronic autoimmune disease.

Advanced Reference: Can involve internal and external structures, including the skin as well as muscles and joints. Causes inflammation and injury to cells and tissues.

Lux   **Quick Reference:** The unit of illumination.

Advanced Reference: Equivalent to one lumen per square metre of surface when measured at right angles to the direction of the light.

Luxation   **Quick Reference:** Dislocation.

Advanced Reference: Subluxation is a partial dislocation of a joint where the bone ends are out of line but still in contact.

LVET   **Quick Reference:** Left ventricular ejection time.

Advanced Reference: The interval from *systole* to closure of the *aortic valve*. It is a measure of the *carotid* pulse tracing from the beginning of the upstroke to the *dicrotic notch*, providing one of the *systolic* time intervals and is measured to assess left ventricular performance.

Lycopene   **Quick Reference:** Red pigment found in blood and the reproductive organs and present in a number of fruits and vegetables, chiefly tomatoes and palm oils.

Advanced Reference: It is an antioxidant that helps prevent cell damage by free radicals and is thought to combat *prostate* cancers and lower *cholesterol* levels.

Lymph   **Quick Reference:** (limf) The slightly yellowish fluid found in the lymph vessels.

Advanced Reference: It originates in the tissue spaces, being derived from the fluid which filters through the walls of the capillary blood vessels. A lymph node is a small collection of lymphoid tissue lying in the course of the lymphatic system and contains *lymphocytes* and antibodies, and acts as a filter to intercept foreign matter and bacteria which may cause it to become enlarged and sometimes painful.

Lymphadenectomy   **Quick Reference:** Surgical excision of lymph nodes.

Advanced Reference: Called also lymph node dissection. Commonly involves axillary, cervical and inguinal lymph nodes.

Lymphatic   **Quick Reference:** (lim-fat-ic) Referring to lymph.

Advanced Reference: Also the lymphatic system and circulation.

Lymphocyte   **Quick Reference:** White blood cells concerned mainly with the immune system.

Advanced Reference: Lymphocytes are formed in the lymph nodes as well as in the reticuloendothelial system. They are divided into two classes, B- and T-cells, the latter being formed in the thymus gland. B-cells produce antibodies.

Lymphoedema   **Quick Reference:** (limf-o-dema) Swelling of the lymph passages. *Lymphatic* obstruction.

Advanced Reference: Swelling is due to accumulation of *lymph* in the tissues. Obstruction may be caused by tumour, inflammation, or injury. Commonly affects the legs and often the arms following mastectomy.

Lymphoma   **Quick Reference:** Condition of the lymph glands.

Advanced Reference: Can be caused by malignant disease or *Hodgkin's disease*. Diagnosis is usually made by lymph node biopsy and treated with radiotherapy or *chemotherapy*.

Lysol   **Quick Reference:** (lie-sol) A soapy solution once used as a household disinfectant.

Advanced Reference: It is caustic and highly irritant, hence its withdrawal from general use.

M

MAC **Quick Reference:** Minimal alveolar concentration.

Advanced Reference: Refers to inhalation/volatile anaesthetic agents and is the minimum concentration of the agent in the alveoli that prevents a response to a surgical stimulus in 50% of subjects. Therefore, it is a measure of the potency/strength of the agent. MAC can be used to compare potencies of different agents, i.e. an agent with a low MAC value will require a lesser concentration than one with a high MAC value.

Macintosh blade **Quick Reference:** A curved laryngoscope blade used for intubation.

Advanced Reference: Refers to the curved adult version designed to pass into the vallecula and lift local structures in order to facilitate intubation.

Macrodex® **Quick Reference:** Proprietary form of dextran 70.

Advanced Reference: Used intravenously as a plasma expander and to help prevent deep vein thrombosis *(DVT)*. Available in dextrose or saline base.

Macrophage **Quick Reference:** Large cells present in connective tissues and in the walls of blood vessels. Also called *phagocytic* cells.

Advanced Reference: They can be fixed or can move around to pick up foreign particles and fragments of broken down cells. They form part of the *reticuloendothelial system*.

Macrosomia **Quick Reference:** Abnormally large body size.

Advanced Reference: Used to describe a fetus that is unusually large. Often due to maternal *diabetes*.

Macula **Quick Reference:** Central area in the *retina* containing the fovea.

Advanced Reference: It is the area where vision is at its clearest.

Magill's forceps **Quick Reference:** Angled forceps for guiding tracheal tubes.

Advanced Reference: Ergonomically designed forceps used for grasping and guiding both endotracheal and nasal tubes towards the larynx. Also useful for retrieving foreign bodies in the pharynx and placement of throat packs.

Magnesium **Quick Reference:** Metallic element, symbol Mg.

Advanced Reference: Used as an antacid and in the treatment of refractory ventricular fibrillation (VF).

Maintelyte® **Quick Reference:** An intravenous maintenance solution.

Advanced Reference: It contains sodium chloride, potassium and magnesium.

Malacia **Quick Reference:** (mal-ace-ea) Denotes abnormal softening in a body part or tissue.

Advanced Reference: Myomalacia indicates the softening of a muscle, osteomalacia is softening of bone.

Malaise **Quick Reference:** (mal-ase) A generalised and sometimes vague feeling of discomfort, illness or lack of well-being.

Advanced Reference: Usually associated with a diseased state and accompanied by exhaustion.

Malignant **Quick Reference:** Term used to distinguish severe or progressive forms of cancer/disease.

Advanced Reference: When used in relation to a tumour, it indicates cancerous as opposed to *benign*.

Malignant hyperthermia **Quick Reference:** Also referred to as malignant hyperpyrexia. Due to an abnormality of the muscle-fibre membrane.

Advanced Reference: Triggered by various drugs and anaesthetic agents, suxamethonium being the most prominent. Others include *halothane*, *lignocaine*, *atropine*, some of the *non-depolarising* muscle relaxants and *benzodiazepines*. Onset commonly begins with a failure to relax and increasing muscle rigidity, followed by a rapid rise in temperature, *tachycardia*, *cyanosis*, *acidosis* and an escalation in serum potassium levels. It is an inherited condition, and if known of all family members should be tested, especially if scheduled for anaesthesia. *Dantrium*® is used for pretreatment as well as following onset. Preplanning for known cases involves preparing an anaesthetic machine and circuitry not previously used with volatile agents, preparing cold IV fluids and cooling mattresses, etc., and the facility for continuous blood-gas monitoring.

Malleable **Quick Reference:** Pliable, able to be formed into different shapes.

Advanced Reference: Substance that is able to be re-shaped without the spontaneous tendency to return to its original shape. In relation to theatres, it includes face masks, intubating *stylettes* and wound retractors.

Malpractice **Quick Reference:** Professional negligence.

Advanced Reference: Involves a failure to exercise reasonable care and judgement which may result in injury or harm. Can be due to a lack of knowledge, experience, skill, care or ability that can be expected of others in the same profession.

Malpresentation **Quick Reference:** Indicates wrongful lie of the *fetus* in the uterus.

Advanced Reference: Any position other than the head presenting first.

Mammography **Quick Reference:** *X-rays* or images of the breast.

Advanced Reference: Used for early detection of breast cancers. A mammogram is a radiological examination of breast tissue in order to identify or exclude tumours.

Mammoplasty **Quick Reference:** Plastic surgery of the breasts.

Advanced Reference: Carried out to alter shape, size and general appearance.

Mandible   Quick Reference: Lower jaw.

Advanced Reference: It is comprised of a single bone that is loosely jointed with the skull at the temporomandibular joint in front of the ear.

Mannitol   Quick Reference: A powerful *diuretic*. *Hypertonic* solution.

Advanced Reference: Therapeutically it is used to treat oedema and decrease pressure in certain body areas when desired, e.g. intracranial during neurosurgery, eyeball during ophthalmic procedures and in *glaucoma*, and to increase renal perfusion during vascular surgery.

Manometer   Quick Reference: Scale used for measuring pressure.

Advanced Reference: The manometer measures *CVP* by the transfer of force/pressure in the veins to a graduated water column. Due to the lower pressure of the venous circulation, water pressure (cmH_2O) is used as opposed to mmHg in the higher pressure arterial system.

Manubrium   Quick Reference: Or manubria. Upper section of the breast-bone (sternum).

Advanced Reference: It articulates with the clavicle and the first costal cartilage.

Marrow   Quick Reference: Soft core of a bone.

Advanced Reference: At birth the bones are filled with red marrow but in adult life the red marrow of the limbs is replaced by yellow marrow, consisting mainly of fat. However, in the rest of the skeleton red marrow persists. Red marrow is actively engaged in producing various blood cells.

Marsupialisation   Quick Reference: To shell out, as from a pouch.

Advanced Reference: Example is shelling out of a cyst or abscess of the Bartholin's gland of the vagina.

Massive transfusion   Quick Reference: Definition involving blood replacement.

Advanced Reference: Although used as a term, it is in fact a calculation/definition of fact, i.e. massive transfusion is the replacement of half the blood volume within one hour.

Mass spectrometry   Quick Reference: Method used to determine the elements in a compound.

Advanced Reference: Can also identify the various isotopes in an element. Works by bombarding the sample with high-energy electrons, producing charged ions which are then separated according to their mass and analysed to give a read-out consisting of peaks where each peak corresponds to a particular ion and its mass.

Mastectomy   Quick Reference: Surgical removal of the breast.

Advanced Reference: Differing forms and grades exist, i.e. simple = the removal of the breast alone, whereas radical indicates removal of the breast as well as associated muscles and lymph nodes. Lumpectomy involves removal of a lump or growth.

Masticate   Quick Reference: To chew food.

Advanced Reference: Involves both upper and lower jaws to break up and mix food with saliva, which aids swallowing.

Mastic(e)   Quick Reference: Plant resin used in medicine for its antibacterial and antifungal properties.

Advanced Reference: A skin adhesive preparation of mastic was used for sticking surgical drapes to skin prior to the availability of mass-produced self-adhesive drapes.

Mastoid   Quick Reference: Bone situated to the rear of the ear.

Advanced Reference: A knob of bone projecting down from the skull behind the ear that attaches to the front part of the *sternomastoid* muscle.

Mastoidectomy   Quick Reference: Surgical removal of diseased bone of the ear.

Advanced Reference: Surgical removal of the diseased bone and drainage of the infected mastoid air cells.

MAST suit   Quick Reference: Military anti-shock trouser. Device used during initial resuscitation and transport which helps to support blood pressure.

Advanced Reference: Theatre staff may encounter these during direct transfer of A&E casualties. The principle is that the suit, once fitted on the patient, can be inflated and, by applying pressure, reduces peripheral venous pooling and therefore aids the transfer of blood to central areas of greater need.

Maternal cardiac output   Quick Reference: Refers to the cardiac output of a pregnant woman.

Advanced Reference: At term, the uterus requires approximately 10%–15% of output.

Matrix   Quick Reference: The place, substance, etc. from which something originates.

Advanced Reference: Examples are: the connective intercellular substance in bone, cartilage or other tissue. Can also refer to a rectangular grid of quantities in rows and columns used in solving certain problems.

Maxilla   Quick Reference: Jaw bone.

Advanced Reference: In particular, used to indicate the upper jaw.

Maxillofacial   Quick Reference: Surgical speciality once termed Facio-maxillary. Referred to colloquially as max-fax.

Advanced Reference: The branch of surgery that deals with facial repair and reconstruction. Has an overlap with dentistry, cosmetic and ENT surgery.

McBurney's point   Quick Reference: Anatomical landmark used in *appendicectomy*.

Advanced Reference: Located at a line on the abdomen connecting the umbilicus and the anterior superior iliac spine (crest) and used as a guide to make an appendicectomy incision.

McCoy   Quick Reference: Laryngoscope blade.

Advanced Reference: The McCoy has a hinged tip which can be manipulated from the handle. This facilitates lifting of the epiglottis and improves visualisation of the larynx during intubation. Useful as an alternative to other blades during difficult intubation situations.

Mean arterial pressure (MAP)   Quick Reference: Term used to denote average arterial blood pressure (BP) throughout the cardiac cycle.

Advanced Reference: It is believed that a MAP of 60 mmHg is sufficient to sustain organ and tissue perfusion. If this falls significantly for an appreciable period of time the tissues will not receive enough oxygen and may become ischaemic. MAP = (CO × SVR) + CVP, where CO = cardiac output, SVR = systemic vascular resistance and CVP = central venous pressure. Mean is an expression of the central tendency of a set of measurements, equal to the sum of all the measurements divided by the number of measurements.

Meatus   Quick Reference: An opening or tunnel.

Advanced Reference: Present in many parts of the body, e.g. the ear (external acoustic meatus), urethral and nasal meatus.

Meckel's diverticulum   Quick Reference: A protrusion from the small intestine.

Advanced Reference: Said to be a vestigial structure representing the yolk stalk. Resembles the appendix and can become inflamed with symptoms similar to those of appendicitis.

Meconium   Quick Reference: Greenish fluid comprised of bile and mucus, present in the intestine of a newborn.

Advanced Reference: It is expelled soon after birth or prior to delivery, if delivery is difficult.

Meconium aspiration syndrome   Quick Reference: (MAS) Also referred to as neonatal aspiration of meconium.

Advanced Reference: Occurs when the baby takes *meconium* into the lungs during or before delivery. Meconium is the product of the baby's first bowel movement and if it is passed into the *amniotic* fluid and the baby takes this in it can lead to respiratory problems.

Median   Quick Reference: In the middle.

Advanced Reference: The median plane divides the body into the left and right halves, whereas medial indicates being towards the midline.

Mediastinum   Quick Reference: Space in the middle of the thorax.

Advanced Reference: A compartment between the lungs containing the heart, major vessels, trachea and oesophagus. Mediastinoscopy is the direct visual examination of the area between the lungs.

Medical air   Quick Reference: Also referred to as compressed air.

Advanced Reference: Can be piped directly into the theatres or provided in cylinders which have a colour coding of a grey body with a white and black shoulder. Used mainly to drive pneumatic drills and ventilators.

The pressure for surgical tools is usually 7.2 bar (= 105 p.s.i) and 4.1 bar (= 60 p.s.i) for patient ventilators.

Medical Devices Agency   Quick Reference: Body responsible for overseeing the safety and quality of all medical-related equipment used in UK hospitals.

Advanced Reference: The agency relies on liaison with all health-care providers as well as manufacturers for information and feedback on safety and quality.

Medic-Alert   Quick Reference: Refers to a database of patients suffering certain conditions and taking necessary medication.

Advanced Reference: Members wear identification bracelets and necklaces indicating condition and contact details for further information.

Medical engineering   Quick Reference: Refers to the department responsible for maintenance of hospital equipment.

Advanced Reference: Also referred to as the Electrical Biomedical Engineering (EBME) department. Besides maintenance responsibilities, these departments are also involved in purchasing and loaning of equipment.

Medicolegal   Quick Reference: Refers to the branch of law that deals with medical litigation.

Advanced Reference: Medical negligence claims rise annually and so either in line with this or because of it, the legal input and involvement has increased to a situation where it has become a separate and specialised branch of law. At one time, except in extreme cases, it involved only doctors but with the emphasis on overall care and individual accountability/registration it can now have an impact on all disciplines of staff.

Medrone®   Quick Reference: Proprietary preparation of the corticosteroid methylprednisolone.

Advanced Reference: Used as an anti-inflammatory mainly for arthritis, joint pain and allergies.

Medulla   Quick Reference: Innermost part of a gland or organ.

Advanced Reference: Examples are the kidney and adrenal glands. Also used to mean the marrow of a bone and spinal cord and the *medulla oblongata* in the hindbrain region. In orthopaedic surgery, an intramedullary nail is one which is inserted lengthwise into the shaft of a bone in order to stabilise a fracture.

Medulla oblongata   Quick Reference: The lowest part of the brain. That portion of the spinal cord positioned inside the skull.

Advanced Reference: It contains the centres which govern the reflexes for breathing, heart rate and blood pressure.

Mefoxin®   Quick Reference: Broad-spectrum antibiotic.

Advanced Reference: Produced in powder form for reconstitution. It is a preparation of the cephalosporin cefoxitin.

Mega   Quick Reference: Huge, great. Alternatively megalo, mego.

Advanced Reference: A quantity of one million times a given unit.

Megacolon   Quick Reference: Abnormal enlargement of the bowel.

Advanced Reference: Condition which may arise due to a number of causes, one being *Hirschsprung's* disease.

Melaena   Quick Reference: (mel-eena) Black tarry faeces.

Advanced Reference: The dark colouring is due to bleeding and partly digested blood from higher up in the digestive tract, i.e. small intestine or upper colon.

Melanin   Quick Reference: Pigment present in the skin, hair, iris and choroid coat of the eye.

Advanced Reference: Ranges in shade from dark brown to black and contained in chromatophore cells. Production of melanin in the skin is increased by exposure to sunlight, which produces tanning that protects the underlying skin from the sun's radiation.

Melanoma   Quick Reference: A tumour of cells containing *melanin*.

Advanced Reference: A malignant tumour that produces secondary deposits, with the skin and eyes most commonly affected. A predominant cause is ultraviolet rays and may arise in a previously existing *mole*, showing signs of growth, change and bleeding.

Melatonin   Quick Reference: Hormone synthesised by the *pineal* gland.

Advanced Reference: Its secretion increases during exposure to light and has an effect on sleep. There are natural and synthetic versions available that are used to treat insomnia and jet-lag.

Membrane   Quick Reference: Thin layer of tissue composed of epithelial cells and connective tissue.

Advanced Reference: Covers surfaces, lines cavities or divides a space within the body. Examples are mucous, serous and synovial membrane.

Mendelson's syndrome   Quick Reference: Also termed aspiration pneumonitis or acid aspiration syndrome.

Advanced Reference: Inflammatory reaction following aspiration of gastric contents into the lungs. First described in 1946 by a New York obstetrician when he discovered an asthma-like condition associated with a mottled appearance on X-ray. He considered this due to gastric acid contents with a pH of less than 2.5 entering the lungs. Associated with induction and recovery from anaesthesia but can happen at any stage if the larynx becomes unprotected and more common, with certain patient groups such as those having emergency surgery and Caesarean section being prominent along with hiatus hernia sufferers.

Meninges   Quick Reference: The membranes surrounding the *brain* and *spinal cord*.

Advanced Reference: There are three layers of connective tissue membranes that line the skull and vertebral canal and enclose the brain and spinal cord: the *dura* mater, *arachnoid* mater and *pia* mater.

Meningitis   **Quick Reference:** Inflammation of the *meninges*.

Advanced Reference: Can become infected as a result of injury to the skull or infection of the middle ear but in general is caused by a variety of *bacteria, viruses* and *fungi*. Symptoms include: headache, fever, *nausea*, vomiting, backache, dislike of light (photo-phobia) and often stiffness in the neck, and in children, *convulsions* and a history of respiratory infection.

Meniscus   **Quick Reference:** Section of cartilage separating joint surfaces.

Advanced Reference: Usually a semicircular or crescent-shaped section of cartilage, as in the knee joint.

Meniscectomy   **Quick Reference:** Removal of a whole or part of a cartilage.

Advanced Reference: The most common being the cartilage of the knee, usually due to sports injury. Is performed via either open or endoscopic technique.

Menopause   **Quick Reference:** Decrease in the capacity for a woman to reproduce.

Advanced Reference: Onset is usually between the ages of 40 and 50 and characterised by the cessation of *menstruation*, reduced ovarian function combined with a decrease in the levels of *oestrogen* in the blood. The hormonal disturbances involved may cause hot flushes, atrophy of the breasts, vaginal dryness, reduced size of the uterus, possible weakening of the muscles of the pelvic floor and a tendency to *osteoporosis*.

Menorrhagia   **Quick Reference:** (Men-or-ag-ea) Excessive blood loss at the monthly period (*menstruation*).

Advanced Reference: Can be due to a number of factors including hormonal imbalance, clotting disorder, irregular ovulation.

Menstruation   **Quick Reference:** Female monthly period.

Advanced Reference: Involves the monthly shedding of the endometrium of the uterus and accompanying blood loss following the preparation for pregnancy which has not occurred.

Menthol   **Quick Reference:** An *alcohol* derived from peppermint oil.

Advanced Reference: It is mildly antiseptic and has a slight effect as a local anaesthetic. Regularly used in inhalations, often with the likes of *eucalyptus* and lotions and ointments.

Mentoplasty   **Quick Reference:** Plastic surgery on the chin. *Augmentation*.

Advanced Reference: Also referred to as genioplasty. The correction of a deformity of the chin.

Mepivacaine   **Quick Reference:** Local anaesthetic agent. Also available as carbocaine and polocaine.

Advanced Reference: Seen mainly in cartridge form for dental work.

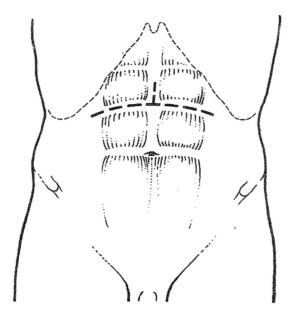

Fig. 14. Mercedes incision. Reprinted with permission from Elsevier.

Mercedes incision   **Quick Reference:** More an anecdotal than formal term for an incision used for liver transplant surgery.

Advanced Reference: So-called because the shape is similar to that of the Mercedes car emblem, composed of an upper midline and two (left and right) lower subcostal incisions.

Mercury   **Quick Reference:** Silvery metallic element. Chemical symbol = Hg.

Advanced Reference: Once widely used in medicine (as an antiseptic) but now reduced because of its toxic properties. Its main use now is in tooth fillings. Metallic mercury is not absorbed but mercury vapour can be inhaled. If digested can cause inflammation of the stomach and intestines in addition to kidney and nerve damage.

Mermaid syndrome   **Quick Reference:** *Congenital* union of the legs with partial or complete fusion of the feet. Also known as Symmelia and Sironomelia.

Advanced Reference: Usually fatal within a short time after birth. It is due to failure of normal vascular supply from the lower *aorta* in utero. Often accompanied by complications with the kidneys and bladder.

Mesentery   **Quick Reference:** A double layer of peritoneum which attaches the intestine to the posterior abdominal wall.

Advanced Reference: Carried within the mesentery are the blood and lymphatic vessels as well as nerves that supply the gut.

Mesothelioma   Quick Reference: A tumour of the pleura, peritoneum or pericardium.

Advanced Reference: Pleural mesothelioma is often due to *asbestos* exposure.

Metabolic syndrome   Quick Reference: Condition related to *chronic obesity*.

Advanced Reference: Characterised by increased abdominal fat, high blood pressure, high blood sugar, and high *cholesterol*. Thought to involve both genetic and lifestyle factors.

Metabolism   Quick Reference: Chemical process by which the substance of the body is produced and maintained.

Advanced Reference: Metabolism consists of catabolism (breakdown of molecules) and anabolism (reconstruction of molecules).

Metabolite   Quick Reference: Any substance that is a product of metabolism.

Advanced Reference: A product of any metabolic process such as digestion, drug breakdown or degradation as in the liver.

Metacarpals   Quick Reference: Bones of the hand and wrist.

Advanced Reference: Comprise the five bones of the hand that connect the wrist (carpus) to the fingers (phalanges).

Metals   Quick Reference: Reference to the various metals used in implants and medical devices.

Advanced Reference: Metals which are used as implants or designed to stay in the body for a short duration require certain properties, i.e. should be insoluble, non-carcinogenic, non-toxic, non-irritant as well as possessing the necessary strength, as in the case of joints and bone plates. The metals involved include: stainless steel, chrome, titanium, molybdenum, alloy, cobalt. Gold and silver could also be used but cost alone excludes them and are usually limited to fillings and replacement teeth.

Metastasis   Quick Reference: (met-ass-ta-sis) Migration of disease from one area of the body to another.

Advanced Reference: Generally used in relation to cancer spread from the primary growth to the secondary site(s).

Metatarsals   Quick Reference: Small bones of the foot.

Advanced Reference: There are five in number and they run between the ankle and the toes.

Methadone   Quick Reference: Powerful narcotic analgesic.

Advanced Reference: Used to relieve severe pain and in the treatment of heroin addiction.

Methaemoglobin   Quick Reference: Substance formed when the iron atoms of the *haemoglobin* have been oxidised. Occurs when there is excessive haemoglobin in the blood.

Advanced Reference: The iron alters to the ferric form from the ferrous form and has the action of preventing oxygen from being transported around the body. Cause can be inherited or due to drugs with an oxidising action. Treatment is with intravenous *methylene blue*, which brings about a conversion to haemoglobin.

Methamphetamine **Quick Reference:** A *sympathomimetic amine* closely related to *amphetamine* and *ephedrine*.

Advanced Reference: Has action similar to amphetamine. Abuse may lead to dependency. Also referred to as crystal meth and P (pure amphetamine).

Methane **Quick Reference:** Odourless, colourless gas (CH_4).

Advanced Reference: A by-product of rotting vegetable matter and component of natural gas and when mixed with air is highly flammable and explosive.

Methanol **Quick Reference:** Methyl alcohol. Better known as wood alcohol and used as a *solvent*.

Advanced Reference: Much more potent than ethyl alcohol, which comprises alcoholic drinks. If ingested, methyl alcohol can cause blindness and death, the blindness being due to damage to the optic nerve. Methylated spirit is a mixture of 5% methanol and 95% ethyl alcohol in combination with other petroleum hydrocarbons. One form is known as surgical spirit or rubbing alcohol.

Methicillin **Quick Reference:** Form of penicillin. A derivative of anti-staphylococcal or penicillinase-resistant penicillin.

Advanced Reference: Main usage is in the treatment of penicillin-resistant *Staphylococcus aureus*. Given only by injection.

Methylene blue **Quick Reference:** A blue dye.

Advanced Reference: Used in staining material for microscopy and intravenously to test renal function, also to identify various structures during surgery. Additionally used in the treatment of methaemoglobinaemia.

Methyl methacrylate **Quick Reference:** Bone cement.

Advanced Reference: Compound formed of two components, powder and liquid. Used for fixation in hip replacements for example. Can produce toxic effects if correct handling procedures are not adhered to.

Metoclopramide **Quick Reference:** An antiemetic/anti-nauseant. Maxolon® and Primperan®.

Advanced Reference: Has a dual action whereby it acts centrally by depressing the vomiting centre and peripherally by stimulating gastrointestinal emptying.

Metric system **Quick Reference:** Decimal system of weights and measures.

Advanced Reference: Based upon the principle that levels of units are related by the factor 10. There are seven basic units of measurement, i.e. metre, second, kilogram, ampere, Kelvin, candela, mole.

Metric tonne **Quick Reference:** Measurement of mass equal to 1000 kg (symbol mT).

Advanced Reference: Ton (UK) = 2240 lbs. Metric tonne (European) = 204.6 lb. Not officially an SI unit; if so, its correct term would be megagram.

Metzenbaum **Quick Reference:** Surgical scissors.

Advanced Reference: Surgeon's dissecting scissors although originally designed as tonsil scissors. Named after American surgeon, they are light, slender and relatively long and available in different sizes.

Microbe **Quick Reference:** A micro-organism.

Advanced Reference: More specifically a micro-organism capable of causing disease.

Microkeratome **Quick Reference:** An ophthalmic surgical instrument used for cutting into the *retina*.

Advanced Reference: It is used for removing a slice or creating a hinged flap with thicknesses in the region of 200 μm.

Micron **Quick Reference:** Micrometre, μm. Plural is micra.

Advanced Reference: One millionth of a metre.

Micro-organism **Quick Reference:** A *microbe*.

Advanced Reference: A minute living organism capable of causing disease.

Microtia **Quick Reference:** Congenital defect of the ear.

Advanced Reference: Involves the absence of all or part of the ear and can affect the inner ear causing deafness.

Microvasculature **Quick Reference:** The portion of the vascular system that is composed of very small vessels.

Advanced Reference: Generally refers to those vessels with an internal diameter of 100 μm or less.

Microwaves **Quick Reference:** Electromagnetic waves with wavelengths of a few centimetres.

Advanced Reference: Used in communication and as they have a shorter wavelength than radiowaves, they are suitable for use in radar systems because they can detect small objects. Heat is produced when microwaves are absorbed, hence in microwave ovens, the energy acts on the water in the food, producing heat and the cooking effect.

Micturition **Quick Reference:** To make water.

Advanced Reference: It is the act of passing urine. Urination.

Midazolam **Quick Reference:** Drug used mainly to induce sedation.

Advanced Reference: One of the benzodiazepine group of drugs. Used for premedication and induction of anaesthesia. Also known as Hypnovel®.

Midbrain **Quick Reference:** A portion of the brainstem.

Advanced Reference: It joins the hindbrain (*cerebellum*) to the forebrain.

Middle ear **Quick Reference:** That part of the ear which separates the ear drum from the inner ear (*labyrinth*).

Advanced Reference: It contains the *ossicles*, the three small bones which transmit vibrations from the ear drum to the nerve mechanisms of the inner ear. It communicates to the nose via the auditory (*Eustachian*) tube.

Mifepristone **Quick Reference:** Synthetic steroid that blocks the actions of *progesterone*. Also commonly referred to as RU-486 and the *morning after pill*.

Advanced Reference: Used as an *abortifacient*, usually in the first 2–3 months of pregnancy. Competes with and inhibits progesterone, encouraging the degeneration and shedding of *endometrium* from the uterus.

Migraine **Quick Reference:** Severe headache, often confined to one side.

Advanced Reference: Often runs in families and proceeded by an *aura* involving flashing lights before the eyes accompanied by vomiting. There is no set time for attacks and frequency also varies. Little is known of the definitive cause but spasm and dilatation of the cerebral arteries is suspected.

Minerva **Quick Reference:** *Plaster of Paris* jacket.

Advanced Reference: When applied includes both the trunk and head (with face and ears free) and is used for fractures of the *cervical* spine.

Minihep® **Quick Reference:** Proprietary anticoagulant.

Advanced Reference: Often used as a subcutaneous injection prior to surgery to help prevent *DVT*.

Minimally vegetative state **Quick Reference:** A condition distinct from *coma* and *vegetative state* (VS).

Advanced Reference: Involves alterations in consciousness which do not meet the criteria for coma (unconscious with eyes closed) or vegetative state (unconscious with eyes open).

Minims® **Quick Reference:** Proprietary anticholinergic preparation.

Advanced Reference: Available in eye-drop form (atropine sulphate). Used to dilate the pupils to aid eye examination.

Minute volume **Quick Reference:** The volume of air breathed or inspired in each minute.

Advanced Reference: Minute volume (MV) equals the *tidal volume* (TV) multiplied by the respiratory rate (RR): $MV = TV \times RR$. Normally 5–7 litres.

Miscarriage **Quick Reference:** An early unintentional end to a pregnancy.

Advanced Reference: The unexpected expulsion of the fetus before it is capable of sustaining independent life.

Mismatched transfusion **Quick Reference:** Indicates giving the wrong blood group to a patient.

Advanced Reference: The effect is that the red cells of the donor will react with the serum of the recipient. In cases of direct incompatibility this can produce serious reactions including intravascular coagulation and capillary blockage due to agglutination, and the subsequent haemolysis can lead to haemoglobinuria (Hb in the urine) and renal failure. Minor reactions include tachycardia, pyrexia and flushing.

Missed abortion Quick Reference: When the fetus dies but is retained within the uterus for over four weeks.

Advanced Reference: The gestation sac can remain in the uterus for weeks or months. If left, would probably be expelled spontaneously but evacuation is commonly achieved with the use of vaginal prostaglandins and intravenous Syntocinon® with vacuum/suction curette.

Mite Quick Reference: Minute *parasite* that lives on the skin.

Advanced Reference: Most common is the *scabies* or itch mite. Their saliva and droppings cause itching which, when scratched, can become infected. They are spread by direct contact, via clothing and bed linen.

Mitral stenosis Quick Reference: Narrowing of the mitral valve.

Advanced Reference: Usually due to inflammation following rheumatic fever in childhood, which leaves the valve shrunken and therefore prone to leakage, reducing the efficiency of the heart generally.

Mitral valve Quick Reference: Shaped like a mitre.

Advanced Reference: Also known as bi-cuspid valve, positioned between the left atrium and left ventricle of the heart.

Mivacurium Quick Reference: Non-depolarising muscle relaxant.

Advanced Reference: Relatively short-acting but with a slow onset of action. It is broken down by plasma (pseudo) cholinesterase in the same way as nitrazepam.

Mobile epidural Quick Reference: Adjusted form of *epidural* used mainly in *obstetrics*.

Advanced Reference: Traditional epidurals require the use of local anaesthetics (LA) in concentrations that may produce significant motor neurone blockade and, therefore, limited mobility. Mobile epidural utilises low concentrations of LA in combination with an opioid. This minimises motor blockade while enhancing analgesia and allowing for improved mobility.

Mogadon® Quick Reference: Tranquilliser and sedative drug.

Advanced Reference: Is a preparation of the long-acting benzodiazepine nitrazepam.

Molar Quick Reference: A back tooth.

Advanced Reference: Specifically indicates the double teeth, also referred to as grinders, of which there are three on either side of the jaw, making a total of twelve.

Mole Quick Reference: A pigmented spot found on the skin.

Advanced Reference: Also a way of determining the amount of one mole is a number equal to the number of atoms in 12 g of carbon-12.

Molecular Quick Reference: Of or inherent in *molecules*.

Advanced Reference: Molecular weight is the total of the *atomic* weights of all the atoms present in a molecule.

Molecule **Quick Reference:** A very small mass of matter. The smallest unit of a substance.

Advanced Reference: A chemical combination of two or more atoms which forms a specific chemical substance.

Molybdenum **Quick Reference:** Chemical symbol = Mo. A greyish metallic element.

Advanced Reference: Used in the manufacture of such things as air/gas cylinders to give extra strength.

Mongolism **Quick Reference:** Down syndrome. Mongol, mongoloid.

Advanced Reference: A congenital defect associated with mental deficiency due to chromosome imbalance in which the person displays a mongoloid appearance. Parents in most cases show no genetic abnormality although the incidence rises with the age of the mother. Female sufferers can become pregnant but males are sterile. Importantly for the anaesthetic/surgery setting, approximately 40% of those with Down syndrome have associated congenital defects of the heart.

Monoamine **Quick Reference:** An amine molecule containing one *amino* group.

Advanced Reference: Includes *serotonin*, *dopamine*, *adrenaline* and *noradrenaline*.

Monoanaesthetic **Quick Reference:** Refers to the possibility of one drug that could supply all the desired components of an anaesthetic.

Advanced Reference: This would be instead of a cocktail of induction agent, analgesic, muscle relaxant and inhalation agent.

Monochorionic **Quick Reference:** Mono = one; chorion = skin or leather. The outermost membrane enclosing the embryo.

Advanced Reference: Monochorionic indicates development in a common chorionic sac, as with twins. The chorion gives rise to the placenta. Diamniotic refers to two amniotic sacs (amnion = innermost).

Monofilament **Quick Reference:** A material comprised of only one strand. Opposite to multifilament, composed of many braided/twisted strands.

Advanced Reference: Term applied to sutures made of silk, cotton, linen, metal or synthetic material. Some are twisted or braided as well as coated for reasons that affect strength, resistance to breakdown/absorption and ease of passage through the tissues.

Monotherapy **Quick Reference:** Treatment of a condition by means of a single drug.

Advanced Reference: The use of a single drug or therapy.

Morbid **Quick Reference:** Pertaining to or inducing disease.

Advanced Reference: Morbid *obesity* (hyper-adiposity) indicates being 2–3 times or 50%–100% above normal weight or having a body mass index (BMI) greater than 39 and is therefore associated with many serious and life-threatening conditions, i.e. **diabetes, hypertension** and often causes **sleep apnoea** in many sufferers. Morbidity indicates a sickness rate, the ratio of sick to well people in any given community.

Moribund Quick Reference: At the point of death.

Advanced Reference: Term used when someone is close to death, fading from life.

Morning after pill Quick Reference: Refers to early non-surgical abortion of pregnancy.

Advanced Reference: Used within the first nine weeks of pregnancy, taken as a combination of pills (**mifepristone**), which prevents the action of **progesterone**, followed two days later by another (misoprostol) a **prostaglandin**, which induces miscarriage. Referred to also as early medical abortion.

Morphine Quick Reference: Narcotic analgesic.

Advanced Reference: An alkaloid of opium used to treat severe pain. May cause nausea and vomiting, reduced peristalsis of the gut and is a respiratory depressant. Also used as a premedication agent.

Mortality Quick Reference: The ratio of deaths to the number of the population in a year.

Advanced Reference: Often expressed as deaths per thousand of the population. The mortality rate of a disease is the ratio of deaths from a disease to the total number of cases.

Motility Quick Reference: Having the ability to move spontaneously.

Advanced Reference: Used in relation to micro-organisms, sperm cells and muscular contraction of the digestive tract.

Mouth Quick Reference: An opening. A gateway.

Advanced Reference: In relation to anatomy, it is the opening on the face to the **alimentary** canal.

Mouth gag Quick Reference: Anaesthetic adjunct used to open the mouth.

Advanced Reference: There are a number of designs, the most common being the Ferguson, which has a ratchet mechanism that holds it open and a fixation screw to maintain the degree of opening.

MRI Quick Reference: Magnetic resonance imaging.

Advanced Reference: Imaging system used for diagnostic purposes and has many benefits over X-ray and the computerised tomography (CT) scan, one being safety from radiation as it uses non-ionising radiation (magnets and radiowaves) to construct a picture. Produces better images when dealing with soft tissue, whereas CT and X-ray are said to be preferable for denser structures such as bone. The magnetism utilised can be a problem with certain implants that are magnetic, i.e. prostheses, vessel clips as well as surgical instruments, but in the latter case machines which limit the problem and have the operating magnet sited remotely are overcoming this problem.

Was originally termed magnetic resonance tomography (MRT) and nuclear magnetic resonance imaging (NMRI) but the use of nuclear created a false impression to patients. Magnetic resonance angiography (MRA) is used for the imaging of arteries (stenosis, aneurysm) and functional MRI refers to brain scanning. MRS (magnetic resonance spectroscopy) is also a related term.

MRSA **Quick Reference:** Methicillin-resistant *Staphylococcus aureus*.

Advanced Reference: Involves this particular bacteria originally becoming resistant to the antibiotic methicillin, hence the term MRSA. At the present time, hospital-acquired MRSA is increasing despite rigorous research and intensive infection control policies. PVL (Panton-Valentine Leukocidin) is a strain of MRSA which attacks white blood cells (WBC) and can be fatal. Other terms and abbreviations associated with MRSA are: CA-MRSA (community-associated MRSA), HA-MRSA (hospital-associated MRSA), MSSA (methicillin-sensitive or -susceptible *Staphylococcus aureus*) and ORSA (oxacillin-resistant *Staphylococcus aureus*).

Mucolytics **Quick Reference:** Substances capable of reducing the viscosity of *mucus*. Also termed expectorants.

Advanced Reference: Taken orally or via the inhalation route in the treatment of respiratory disorders characterised by the production of excess mucus.

Mucous membrane **Quick Reference:** Membrane that secretes mucus.

Advanced Reference: A layer of delicate tissue which contains glands that secrete mucus. Examples are the linings of the air passages and digestive tract, i.e. areas that have contact with the exterior.

Mucus **Quick Reference:** Fluid secreted by *mucous membranes*.

Advanced Reference: Acts as a lubricant, protective barrier and transport medium for such things as *enzymes*.

Muir and Barclay formula **Quick Reference:** Fluid regime formula used for burns patients.

Advanced Reference: It estimates the amount of fluid that needs to be infused during the first 36 hours after a major burn by dividing the total time into three periods. The formula is: *weight in kilograms multiplied by % of total body surface area of burn divided by 2.*

This formula was originally described for use with *albumin* as the resuscitation fluid.

Multi-organ (system) failure **Quick Reference:** Also known as multisystem failure but now more often termed multiple organ dysfunction syndrome (MODS).

Advanced Reference: May be due to sepsis, injury, *hypoperfusion* or *hypermetabolism* and by definition involves the failure of at least two systems, i.e. cardiovascular and renal. It is said to be a process more than an event, when *homeostasis* cannot be maintained without intervention. Commonly occurs as a result of *septic shock*.

Multifocal **Quick Reference:** Term applied to abnormal heartbeat grouping.
Advanced Reference: Multifocal ectopic beats stem from different areas (foci) of the heart, while multi-formed indicates runs of ectopic beats with more than one shape.

Multiple sclerosis **Quick Reference:** Disease of the *central nervous system*.
Advanced Reference: Involves the loss of the sheath which normally surrounds the nerve fibres, leading to loss of function. Cause is unknown but suggestions include autoimmune disease and infection. Affects mainly those in their teens and early twenties.

Munchausen's **Quick Reference:** (munch-house-ons) When an individual inflicts harm on themselves.
Advanced Reference: A mental disorder. The patient tries to receive hospital treatment for a non-existent, imaginary illness. Common for the individual to be extremely knowledgeable of the condition of which they are complaining. Self-inflicted injuries are common in an attempt at authenticity. Munchausen's syndrome by proxy (MSbP) involves inflicting harm on others.

Murmur **Quick Reference:** Heart sounds heard through a stethoscope in addition to the normal heart sounds.
Advanced Reference: These sounds may be due to vibrations and turbulence as the blood passes through the chambers and valves of the heart. Their presence does not necessarily indicate a disease state.

Muscle **Quick Reference:** The most abundant tissue in the human body. Responsible for various types of movement/motion.
Advanced Reference: There are three types of muscle in the human body, which differ in structure and function, i.e. striated (striped), smooth (involuntary) and cardiac.

Muscle relaxant **Quick Reference:** Drug that prevents muscle contraction.
Advanced Reference: There are two main types, i.e. *depolarising* and *non-depolarising*, which have different actions at the neuromuscular junction (end-plate).

Muscular dystrophy **Quick Reference:** (dis-tro-fee) A group of genetic *degenerative myopathies*.
Advanced Reference: Characterised by progressive weakness and *atrophy* of muscle without involvement of the nervous system.

Mutans **Quick Reference:** Species of *Streptococcus* bacterium.
Advanced Reference: Associated most commonly with the production of dental *caries*.

Mutation **Quick Reference:** A significant and basic alteration.
Advanced Reference: A permanent physical, chromosomal or biochemical change in hereditary material.

Myasthenia gravis **Quick Reference:** A condition in which the muscles become quickly fatigued.

Advanced Reference: It occurs in women more than men and may be associated with **thyrotoxicosis**. It has been found to be an **autoimmune** response. Diagnosis can be confirmed with the use of the drug **edrophonium**, which has an **anticholinesterase** action and therefore helps the action of **acetylcholine** at the neuromuscular end-plate. Treatment can be with **neostigmine**, which has a longer action than edrophonium.

Myelin   Quick Reference: An insulating layer around nerve fibres.

Advanced Reference: Myelinated = having a myelin sheath. Made up of **protein** and fatty substances. Myelin fibres form the greater part of the **white matter** of the **brain**, **spinal cord** and peripheral nerves.

Myelography   Quick Reference: X-ray examination of the spinal cord.

Advanced Reference: Involves the introduction of a **radio-opaque** medium via **lumbar puncture** into the **subarachnoid** space. The medium is 'heavier' than the spinal fluid so that it can reach all desired levels.

Myelotomy   Quick Reference: Incision of the spinal cord.

Advanced Reference: Involves severing tracts of the spinal cord.

Mycobacterial infection   Quick Reference: A **genus** of **aerobic** bacteria.

Advanced Reference: Responsible for such diseases as **tuberculosis** and leprosy.

Myocardial infarct(ion)   Quick Reference: The result of blockage of the blood supply to a part of the heart.

Advanced Reference: The blockage involves the coronary arteries and affects the **myocardium** causing death of the area starved of a blood supply.

Myocarditis   Quick Reference: Inflammation of the heart muscle.

Advanced Reference: May be caused by a virus, bacteria or an immunological reaction following infection.

Myocardium   Quick Reference: Myo = muscle, cardium refers to the heart.

Advanced Reference: It is the middle of the three layers of the heart wall, the others being the endocardium (inner lining) and pericardium/epicardium (outer layer).

Myoglobin   Quick Reference: The oxygen-transporting pigment of muscle. Iron containing, it resembles **haemoglobin**.

Advanced Reference: It combines with oxygen released by erythrocytes, stores it and transports it to the mitochondria (the powerhouse of a cell) of muscle cells where it generates energy.

Myoma   Quick Reference: A tumour.

Advanced Reference: Usually benign and grows from muscle fibres. Common in the uterus as **fibroids**.

Myometrium   Quick Reference: Muscular layer of the uterine wall.

Advanced Reference: Smooth muscle fibres of the myometrium curve around the uterus horizontally, vertically and diagonally.

Myopathy   Quick Reference: Indicates any disease of a muscle.

Advanced Reference: Can affect any muscles and in the heart it is termed cardiac myopathy. All involve wasting and weakness in the muscle. Neither of these is due to defects in the related nervous system.

Myopia   **Quick Reference:** Short-sightedness.

Advanced Reference: Also referred to as near-sightedness. Correction involves changes to the focusing of the eye.

Myositis   **Quick Reference:** Inflammation of the muscles.

Advanced Reference: Usually due to infection. Polymyositis is an **auto-immune disease** where **lymphocytes** become sensitised against muscle tissue causing inflammation and weakness.

Myotome   **Quick Reference:** A surgical instrument used for dividing muscle (myotomy).

Advanced Reference: With reference to anatomy myotome indicates a muscle or group of muscles innervated by a single segment of a spinal nerve, i.e. the relationship between a spinal nerve and muscle.

N

Naevus **Quick Reference:** (nevus) A birthmark.

Advanced Reference: Area of pigmentation on the skin due to dilated blood vessels.

Nail brush **Quick Reference:** Small, stiff-bristled brush used during the scrub-up procedure.

Advanced Reference: Available as a disposable presterilised item and in some designs impregnated with antiseptic/antibacterial solution. Not recommended by all authorities: some consider brushing too harsh and may cause skin injury as well as disturb resident flora and so create a more suitable environment for bacteria to prosper; some recommend a softer sponge alternative. However, used as originally intended for nail cleaning, it has undoubted benefits.

Naloxone **Quick Reference:** Opiate antagonist. Narcan®.

Advanced Reference: Used as an antidote to narcotic analgesics and in situations of overdose.

Nanogram **Quick Reference:** Indicates one-thousandth millionth of a gram. Abbreviation = ng.

Advanced Reference: A nanogram is one-thousandth millionth of a gram or one-billionth (10^{-9}) of a gram.

Nanometre **Quick Reference:** One-millionth of a millimetre. One-billionth of a metre. One-thousandth of a *micron*.

Advanced Reference: Abbreviation = nm.

Narcolepsy **Quick Reference:** A condition which produces an uncontrollable desire to sleep.

Advanced Reference: Those suffering the condition experience excessive daytime sleepiness and often at the most inappropriate times.

Narcosis **Quick Reference:** Dulling of consciousness.

Advanced Reference: A state of unconsciousness usually produced by drugs of the narcotic category.

Narcotic **Quick Reference:** Any drug that produces *narcosis.*

Advanced Reference: Usually refers to morphine-like drugs. Related terms are *opiate* and *opioid.*

Nares **Quick Reference:** The nostrils.

Advanced Reference: The nares reach from the outside of the nose to the *nasopharynx.* The two nostrils are separated at the entrance by the columella and within the nasal passage by the nasal *septum.*

Nasal prongs/specs Quick Reference: Patient oxygen delivery system.

Advanced Reference: Designed to be inserted with one prong in each nostril for the delivery of oxygen. Inaccurate in percentage delivery as factors such as depth of insertion and degree of mouth opening have a bearing on functional oxygen, therefore values of 40% are quoted but cannot be taken as accurate in all situations. Intended in the ideal setting to deliver 4% for each litre of oxygen flow, [therefore a 6-l flow would provide 24% + 21% (room air) = 45%]. There is an alternative version available with one nostril prong. Often referred to as oxygen 'specs' due to the design which loops over the ears in the manner of spectacles.

Nasogastric tube Quick Reference: Tube (usually plastic/*PVC*) passed via the mouth/nose into the stomach.

Advanced Reference: Usually inserted for suction, lavage or feeding. Available in a number of bores, e.g. 10 g through to 18 g. Also referred to as Ryle's tube, which is a nasogastric tube with a weighted tip. It has an integral radio-opaque line for placement detection by X-ray when *in situ*. In order to maintain some degree of rigidity, they are often stored in the fridge.

Nasopharyngeal airway Quick Reference: Airway used primarily in anaesthesia.

Advanced Reference: Inserted via the nostrils with the distal tip sitting in the pharynx. Available in plastic, latex and in various diameters from neonate to large adult. Lengths also vary accordingly and may be assessed by using the distance from *nares* to ear as a guide.

Nausea Quick Reference: Sensation of imminent vomiting.

Advanced Reference: Can indicate the feeling of sickness without vomiting actually occurring.

Navel Quick Reference: The umbilicus.

Advanced Reference: The indentation, scar or tissue residue in the centre of the abdominal wall which is the junction of where the umbilical cord joined the fetus, with the other end attached to the *placenta.*

Nebuliser Quick Reference: Device that converts a liquid into a vapour.

Advanced Reference: Used for the purpose of humidification in oxygen delivery systems and ventilators as well as a method of medicine delivery. Also referred to as an atomiser.

Necrosis Quick Reference: Death of tissue.

Advanced Reference: Can involve tissue or an entire organ usually due to interruption in the blood supply or because of infection.

Necrotising fasciitis Quick Reference: Flesh-eating condition due to bacterial infection.

Advanced Reference: Affects the deeper layers of the skin and subcutaneous tissues. Involves many types of bacteria including *Streptococcus, Clostridium* but most commonly the *Streptococcus* A group. The actual cause is due to toxins released by the bacteria rather than actual flesh-eating activity. Although it can start without apparent cause, trauma is usually the reason, even following surgery. Begins with pain, swelling and typically fever, followed by discoloration and blistering which leads to necrosis. Treatment is with intravenous antibiotics and if necessary debridement of the area and sometimes amputation.

Needle biopsy **Quick Reference:** Removal of a tissue specimen (via the exterior of an organ) for biopsy by aspiration through a hollow needle.

Advanced Reference: The device is usually spring-loaded and often guided into the target tissue using *CT scan* or *ultrasound.* Also called aspiration biopsy.

Needle holder **Quick Reference:** Instrument for holding sutures/needles during surgery.

Advanced Reference: Available in various designs and sizes depending on need and speciality. Examples are Mayo, Gillies, Castroviejo, Crile-Wood, DeBakey.

Needle-stick injury **Quick Reference:** Injury from a hypodermic needle or other sharp implement used on a patient.

Advanced Reference: Can be a route of cross infection and due to its potential seriousness many policies, procedures and devices have been introduced in an attempt to lower incidence.

Needle valve **Quick Reference:** The control mechanism of a *flowmeter*, such as that controlling the delivery of oxygen or nitrous oxide from an anaesthetic machine.

Advanced Reference: The valve increases or decreases the flow of gas as it is turned clockwise or anti-clockwise.

Neighbour strapping **Quick Reference:** Refers to the technique of fixing a finger or toe to the next as a form of splinting.

Advanced Reference: Usually done in the situation of fracture when the affected digit is taped to its neighbouring digit and so using it as a splint. The term is also used in relation to fixing a fractured or injured leg to the other often with figure of eight bandaging.

Neodymium **Quick Reference:** Silvery metallic rare element used in the manufacture of extremely strong magnets.

Advanced Reference: A component of many electronic devices such as computers, mobile phones and headphones and can interfere with the functioning of implanted heart devices.

Neomycin **Quick Reference:** Broad-spectrum antibiotic.

Advanced Reference: Effective against topical bacteria but too toxic to be used via the intravascular or intramuscular routes.

Neonatal **Quick Reference:** Of newborn baby, neonate.

Advanced Reference: Term used conventionally to indicate the first four weeks of life.

Neoplasm **Quick Reference:** New growth or *tumour.*

Advanced Reference: A tumour may be *benign* or *malignant.*

Neoprene® **Quick Reference:** Trade name for a family of rubbers.

Advanced Reference: Originally called Duprene®, it was the first mass-produced synthetic rubber compound. It is waterproof and chemically inert and therefore useful for many hospital-based products, i.e. gloves, washers and gaskets, which come into contact with chemicals and gases.

Neostigmine **Quick Reference:** An *anticholinesterase* drug.

Advanced Reference: Increases the activity of the neurotransmitter *acetylcholine,* which transmits instructions from the brain to skeletal muscle. Used as a reversal to non-depolarising muscle relaxants.

Nephrectomy **Quick Reference:** Surgical removal of the kidney.

Advanced Reference: Removal of one or both kidneys due to a variety of diseases and conditions. A graft nephrectomy is the surgical removal of a previously transplanted kidney.

Nephritis **Quick Reference:** Inflammation of the kidneys.

Advanced Reference: A non-specific term that may be used to describe a wide variety of diseases of the kidney.

Nephrocalcinosis **Quick Reference:** Condition characterised by precipitation of calcium salts.

Advanced Reference: Due to excess calcium (mainly calcium phosphate and oxalate) in the blood. Causes a build-up in the renal tubules resulting in renal insufficiency and polyuria.

Nephrostomy **Quick Reference:** Draining of the kidney directly to the exterior.

Advanced Reference: Involves the insertion of a self-retaining catheter through a small incision in the cortex of the kidney. The most common reason for this procedure is bilateral ureteric obstruction.

Nerve **Quick Reference:** A bundle of conducting fibres.

Advanced Reference: Nerve fibres are contained in a sheath of connective tissue and they run from the central nervous system (CNS) to the muscles, skin and other organs, conveying either motor or sensory impulses. The nervous system is divided into the CNS (which includes the brain and spinal cord), the peripheral nervous system, and the *autonomic* system, which includes the sympathetic and parasympathetic systems.

Nerve block **Quick Reference:** Indicates blocking nerve pathways to prevent pain.

Advanced Reference: Carried out using local anaesthetic (LA) agents. Examples are wound infiltration (following surgery), digital block (provides operating conditions as well as postoperative pain relief following surgery on toes and fingers), femoral block (useful in patients with fractured neck of femur) or ankle block (following surgery). In addition to LAs for this purpose, electrical nerve stimulation, acupuncture, cryotherapy as well as drugs and inhalation agents are all used as pain-blocking techniques.

Nerve stimulator   **Quick Reference:** Peripheral stimulator used to assess neuromuscular blockade induced with muscle relaxants.

Advanced Reference: Used to monitor transmission across the neuromuscular junction with reference to reversal of muscle relaxants. Also used during nerve blocks to produce muscular contractions when locating a nerve plexus.

Neuralgia   **Quick Reference:** Pain extending along a nerve.

Advanced Reference: Can affect many nerves, e.g. facial, brachial, occipital.

Neuritis   **Quick Reference:** Inflammation of a nerve.

Advanced Reference: May lead to pain, tenderness, anaesthesia, paralysis, wasting and eventual disappearance of the reflexes.

Neurofibroma   **Quick Reference:** Benign tumour.

Advanced Reference: A benign tumour arising from the sheath of a nerve.

Neuroleptic   **Quick Reference:** (nuro-leptic) Category of drugs which affect the nervous system in the manner of dulling emotional behaviour and slowing psychomotor activity.

Advanced Reference: Term applied to a technique of anaesthesia which involves using opioid analgesics such as *fentanyl* and *phenoperidine* in combination with, for example, droperidol. Produces neurolepsis and a reduction in motor activity.

Neurolysis   **Quick Reference:** Release of a nerve sheath by cutting it longitudinally.

Advanced Reference: Carried out for a number of reasons including perineural adhesions, relief of tension upon a nerve and destruction of a nerve for the relief of pain.

Neuroma   **Quick Reference:** A tumour consisting of nerve fibres.

Advanced Reference: A tumour growing from a nerve.

Neurones   **Quick Reference:** Or neurones. Nerve cell.

Advanced Reference: A nerve cell with conducting fibres.

Neuropathy   **Quick Reference:** Disease of the peripheral nerves causing numbness and weakness.

Advanced Reference: Mononeuropathy affects single nerves and polyneuropathy many or all of the associated nerves.

Neurosis   **Quick Reference:** Mental illness. Unlike *psychosis* those affected retain insight and are aware of their condition.

Advanced Reference: Sufferers can display signs of anxiety, hysteria and obsessional behaviour.

Neurotransmitter   **Quick Reference:** A chemical substance which transmits impulses across nerve synapses.

Advanced Reference: Released from nerve endings; includes *acetylcholine, noradrenaline, dopamine and serotonin.*

Niacin   **Quick Reference:** Nicotinic acid, nicotinamide.

Advanced Reference: A B-complex *vitamin.*

Nicotine   **Quick Reference:** An *alkaloid* present in tobacco.

Advanced Reference: Has the effects of firstly stimulating then to a degree paralysing the *autonomic nervous system.*

Nifedipine   **Quick Reference:** A calcium antagonist. Antihypertensive.

Advanced Reference: Used in the treatment of hypertension and angina.

Nikethamide   **Quick Reference:** Respiratory stimulant.

Advanced Reference: Used to relieve severe respiratory difficulties, e.g. respiratory depression, chronic respiratory disease.

Nipple   **Quick Reference:** Projection of the breast.

Advanced Reference: Structure through which a baby/offspring withdraws mother's milk. Can also refer to rubber/plastic covers through which fluids are fed and so named for their shape and function, which resembles a human nipple.

Nipride®   **Quick Reference:** Proprietary form of the antihypertensive drug sodium nitroprusside.

Advanced Reference: Used to treat hypertension and in an infusion during surgery to induce hypotension by vasodilatation. Short-acting, used in theatres as a preparation for reconstitution in 5% dextrose. Should be protected from light as it decomposes to form unstable solutions which may form cyanide toxicity.

Nitric oxide   **Quick Reference:** Chemical formula $= NO$.

Advanced Reference: Used in inhalant form as a pulmonary vasodilator, mainly in intensive care units (ICU).

Nitrile   **Quick Reference:** A synthetic rubber.

Advanced Reference: An organic compound produced in many forms. Most commonly in health care as disposable gloves. It is more resistant to oils and acids than natural rubber but has less strength and flexibility.

Nitrogen   **Quick Reference:** Inert colourless gas. Chemical symbol $= N_2$.

Advanced Reference: Present at a level of 78% in atmospheric air. Not able to support life on its own but plays a part in supporting the alveoli of the lungs. The term *nitrogen splint* is often used in anaesthesia and refers to the period of emergence when a patient who has been ventilated is allowed to breath room air via the endotracheal tube (ETT) so as to take in nitrogen which assists in opening up and supporting the alveoli prior to extubation.

Nitrous oxide   **Quick Reference:** N_2O. Has the lay name of laughing gas.

Advanced Reference: Weak analgesic and anaesthetic. Given in combination with oxygen during general anaesthesia and as a gas/air mixture for pain relief in A&E departments, etc.

Noble gases   **Quick Reference:** *Inert* gases such as helium, neon, argon, krypton, *xenon* and usually *radon.*

Advanced Reference: They display great stability and low reaction rates, i.e. they do not react chemically with other constituents of a system.

Nocturnal enuresis **Quick Reference:** Bed wetting.

Advanced Reference: Voiding of the bladder during (night-time) sleep. May be due to small bladder capacity and failure to wake when the bladder fills. Often linked with daytime incontinence and affecting the young and adolescent, when it is termed primary nocturnal enuresis.

Node **Quick Reference:** (or nodule) A protuberance or swelling.

Advanced Reference: There are various nodes found throughout the body, e.g. atrioventricular (AV) node and sinoatrial (SA) node in the heart, which are responsible for impulse transmission; the nodes of Ranvier are present in nerve fibres. Also, *lymph* nodes.

Nodule **Quick Reference:** A small swelling.

Advanced Reference: A small mass of rounded or irregular shape, as a tumour growth or calcification near an arthritic joint.

Nomenclature **Quick Reference:** A system of names and terminology used in the sciences.

Advanced Reference: As with anatomical structures and biological organisms.

Nominal hazard zone **Quick Reference:** (NHZ) The space in which direct, reflected or scattered laser radiation exceeds the maximum permitted exposure (MPE).

Advanced Reference: Inside of this area laser safety eyewear (LSE) must be worn.

Non-depolariser **Quick Reference:** Refers to a specific group of muscle relaxants which act at the neuromuscular junction.

Advanced Reference: The drugs attach themselves to receptor sites on the postsynaptic membrane of the neuromuscular junction and prevent acetylcholine reaching the end-plate and producing depolarisation, whereas depolarising muscle relaxants produce their effect (prolonged contraction and paralysis) at the membrane in the same way as acetylcholine.

Non-invasive **Quick Reference:** Indicates not entering inside the body.

Advanced Reference: As opposed to invasive, when devices are placed inside the body or through the skin. An example is non-invasive blood pressure (BP) measurement using a limb cuff whereas invasive BP measurement would involve cannulating an artery to obtain a direct reading.

Non-invasive ventilation **Quick Reference:** NIV. Also referred to as non-invasive positive pressure ventilation (NPPV). Patient ventilation without tracheal intubation.

Advanced Reference: Positive pressure ventilation delivered via a mask (oral, nasal) in the treatment of *sleep apnoea*, neuromuscular diseases, certain pulmonary and cardiac conditions and most forms of chronic obstructive pulmonary disease (*COPD*).

Non-medical anaesthetist Quick Reference: Health-care professional trained to deliver anaesthesia.

Advanced Reference: Traditionally only trained medical doctors delivered anaesthesia. This discipline, also termed Advanced Anaesthetic Practitioner (AAP), has comparisons with the USA-based Nurse Anaesthetist in that they are usually an established health-care professional who has undergone further training in anaesthesia and works in a semi-autonomous role performing a number of duties which were previously unique to the anaesthetist.

Non-rebreathing Quick Reference: Refers to types of breathing circuits and the valves within them.

Advanced Reference: With these circuits the patient continually receives a fresh flow of gas. Examples in common use are the Ruben valve and those incorporated into the bag-valve-mask (*BVM*) used mainly during resuscitation.

Non-steroidal anti-inflammatory drugs Quick Reference: NSAIDs. Group of drugs with analgesic, anti-inflammatory and antipyretic actions.

Advanced Reference: Act by inhibiting prostaglandin synthesis and so decreasing the inflammatory response to surgery and associated pain. Commonly used examples are diclofenac and ketorolac. On a more basic and everyday level, *aspirin* is also a member of this group.

Noradrenaline Quick Reference: A *catecholamine*, a *hormone* secreted by the medulla of the adrenal glands.

Advanced Reference: Closely related to adrenaline but not as selective in its actions. Also a neurotransmitter of the sympathetic nervous system. Noradrenaline is almost entirely concerned with contraction of the arteries and supporting blood pressure.

Normal saline Quick Reference: Indicates an isotonic solution of sodium chloride. Normal in terms of physiological rather than chemistry terms.

Advanced Reference: Is a 0.9% solution used as an intravenous maintenance and replacement fluid as well as a vehicle for medications.

Normal value(s) Quick Reference: A set of laboratory tests.

Advanced Reference: Values used to characterise (apparently) healthy individuals.

Normasol® Quick Reference: Proprietary saline solution.

Advanced Reference: Produced in the form of a sterile solution and used to flush wounds. Also available in ophthalmic form as an eye wash.

Normothermic/normothermia Quick Reference: Normal body temperature.

Advanced Reference: When the core body temperature is between 36.5°C and 37.2 °C.

Normovolaemic Quick Reference: Normal fluid balance.

Advanced Reference: Adequate circulating volume. Indicates the opposite of hypovolaemic or a patient who has been over-perfused.

Nose Quick Reference: Organ of smell and air passage.

Advanced Reference: Air is drawn from the exterior via the two nostrils which are separated by the septum, it is then warmed, humidified and filtered before progressing to the respiratory tract. The lower septum is comprised of cartilage and the upper part of bone. The *olfactory* nerve conveys sense of smell to the brain.

Nosocomial   **Quick Reference:** Refers to infections that are acquired during hospitalisation.

Advanced Reference: Acquired from either a patient or staff source and include bacterial and fungal infections and may be due to an already reduced resistance.

Nosworthy   **Quick Reference:** (nose-worthy) Type of endotracheal tube connector.

Advanced Reference: Of metal design and now replaced by the standard fittings which are made from plastic/PVC.

Noxyflex®   **Quick Reference:** A proprietary antimicrobial agent.

Advanced Reference: Produced in the form of a powder for reconstitution and often used for wound and cavity washout.

Nubain   **Quick Reference:** Narcotic analgesic drug.

Advanced Reference: Used to treat moderate to severe pain. A preparation of the opiate nalbuphine.

Nuclear   **Quick Reference:** Of or relating to a nucleus (the central part or core around which something may develop).

Advanced Reference: Nucleic acid = *DNA, RNA* or similar complex present in all living cells. Nuclear fission = the splitting of a nucleus of an atom. Nuclear fusion = the combining of two nuclei into a heavier nucleus releasing energy in the process.

Nuclear stress testing   **Quick Reference:** Diagnostic cardiac investigation involving oxygen saturation.

Advanced Reference: Involves injection of a radioactive substance which is then tracked by a gamma-ray camera as blood moves through the heart.

Nulliparous   **Quick Reference:** Having borne no children. Or more precisely, having never given birth to a viable infant. Also shortened to para: 0.

Advanced Reference: In medical terminology parity refers to the number of times a woman has given birth, i.e. para: 1, 2, 3. Biparous indicates two births and multiparous refers to two or more births. Grand multipara indicates more than five births. Parity is recorded in the format, T-P-A-L; T = number of full-time births, P = the number of *premature* births, A = number of abortions, L = number of living children.

Nystagmus   **Quick Reference:** (nye-stag-mus) Involuntary eyeball movement.

Advanced Reference: Both side-to-side and less commonly up and down movement are involved or a combination of both when a rotary movement occurs. May be due to CNS disease.

O

Obesity **Quick Reference:** An excess of body fat.

Advanced Reference: Generally indicates an overweight condition, with excess fat spread anywhere throughout the body. Confirmation of excess fat can be assessed using the body mass index (**BMI**) formula.

Oblique **Quick Reference:** Indicates slanting, declining from the vertical or horizontal, diverging from a straight line.

Advanced Reference: Term used when relating to muscles, i.e. those of the wall of the abdomen which slant from side to centre (obliques) and the two muscles which are responsible for turning the eye upwards/downwards and inwards/outwards.

Obstetrics **Quick Reference:** Medical care in pregnancy and childbirth.

Advanced Reference: Involves both a specialist doctor and midwives.

Obstruction **Quick Reference:** Blockage, preventing the normal flow, as with gas flow in anaesthetics or normal body function in the gastrointestinal tract.

Advanced Reference: With reference to surgery can indicate bowel obstruction due to many causes, e.g. tumours, twisting, strangulation, and obstruction to blood flow through the coronary arteries (coronary thrombosis). In anaesthesia it can involve the airway itself obstructed by a foreign body, the tongue, vomit and the circuitry becoming kinked or blocked by foreign objects. Also, intravenous flow can be prevented by blood clots in the cannula/catheter.

Obtund **Quick Reference:** To blunt. To deaden pain.

Advanced Reference: To render insensitive to painful stimuli by reducing the level of consciousness, as in anaesthesia or with the use of analgesics.

Obturator **Quick Reference:** Something which occludes an opening.

Advanced Reference: Many examination scopes have an obturator for use when being inserted. An *oesophageal obturator* airway has two lumens, of which one is occluded and is intended to block the oesophagus and leave the trachea open. An obturator nerve block targets the obturator nerve which supplies the muscles of the thigh/hip.

Occipital **Quick Reference:** Indicates the back of the head.

Advanced Reference: The occipital bone is the back of the floor of the skull and forms a moveable joint with the spine. The brainstem passes through a hole in the occipital bone and becomes the spinal cord. The occipital lobe of the brain is at the back of the skull above the *cerebellum*; it receives visual input and interprets vision.

Occult   Quick Reference: Concealed, cut off from view.

Advanced Reference: Occult blood refers to blood that is not evident to the naked eye. A common example is blood in stools that is not visible but can be detected with laboratory examination.

Oculocardiac reflex   Quick Reference: (OCR) Reflex common during ophthalmic procedures such as correction of squint (*strabismus*).

Advanced Reference: The reaction is marked by a slowing heart rate and *dysrhythmias* in response to traction on extra-ocular muscles or pressure on the globe. Involves the trigeminal vagal reflex arc.

Oculogyric   Quick Reference: Relates to turning of the eyeballs in the sockets.

Advanced Reference: Spasmodic movements of the eyeballs into a fixed position, usually upwards, but can be in the opposite direction or to either side. Most commonly due to the effects of certain drugs or medical conditions.

Odontoid   Quick Reference: Tooth-like.

Advanced Reference: Resembling a tooth.

Oedema   Quick Reference: Accumulation of excess fluid.

Advanced Reference: May have a localised cause, such as interference with *lymphatic* or venous drainage, or be a generalised condition due to cardiac or renal failure. *Pulmonary oedema* is the accumulation of fluid in the lungs. Oedematous indicates being affected by oedema.

Oesophageal detector device   Quick Reference: (ODD) Method of differentiating oesophageal from tracheal intubation.

Advanced Reference: Not a replacement for a *capnograph* but useful in settings where the latter may not be available and for those unaccustomed to carrying out regular intubation. There are many devices, both manufactured and 'home-made', however all are designed to aspirate air via the endotracheal tube whether utilising a self-inflating bulb (SIB) or a syringe aspiration technique (SAT), and depend on the structural difference between the oesophagus and trachea to confirm tube position. Being able to aspirate air confirms tracheal intubation because of the rigid structure of the trachea; failure indicates oesophageal placement as it collapses around the end of the tube.

Oesophageal obturator   Quick Reference: A type of airway with an attached face mask.

Advanced Reference: Used in emergency resuscitation situations and when intubation with an endotracheal tube (ETT) is not possible. These devices are designed to be inserted blindly (without a laryngoscope) with the intention of entering the oesophagus, blocking it off and thus allowing for tracheal ventilation with oxygen via a second lumen which opens higher up the tube. A number of designs and variations on the theme have been available and it is maybe this fact that has deterred popularity. Besides the intended scenarios already mentioned, it is intended for use by those not familiar with ETT intubation.

Oesophageal stethoscope **Quick Reference:** Multi-lumen device that is placed in the oesophagus during anaesthesia.

Advanced Reference: Single-use item made of plastic/PVC inserted into the oesophagus during anaesthesia or long-term ventilation to provide continuous monitoring of breath sounds, temperature and heart beat.

Oesophagectomy **Quick Reference:** Surgical removal of the whole or a portion of the oesophagus.

Advanced Reference: May be performed for carcinoma of the oesophagus and often combined with a partial or total *gastrectomy*.

Oesophago-gastrectomy **Quick Reference:** Removal of part of the oesophagus and stomach.

Advanced Reference: Excision of the lower third of the oesophagus and all of the stomach, usually carried out because of tumours at or near the oesophago-gastric junction. An anastomosis is made between the jejunum and oesophagus.

Oesophagoscopy **Quick Reference:** Examination of the oesophagus with an oesophagoscope.

Advanced Reference: Originally rigid scopes were used which had a detachable light source, however flexible scopes with an integral light source have mostly replaced use of the rigid variety.

Oesophagus **Quick Reference:** Food canal, the gullet.

Advanced Reference: The oesophagus extends from the *pharynx* to the stomach, passing through the chest cavity and *diaphragm*. In the adult it is approximately 23–25 cm in length. Oesophagitis is inflammation of the oesophagus.

Oestrogen **Quick Reference:** (east-ro-gen) Female sex *hormone*.

Advanced Reference: Oestradiol is the hormone naturally secreted by the ovaries and any substance which has a similar action to this hormone is called oestrogen. Oestrogen is involved in the development of the secondary sexual characteristics at *puberty*, stimulation of *menstruation* and suppression of ovulation. Oestrogens can be natural or synthetic and are used in the contraceptive pill and for treating certain menstrual disorders. Oestrogens can be associated with an increased risk of intravascular clotting, a risk that could be heightened during surgery and anaesthesia.

Ohm **Quick Reference:** SI unit of electrical resistance.

Advanced Reference: Ohm's law involves the resistance to a current of electricity passing through a conductor:

Voltage = current (amperes) × resistance (ohms)

Or, with reference to the flow of fluids:

Pressure = flow × resistance.

Olecranon **Quick Reference:** Upper end of the *ulna* bone of the arm.

Advanced Reference: Forms the point or prominence at the elbow.

Olfactory   **Quick Reference:** Concerned with the sense of smell.

Advanced Reference: The olfactory nerve conveys the sensations of smell from the nose to the brain. It is in fact the first cranial nerve and runs from the upper part of the nose, through the **ethmoid** bone and into the brain. Injury or disease to this nerve brings about a loss of smell.

Oliguria   **Quick Reference:** Diminished flow of urine.

Advanced Reference: Can be due to severe dehydration or renal failure.

Omentum   **Quick Reference:** Apron of **peritoneum** which hangs from the stomach and colon to lie in front of the intestines.

Advanced Reference: Referred to as the abdominal policeman, as it watches over the organs and attempts to stop injury and infection by enfolding the affected part. It may adhere to inflamed areas in an attempt to separate them off from the rest of the abdominal cavity. There are in fact two separate areas of omentum: the greater, which hangs from the greater curvature of the stomach and in front of the intestine, and the lesser, which is attached to the lesser curvature of the stomach and attaches to the under surface of the **liver**.

Oncology   **Quick Reference:** The study of malignant tumours.

Advanced Reference: An oncologist is a specialist in the diagnosis and treatment of cancer. Also used as a second title for surgeons who deal with cancer treatment within their particular speciality.

Ondansetron   **Quick Reference:** Antiemetic drug.

Advanced Reference: Developed to treat the severe nausea associated with chemotherapy. In relation to surgery and anaesthesia, often given pre-operatively then at intervals during and after surgery. Proprietary name – Zofran®.

One-lung anaesthesia   **Quick Reference:** Anaesthesia technique used for thoracic surgery.

Advanced Reference: Involves the deliberate collapse of one lung with a specialised tube such as a bronchial blocker or endobronchial tube so as to gain improved visualisation and access during surgery.

Oopherectomy   **Quick Reference:** Removal of one or both ovaries. Oophero = ovary.

Advanced Reference: Oophoropexy is the surgical fixation to the pelvic wall of a displaced ovary. An oophorosalpingectomy is the removal of an ovary and its associated uterine **(Fallopian)** tube.

Opacity   **Quick Reference:** Pertaining to an opaque quality.

Advanced Reference: An opaque substance neither transmits nor allows the passage of light; it is neither transparent nor **translucent**. A **cataract** is an opacity of the lens of the eye.

Ophthalmic   **Quick Reference:** Relating to the eye.

Advanced Reference: Ophthalmology indicates medical and surgical care of the eyes. An ophthalmologist is a medical practitioner specialising in this branch. An ophthalmoscope is an illuminated instrument used for examining the interior of the eye.

Opiate   **Quick Reference:** A drug of the narcotic category.

Advanced Reference: Indicates a drug that is derived from opium, e.g. morphine.

Opioid   **Quick Reference:** Any synthetic narcotic that has opiate action but is not a derivative of opium.

Advanced Reference: Drugs derived from opium are opiates.

Opiorphin   **Quick Reference:** Painkiller naturally produced in the body.

Advanced Reference: Said to be approximately six times more powerful than *morphine*.

Opium   **Quick Reference:** The dried juice of the unripe seed capsule of the poppy.

Advanced Reference: Many *alkaloids* are contained in it, the principal ones being *morphine, codeine*, noscapine and *papaverine*. Together they may be used under the name papaveretum.

Orbit   **Quick Reference:** Bony cavity containing the eye ball.

Advanced Reference: The orbit is made up of eight bones. Orbitopalpebral indicates the region of the orbit or eye and surgical procedures carried out on this area. Orbit refers to the eye socket and palpebral to the eyelid.

Orcadian (operation)   **Quick Reference:** UK police operation looking into deaths under anaesthesia.

Advanced Reference: Set up in 2001–2002 to look into the deaths under anaesthesia caused by blockage of breathing circuits.

Orchidectomy   **Quick Reference:** Removal of one or both testicles.

Advanced Reference: The testicles are referred to as orchids. The prefix orchi(o) indicates the testis or of the testicles. Orchitis is inflammation of the testis.

Orchidopexy   **Quick Reference:** Fixation or anchoring of the testis inside the *scrotum*.

Advanced Reference: Commonly carried out because of torsion of the testis. After correction the testicle is fixed by suture to the inside wall of the scrotum in an attempt to prevent repeat torsion.

Organ donation   **Quick Reference:** Refers to giving (donating) a body organ or part for transplantation. Usually involves heart, liver, lungs, or cornea. Donation can be from both living and *cadaver* sources.

Advanced Reference: In the UK those wishing to donate organs in the event of their death carry a donor card, whereas in some countries the right to take organs from a body is assumed unless the person (or relatives) has expressed otherwise. The term harvesting is used to indicate the removal of a number of organs to be retrieved from a cadaver. 'Live-related donor' is used to describe the situation when organs, such as kidney, are donated by a living relative.

Organ of Corti Quick Reference: The true organ of hearing.
Advanced Reference: The organ of Corti is situated within the membranous labyrinth of the **cochlea**.

Orifice Quick Reference: An opening.
Advanced Reference: Can be applied to a number of bodily openings including the mouth, anus and ear.

Oropharyngeal Quick Reference: (oro-farin-geal) Indicates the oral aspect of the pharynx.
Advanced Reference: Used in reference to airways, i.e. oropharyngeal, an airway that is placed in the mouth and reaches back into the pharynx. A nasopharyngeal airway is inserted in one nostril and also reaches back into the pharynx. With an oropharyngeal airway, determination of suitable size is assessed by measuring the distance from the ear to the corner of the mouth.

Oropharynx Quick Reference: (oro-farinx) The lower portion of the **pharynx**.
Advanced Reference: Situated below the nasopharynx, behind the tongue.

Orthodromic Quick Reference: Conducting impulses in the normal direction.
Advanced Reference: As with heart and nerve fibres in normal physiology.

Orthopaedics Quick Reference: Involves and indicates the treatment of bones, joints and related muscles.
Advanced Reference: The branch of surgery related to disease, injuries and distortion of the bones, joints and/or muscles. The word orthopaedics means 'straight children' and refers back to the times when children suffered rickets and the treatment was to attempt straightening of their bones.

Orthopnoea Quick Reference: The effects of body position on the ability to breathe normally, i.e. otherwise than in an upright position.
Advanced Reference: Most commonly refers to when a patient may have difficulty in breathing when laying flat. Most important in patients with heart and lung conditions.

Orthostatic hypotension Quick Reference: Drop in blood pressure when a person is in the standing position.
Advanced Reference: Happens when the compensatory mechanisms, particularly **vasoconstriction** and increased heart rate, do not adequately restore blood pressure when a person is standing. Due mainly to gravity and pooling of blood in the leg veins.

Os Quick Reference: An opening.
Advanced Reference: There are two in the **birth canal**: the external os is the opening of the cervix into the **vagina** and the internal os is the junction of the **cervical** canal and uterus.

Oscillate Quick Reference: To swing back and forth as a pendulum.
Advanced Reference: To move between extremes.

Oscilloscope Quick Reference: Apparatus which displays recorded signals, usually on a screen.

Advanced Reference: Regular use is made of oscilloscopes with *ECG* reading and recording.

Oscillotonometer   **Quick Reference:** Non-invasive apparatus for measuring blood pressure.

Advanced Reference: Alternatively titled the Von Recklinghausen oscillotonometer, it consists of a double cuff, one for occluding the artery and the other, a sensing cuff, attached to an inflating bulb and reading dial. Following inflation, slow release of pressure allows for deflections of the pointer as systolic then diastolic readings are taken.

Osculate   **Quick Reference:** To touch.

Advanced Reference: To make contact with, bring together. Also used in relation to focusing and tuning of monitors.

Osmolality   **Quick Reference:** The concentration of osmotically active particles in solution.

Advanced Reference: Expressed in terms of osmoles of solution per kilogram of solvent.

Osmosis   **Quick Reference:** Selective migration of molecules through a semi-permeable membrane.

Advanced Reference: The passage of fluid from a solution of low concentration to one of a higher concentration, passing through a semi-permeable membrane. Osmotic pressure refers to the pressure exerted by large molecules such as *globulin* proteins in the blood, which assist in drawing fluid into the circulation from surrounding tissues.

Osseous   **Quick Reference:** Pertaining to bone.

Advanced Reference: Consisting of or resembling bone.

Ossicles   **Quick Reference:** Small bones of the middle ear.

Advanced Reference: The ossicles are comprised of the malleus, incus and stapes, which are all involved in the relay and passage of sound waves.

Osteo   **Quick Reference:** Refers to bone.

Advanced Reference: Used as a prefix when referring to a bone, related condition or procedure, e.g. *osteotomy* and osteotome.

Osteoarthritis   **Quick Reference:** A condition of the synovial joints in which there is a loss of the articular cartilage and change in the underlying bone.

Advanced Reference: Affects women more than men and worsens with age and can run in families. The underlying cause is not fully known but stress is often quoted as a trigger. Therefore, treatment is limited and consists of painkillers (*NSAIDs*), anti-inflammatory drugs and physiotherapy, while in severe cases, such as those affecting the hip, joint replacement is often the last resort.

Osteoblast   **Quick Reference:** Cells associated with the production and build-up of bone, e.g. following fracture.

Advanced Reference: Ossification is the formation of bone. It occurs in three stages involving the action of osteoblast cells: firstly the laying down of collagen fibres, followed by cementing and finally impregnation with calcium salts.

Osteoclast **Quick Reference:** Cells associated with the absorption and removal of bone. Also referred to as osteophage.

Advanced Reference: The cells are active in reshaping a bone following fracture. There is a surgical instrument of the same name used for therapeutic fracturing of bone.

Osteogenesis imperfecta **Quick Reference:** Genetic bone disorder.

Advanced Reference: Due to sufferers having less collagen, or poorer quality collagen, in their bone structure.

Osteology **Quick Reference:** The study of the bony skeleton.

Advanced Reference: The study of the structure and function of the entire framework of bones and *cartilage*, including the treatment of related diseases and disorders.

Osteolysis **Quick Reference:** Dissolution of bone.

Advanced Reference: Term used mainly to indicate loss of calcium from the bone. Can happen in many disease states but also with prosthetic implants such as hips, knees and shoulders. As particles from the prostheses wear away, the bone tends to recede from the area leading to loosening of the implant.

Osteoma **Quick Reference:** A *benign* bone tumour.

Advanced Reference: Usually occurs in the end of long bones, extremities and vertebrae.

Osteomalacia **Quick Reference:** Softening of the bones.

Advanced Reference: Usually due to lack of vitamin D. In children is called rickets. Can lead to pain and deformity.

Osteomyelitis **Quick Reference:** Inflammation of the bone marrow.

Advanced Reference: May be due to *Staphylococcus* and *Streptococcus* infection.

Osteoporosis **Quick Reference:** Reduction in bone mass. Literally means porous bone.

Advanced Reference: More marked in women and over the age of 50. It is not so much an alteration in the bone's chemical composition but an imbalance between the processes of absorption and formation of bone. As the cortex becomes thinner, the bones are more susceptible to fracture and vertebrae to collapse. In women the main cause is reduction in oestrogen levels after the menopause.

Osteotomy **Quick Reference:** To cut bone (surgically).

Advanced Reference: Cutting into or through a bone, usually to correct a deformity or replace with a prosthesis.

Otitis media **Quick Reference:** Inflammation of the middle ear.

Advanced Reference: Infection within the eardrum which commonly arises in the back of the nose and progresses to the ear via the *Eustachian tube*.

Otoplastia   Quick Reference: Surgery to pin back ears that stick out.
   Advanced Reference: An otoplasty is the surgical repair or reconstruction of the ears, involves the congenital defect known as 'bat ears'.

Otorrhoea   Quick Reference: (ot-or-ear) A watery discharge from the ear.
   Advanced Reference: Often caused by an ear infection such as *otitis media*.

Otrivine®   Quick Reference: A proprietary nasal decongestant.
   Advanced Reference: A *sympathomimetic* in the form of drops and spray which is often used during surgery.

Oubaine   Quick Reference: (wa-bane) A cardiac glycoside to stimulate the heart.
   Advanced Reference: Used in the treatment of atrial fibrillation and congestive heart failure, often as an alternative to digoxin but has more recently been found to have differing properties.

Oval window   Quick Reference: Oval-shaped aperture in the wall of the middle ear.
   Advanced Reference: Leads through to the inner ear.

Ovarian hyperstimulation syndrome   Quick Reference: (OHSS) Often results from complications with forms of fertility medication that stimulate *follicle* development from the *ovaries*.
   Advanced Reference: Presents with varying degrees of torsion and/or rupture of the ovaries, cysts and *ascites*.

Ovaries   Quick Reference: Female sex glands.
   Advanced Reference: Two almond-shaped glands situated in the pelvis of the female. They are responsible for producing *ova* (mature female sex cell or ovum), which pass down the *Fallopian* tubes into the uterus, as well as hormones that help control the *menstrual* cycle.

Ovulation   Quick Reference: The shedding of an *ovum*.
   Advanced Reference: The ovum, or germ cell, is shed from the ovary each month on or about the 15th day of the menstrual cycle.

Ovum   Quick Reference: Egg cell, or germ cell.
   Advanced Reference: The mature female sex cell (gamete).

Oxford   Quick Reference: Refers to a number of anaesthetic-related adjuncts.
   Advanced Reference: There are Oxford types of ventilator, endotracheal tube, airway, vaporiser and infant laryngoscope blade.

Oxidation   Quick Reference: Rust is a form of oxidation.
   Advanced Reference: Combination/reaction of a substance with oxygen.

Oxidative stress   Quick Reference: Any of a number of *pathological* changes seen in living organisms.
   Advanced Reference: Usually due to free radicals in the environment and toxic (cytotoxic) effects on cells.

Oximeter   Quick Reference: Monitoring equipment used to determine the oxygen saturation of the blood.

Advanced Reference: The oximeter probe can be attached to an ear or digit (usually finger) to measure oxygen saturation in the blood. Usually available as a pulse oximeter which has the added facility of recording pulse rate.

Oxinium Quick Reference: Material used for prosthetic implants.

Advanced Reference: Produced from a process that allows oxygen to absorb into *zirconium* metal, which changes only its surface from a metal to ceramic. It is a hard, smooth material producing reduced friction and is resistant to scratching.

Oxycodone Quick Reference: A *narcotic* alkaloid related to *codeine*.

Advanced Reference: Used as an analgesic and sedative.

Oxygen Quick Reference: Colourless, odourless gas necessary to support life.

Advanced Reference: Oxygen is transported to the tissues from the lungs in combination with *haemoglobin*.

Oxygen bypass Quick Reference: System which allows for direct oxygen delivery on anaesthetic machines.

Advanced Reference: When utilised, this system bypasses oxygen from going through the *flowmeter* and directly to the fresh gas flow (FGF) outlet, usually activated by a push-button or swivel-switch device: mounted conveniently on the anaesthetic machine.

Oxygen failure device Quick Reference: Safety device fitted into anaesthetic machines.

Advanced Reference: Similar systems were fitted into early anaesthetic machines and were called a Bowson's whistle. Although differing in function, the more modern arrangement remains to provide an audible warning when oxygen availability and delivery cease.

Oxyhaemoglobin Quick Reference. Haemoglobin which has been oxygenated, or taken up oxygen.

Advanced Reference: Oxygenated haemoglobin is present in arterial blood and deoxygenated haemoglobin in veins.

Oxytocin Quick Reference: A hormone of the *pituitary* gland.

Advanced Reference: Oxytocin stimulates contraction of the uterus, which is especially sensitive to its action in the latter stage of pregnancy. Used to instigate contractions of the uterus when labour is delayed.

Ozone Quick Reference: A more active form of oxygen, having three atoms instead of two.

Advanced Reference: Its chemical formula is O_3. In large quantities or high levels it acts as an irritant to the lungs.

P

P wave   **Quick Reference:** Part of the *ECG* trace.

Advanced Reference: It is the first wave or deflection of the trace and indicates depolarisation of the atria.

Pacemaker   **Quick Reference:** Refers to the natural pacemaker of the heart and not the mechanical and electronic devices, such as the *demand pacemaker.*

Advanced Reference: The sinoatrial or *SA node* is the primary natural pacemaker but under various circumstances another pacemaker (atrioventricular or AV node/junction, ventricles) may become dominant. All have their own inherent rate and in general the pacemaker with the fastest rate is dominant and this situation can develop in certain diseases and cardiac conditions. The SA node rate $= 60$–100 beats per minute or bpm. *AV node*/junction rate $= 40$–60 bpm, ventricular rate $= 20$–40 bpm. It is a protective mechanism that keeps the heart beating even in the event of abnormal function.

Packed red cells   **Quick Reference:** Intravenous blood preparation.

Advanced Reference: Also termed *plasma*-reduced blood. Indicates whole blood with a volume of plasma removed and so concentrates the red cells within a lesser volume of fluid. The extracted plasma is then used in the production of alternative blood products.

PaCO$_2$ **Quick Reference:** Symbol for arterial carbon dioxide level.

Advanced Reference: Indicates partial pressure of carbon dioxide in arterial blood.

Paget's disease   **Quick Reference:** Chronic disease of bone. Also referred to as osteitis deformans.

Advanced Reference: Occurs mainly in middle-aged men affecting the bones of the skull, spine and pelvis and long bones. Characterised by thickening and deformity of the bone.

Palliative care   **Quick Reference:** Treatment designed to relieve pain and distress but not cure.

Advanced Reference: Treatment intended to soothe the symptoms of a disease when a cure is not possible, as with many types of cancer which are inoperable or have progressed too far for intervention with radiation or chemotherapy.

Pallor   **Quick Reference:** Unusual paleness of the skin.

Advanced Reference: Caused by a reduced flow of blood to the skin, as happens in shock, or can be due to a deficiency in normal pigments.

Palmar   Quick Reference: Relating to the palm of the hand.

Advanced Reference: Also the palmar arch, i.e. the *anastomosis* in the hand of the *radial* and *ulnar* arteries.

Palmar fasciectomy   Quick Reference: (fas-she-ec-tommy) Operation to remove abnormal, thickened tissue from the palm of the hand.

Advanced Reference: Also known as *Dupuytren's* contracture. The condition is produced by a progressive thickening and contraction of the palmar aponeurosis, resulting in flexion of the ring, middle and little fingers. *Excision* of abnormal tissue (fasciectomy) allows return of finger movement.

Palpate   Quick Reference: To palpate, to feel with the hands. Palpation.

Advanced Reference: Examination via the surface of the body of the position, size and shape of internal organs.

Palpitation   Quick Reference: An awareness of the heart beat, felt in the chest or neck.

Advanced Reference: The action of the heart is not normally felt but does occur if beat is increased in force or speed. Can be due to anxiety, emotion, exercise, cardiac irregularities such as *extrasystoles* and excessive intake of stimulants, e.g. *caffeine, nicotine*.

Palsy   Quick Reference: Indicates paralysis.

Advanced Reference: Including cerebral palsy, caused by brain damage during birth; and Bell's palsy, paralysis of the facial muscles on one side.

Pan   Quick Reference: All, entire.

Advanced Reference: Examples of its use are: pandemic (affecting all of the population), pan-procto-colectomy (removal of all of the colon).

Pancreas   Quick Reference: Large gland situated across the back wall of the upper abdominal cavity and behind the stomach.

Advanced Reference: Is a dual-purpose gland which forms part of the digestive system. Its *exocrine* secretions help to neutralise digestive acid while its *endocrine* secretion, insulin, passes directly into the bloodstream and is involved in the chemical control of sugar in the blood.

Pancuronium   Quick Reference: Non-depolarising muscle relaxant. Pavulon®.

Advanced Reference: A synthetic non-depolariser with an approximate duration of action of 30 min. May produce slight *tachycardia* and a rise in blood pressure. Not thought to cause *histamine* release and does not cross the *placenta* in significant amounts. Metabolised in the liver.

Pandemic   Quick Reference: Pan = all, entire, demic = epidemic.

Advanced Reference: A widespread *epidemic* of a disease over a large geographical area affecting a large proportion of the population.

PaO₂   Quick Reference: Symbol to indicate arterial oxygen level.

Advanced Reference: Partial pressure of O_2 in arterial blood.

Papaveretum   Quick Reference: Compound preparation of *alkaloids* of *opium*. Previously named Omnopon®.

Advanced Reference: Composed of mainly *morphine* plus *codeine*, noscapine and *papaverine*. Used as a narcotic analgesic for both *premedication* and postoperative pain relief.

Papaverine   **Quick Reference:** A smooth-muscle relaxant.

Advanced Reference: It is technically an opiate but possesses little or no analgesic effect. Used in the treatment of *bronchospasm* in *asthma*. In relation to theatres, used sometimes in vascular procedures to relax vessel ends to enable easier anastomosis and for vasodilatation in the event of inadvertent arterial injection of an agent that causes spasm.

Pap (smear)   **Quick Reference:** Papanicolaou test.

Advanced Reference: Smear test. Microscopic examination of cells scraped from the cervix.

Papovavirus   **Quick Reference:** Any virus of the family Papovaviridae.

Advanced Reference: Name derived from the following abbreviations: Pa = papillomavirus, Po = polyomavirus and V = vacuolation. The human papilloma virus is the one that most commonly causes disease (e.g. *verruca*).

Para   **Quick Reference:** Next to or to the side of.

Advanced Reference: Examples are paramedian (incision) and para-medical (professions and services that work alongside and support medical staff).

Paracentesis   **Quick Reference:** (para-sen-tee-sis) The puncturing with a hollow needle of a body cavity to draw off excess fluid.

Advanced Reference: Carried out in order to withdraw abnormal fluid for the relief of symptoms or for pathological examination.

Paracetamol   **Quick Reference:** Analgesic and antipyretic. Acetaminophen. Trade names include Panadol® and Tylenol®.

Advanced Reference: Popular in the treatment of headaches and fever but known to be most effective on musculoskeletal pain. Has little anti-inflammatory action but is used in combination with many other drugs. Overdose leads to kidney and liver damage.

Paraesthesia   **Quick Reference:** An abnormal touch sensation.

Advanced Reference: Examples are prickling and burning often in the absence of external stimulus.

Paraldehyde   **Quick Reference:** Sedative with rapid onset.

Advanced Reference: Used in the treatment of severe and continuous epileptic seizures. Administered by injection but may be given rectally. Recognised by its distinctive and strong smell.

Paralytic ileus   **Quick Reference:** Non-mechanical obstruction of the bowel. Also termed adynamic ileus and enteroplegia.

Advanced Reference: Prominent causes are localised or generalised *peritonitis* and shock. Surgery is usually contraindicated unless mechanical obstruction, strangulation or sepsis is suspected.

Paramedian   Quick Reference: To the side of the median plane.

Advanced Reference: A paramedian incision is one made to the side of the midline.

Parameter   Quick Reference: A set of measurements. A factor that determines a range of variations.

Advanced Reference: In relation to medicine could be temperature, blood pressure and so on.

Parametrium   Quick Reference: To the side of the endometrium (uterus). The layer of tissue surrounding the uterus.

Advanced Reference: Term referred to in relation to hysterectomy, when surrounding tissues are also removed in the more radical versions of this procedure.

Paranoia   Quick Reference: (par-a-noy-a) Term used to describe behaviour characterised by delusions of grandeur and persecution.

Advanced Reference: Can manifest in a number of conditions including psychotic disorder and paranoid *schizophrenia*.

Para-phenylenediamine   Quick Reference: A derivative of benzine used as a dye in many industrial processes as well as being used in conjunction with henna for tattoos.

Advanced Reference: Is a strong allergen which causes contact dermatitis and bronchial asthma.

Paraphimosis   Quick Reference: (para-fie-mosis) Tight *foreskin* of the penis.

Advanced Reference: Occurs when a tight foreskin is drawn back behind the glans of the penis and swelling or engorgement prevents return to normal position/state. If persistent, a *circumcision* is performed.

Paraplegia   Quick Reference: Paralysis of both sides of the body from the waist down.

Advanced Reference: Usually due to disease or injury of the spinal cord.

Parasite   Quick Reference: Creature that lives at the expense of another.

Advanced Reference: These can include *viruses, bacteria, fungi, protozoa* and *worms*.

Parasympathetic   Quick Reference: Part of the *autonomic nervous system*.

Advanced Reference: The parasympathetic system works in balance with and sometimes in opposition to the *sympathetic* system.

Parathyroidectomy   Quick Reference: Surgical excision/removal of the *parathyroid glands*.

Advanced Reference: Carried out because of hyperparathyroidism, when usually all four glands are removed. Overactivity causes an increased level of calcium in the blood which can result in stone formation in the renal tract.

Parathyroid glands   Quick Reference: Group of small yellow-coloured glands situated behind or attached to the thyroid glands.

Advanced Reference: Their function is to secrete the hormone parathormone, which regulates the availability and use of calcium in the body. If the blood concentration of calcium falls, the parathyroids are stimulated to produce more of the hormone and this increases the solubility of calcium in the bones and restores the blood levels to normal. Overactivity or stimulation of the parathyroids is often due to a tumour, which can cause an increase of parathormone and consequently too much calcium is then withdrawn from the bones, increasing their fragility. Any surplus calcium is excreted in the urine and can lead to kidney stones. If the condition warrants, surgical removal is carried out, sometimes requiring splitting of the *sternum* to access the glands.

Parenteral **Quick Reference:** Indicates outside of or away from the *enteral* route, i.e. not via the mouth or bowel.

Advanced Reference: Total parenteral nutrition (TPN) indicates a feeding process other than the alimentary route. TPN involves intravenous feeding for patients unable to take food orally (e.g. ventilated on ICU) or to absorb through the gut due to disease.

Parietal **Quick Reference:** (par-e-atal) Indicates the inner walls of a body cavity.

Advanced Reference: A common example is the parietal *pleura*, which is attached to the inner chest wall.

Parkland formula **Quick Reference:** Fluid regime designed for use with burns patients.

Advanced Reference: It is just one means of estimating the volume (crystalloids) to be administered to make up losses in this category of patient. Parkland formula is $V = A(\%) \times M(\text{kg}) \times 4$ ($V =$ volume of crystalloid, $A =$ total body surface area, M is mass).

Parotid **Quick Reference:** Salivary gland sited in front of the ear and the angle of the jaw.

Advanced Reference: It has a duct which opens into the mouth which can become enlarged by inflammation, infection or the presence of a stone.

Paroxysmal **Quick Reference:** An outburst. Sudden attack of a disease, convulsion or pain.

Advanced Reference: Paroxysmal supraventricular tachycardia (PSVT) involves repeated episodes (paroxysms) of *tachycardia* characterised by an abrupt onset and equally abrupt end, although they can last for a period of seconds or hours.

Parturition **Quick Reference:** The act of giving birth.

Advanced Reference: The actual function of expelling the products of conception (fetus and placenta) from the uterus.

Pascal **Quick Reference:** The SI unit for pressure. Abbreviated to Pa.

Advanced Reference: Due to the relative small size of the Pascal, pressure is usually measured in kilopascals (kPa) $= 1000\,\text{Pa}$, where $1\,\text{kPa}$ converts to approximately 1% of atmospheric pressure (at sea level).

Bar and millimetres of mercury (mmHg) are also used to measure pressure, where 1 atmosphere (atm) $= 760\,\text{mmHg} = 1\,\text{bar} = 100\,000\,\text{Pa} = 100\,\text{kPa} = 15\,\text{lb/in}^2$.

Passive **Quick Reference:** Indicates inactivity, lack of movement.

Advanced Reference: An example in relation to theatres is a passive *scavenging system* which involves the diversion of expired gases into a container where volatile agents adhere to an agent such as carbon/charcoal granules. A passive wound drain is one that functions without the aid of suction or vacuum.

Pasteurisation **Quick Reference:** (past-your-eye-sashun) Disinfection process.

Advanced Reference: Involves the use of heat (hot water) at a temperature of between 60 °C and 80 °C. Not a sterilising process. At one time it was suitable for surgical instruments, rigid scopes and anaesthetic equipment that were required to be 'clean' rather than sterile.

Patch test **Quick Reference:** Skin test for identifying allergy reactions.

Advanced Reference: Used to test for allergies, such as those to foodstuffs, pollen and animal fur, but can also be used to identify sensitivity to chemicals such as surgical skin preps.

Patent **Quick Reference:** Open, clear.

Advanced Reference: Not occluded. May be used in relation to vessels such as Fallopian tubes and blood vessels.

Pathema **Quick Reference:** Path = disease, Em = inside.

Advanced Reference: Any disease state or *morbid* condition.

Pathogenic **Quick Reference:** A disease-producing agent.

Advanced Reference: Pathogenic organisms are capable of causing disease.

Pathological **Quick Reference:** Relating to, arising from or caused by disease. A pathological fracture is one that is due to disease of the bone.

Advanced Reference: Pathology is the branch of medicine that deals with the nature of disease. Pathogenesis indicates the origin and development of a disease whereas pathognomonic relates to the characteristics of a particular disease.

Patient positioning **Quick Reference:** The position on the operating table required for the procedure in question.

Advanced Reference: Also termed table position and surgical position. There are a number of standard positions, e.g. *Trendelenburg and lithotomy*, as well as regional and personal variations and differences demanded by various table designs.

Patient State Index **Quick Reference:** Quantitative electroencephalographic (EEG) index.

Advanced Reference: Used for the assessment of consciousness during sedation and general anaesthesia.

Patties **Quick Reference:** A small swab used in neurosurgery.

Advanced Reference: Small piece of lint with an attached length of cotton, usually used moist so as to absorb blood and cover delicate exposed tissue during craniotomy.

PCA **Quick Reference:** Patient-controlled analgesia.

Advanced Reference: System in which small doses of analgesic are administered by the patient themselves as and when required, usually into the postoperative period. An *antiemetic* is sometimes combined with the analgesic drug. The delivery of the drug(s) involves an infusion device pre-programmed to deliver set doses. The machines have many in-built safety features to prevent over-dosage and tampering.

Pedicle **Quick Reference:** A stalk of tissue that connects parts of the body together. Also termed peduncle.

Advanced Reference: A narrow strip or stalk by which a tumour is attached to normal tissue and through which the blood supply runs. A pedicle graft is one that is set in its intended place but left with a pedicle containing blood supply until it can survive independently.

PEG tube **Quick Reference:** Percutaneous endoscopic gastrostomy tube.

Advanced Reference: Feeding tube inserted directly into the stomach and used when a patient is unable to take nutrition orally.

Pelvis **Quick Reference:** Lower limb girdle composed of the lower portion of the backbone and the two hip bones.

Advanced Reference: The pelvis is the large complex of bones shaped like a basin which connects the spine with the legs and contains the lower part of the abdominal cavity. It comprises the two hip bones, namely *sacrum* and *coccyx*. In front the two hip bones meet at the *symphysis pubis* and behind they join the sacrum.

Penbritin® **Quick Reference:** Broad-spectrum antibiotic.

Advanced Reference: Proprietary form of ampicillin. Used to treat respiratory infections and those of the urinary tract and middle ear.

Penicillin **Quick Reference:** First widely used *antibiotic*.

Advanced Reference: First reported use was in 1941 but since there have followed numerous closely related antibiotics which are mostly compounds of aminopenicillanic acid. The acid itself is the first extracted from moulds.

Penis **Quick Reference:** The male sex organ.

Advanced Reference: Both urine and semen are discharged through it via the urethra. The shaft of the penis contains spongy tissue (corpus spongiosum) which fills with blood during sexual excitement making the organ erect.

Pentaspan® **Quick Reference:** Pentastarch, a synthetic colloid.

Advanced Reference: Plasma expander that increases plasma volume by 1.5 times. Does not interfere with clotting in the manner of some alternatives.

Penthrane   Quick Reference: Volatile anaesthetic agent.

Advanced Reference: Now withdrawn mainly due to its potential toxic effects on the kidneys.

Pepsin   Quick Reference: A stomach *enzyme* that begins the digestion of proteins by splitting them into peptones.

Advanced Reference: Pepsinogen is secreted by the gastric glands and this is acted upon by *hydrochloric acid* to produce pepsin.

Peptic (ulcer)   Quick Reference: Ulceration in either *stomach* or *duodenum*.

Advanced Reference: Causes include overproduction of acid and *pepsin*, stress and bacteria.

Peracetic acid   Quick Reference: Also known as peroxyacetic acid ($C_2H_4O_3$). Strong oxidising agent used for sterilising.

Advanced Reference: A peroxide that when mixed with water will kill *bacteria, fungi and viruses*.

Percutaneous   Quick Reference: Per indicates through, by way of, and cutaneous means pertaining to the skin or via the skin.

Advanced Reference: Percutaneous indicates to pass through the skin in order to reach an inner area for treatment, e.g. percutaneous *lithotripsy*, percutaneous *tracheostomy*.

Perfluorocarbons   Quick Reference: (PFCs) Group of chemical compounds derived from hydrocarbons and composed of carbon, fluorine and sulphur; used increasingly in many areas of medicine.

Advanced Reference: It is as a blood substitute that this group is most prominent. Besides being biologically *inert*, oxygen is 100 times more soluble in perfluorocarbons than in plasma, and carbon dioxide also readily dissolves in them. Perfluorocarbons are already used as a temporary substitute for *vitreous humour* in *retinal detachment* surgery. Other potential uses are as an oxygen carrier in lung injury and in contrast media.

Perfuse (perfusion)   Quick Reference: Passage of a liquid through/into body tissues or an organ.

Advanced Reference: Tissue perfusion indicates when fluid accesses, reaches or passes through an area, as with IV fluid reaching the tissues of a dehydrated patient, cerebral perfusion, or perfusion of a graft kidney prior to transplantation.

Perinatal   Quick Reference: Pertaining to birth, being born.

Advanced Reference: Indicates the time and process of giving birth.

Perineal post   Quick Reference: Table attachment involved in patient positioning.

Advanced Reference: It is a limiting device which sits up against the perineal area between the thighs on a number of orthopaedic tables for such procedures as hip replacement and fractured femur repair. It has the potential to cause injury to the genitalia and *pudendal* nerve.

Perineoplasty **Quick Reference:** An operation to enlarge the vaginal opening.

Advanced Reference: This involves incising the hymen and a portion of the *perineum*.

Perineorrhaphy **Quick Reference:** (perin-e-orafy) Surgical repair of the *perineum*.

Advanced Reference: Often carried out to repair a tear following vaginal childbirth.

Perinephric **Quick Reference:** Surrounding the kidney.

Advanced Reference: Perinephric or peri-renal fat is the protective capsule of fat surrounding the kidney. Perinephritis is inflammation of tissues around the kidney.

Perineum **Quick Reference:** The region between the *genital* organs in front and the *anus* behind.

Advanced Reference: Regularly extended to indicate the area bounded by the pubic *symphysis*, the ischial *tuberosities* and the *coccyx*.

Perineural **Quick Reference:** Surrounding a nerve or nerve fibre.

Advanced Reference: Term often used in relation to nerve blocks when the analgesic agent is injected so as to surround the nerve.

Periodontal **Quick Reference:** Surrounding or encasing a tooth.

Advanced Reference: Also relates to the tissues and structures surrounding and supporting teeth.

Perioperative **Quick Reference:** Indicates the entire operative period.

Advanced Reference: Usually used to mean the pre-, intra- and post-operative phases of a patient's surgical treatment in one term.

Periosteum **Quick Reference:** The layer of *connective tissue* covering bone but not the articular surfaces.

Advanced Reference: The periosteum provides attachment for *tendons, ligaments* and *muscles*. Its outer layer contains blood vessels and the inner layer mainly *osteoblasts*.

Peripheral **Quick Reference:** (per-if-eral) Towards the surface of the body.

Advanced Reference: Applies to structures close to the surface as opposed to central, as with blood vessels.

Peripheral vascular disease **Quick Reference:** A circulatory disorder.

Advanced Reference: A disorder that reduces the amount of blood and oxygen reaching the periphery and so causes death of associated tissues. Particularly affects those suffering from *type 2 diabetes*.

Peristalsis **Quick Reference:** Wave of contraction followed by period of relaxation as in the intestinal tract.

Advanced Reference: The wave-like motion produced in some body organs to move contents onward. Alternative contraction and relaxation produced by the action of circular and longitudinal muscles.

Peritomy Quick Reference: Surgical incision of the *conjunctiva* and subconjunctival tissue around the entire circumference of the *cornea*.

Advanced Reference: Usually done as part of an *enucleation* or *detachment of retina*.

Peritoneum Quick Reference: Membrane covering the inner walls of the abdominal cavity.

Advanced Reference: The peritoneum is a *serous* membrane and comprises two layers, i.e. the *parietal* layer, which covers the wall of the cavity, and the visceral layer, which covers the abdominal organs.

Peritonitis Quick Reference: Inflammation of the peritoneum.

Advanced Reference: In the acute form, most cases are as a result of disease of an abdominal organ, e.g. *appendicitis*, *diverticulitis*, perforated bowel. Symptoms include *exudate* from the peritoneum, bowel paralysis, pain and vomiting. The chronic form may be a result of *tuberculosis* causing fluid collection within the peritoneal cavity, associated swelling and pain. Treatment is with antibiotics.

Pernicious Quick Reference: Highly injurious, destructive or deadly.

Advanced Reference: Commonly used when describing diseases or conditions that may be fatal if untreated, e.g. pernicious anaemia, pernicious vomiting.

Peroneal Quick Reference: Relating to the fibula and structures on the outer side of the leg.

Advanced Reference: Involves muscles and nerves on the fibular side of the lower leg and the peroneal artery is of significance when placing patients in the lithotomy position, i.e. placing legs on either the inside or outside of the stirrups has potential for pressure-induced injury.

Petri dish Quick Reference: Glass container used in hospital laboratories.

Advanced Reference: A shallow glass dish in which organisms are grown on a culture medium, usually *agar*.

Petrochemicals Quick Reference: Chemicals derived from crude oil and natural gas.

Advanced Reference: They are used in the manufacture of a range of compounds and materials including plastics, drugs, solvents and detergents.

Pexy Quick Reference: Indicates to fix or suture in place.

Advanced Reference: Common example is *orchidopexy*, i.e. securing the testicle within the *scrotum*.

Peyronie's disease Quick Reference: Curvature of the penis.

Advanced Reference: Due to the build-up of fibrous tissue in the erectile body and causes the penis to angulate on erection. Cause is unknown.

Pfannenstiel Quick Reference: (fan-en-steel) Surgical incision.

Advanced Reference: Alternative name for *transverse* incision. Used for the likes of *Caesarean section*, *hysterectomy* and open *prostatectomy*.

pH   Quick Reference: Indication of the acid/alkali balance.

Advanced Reference: pH measures the concentration of hydrogen ions in a solution on a scale. Below 7 indicates acidity that becomes stronger as the number decreases; greater than 7 indicates increasing alkalinity. Normal pH is in the range of 7.38 to 7.42.

Phagocyte   Quick Reference: (fage-o-site) Cells that envelop and digest bacteria.

Advanced Reference: Includes the destruction of white blood cells, macrophages and debris. They are a vital part of the body's defence system.

Phakoemulsification   Quick Reference: (Also termed as phacoemulsification). Phaco = lens of the eye. A method of **cataract** extraction.

Advanced Reference: The lens is fragmented by **ultrasonic** vibration followed by irrigation and aspiration.

Phalanges   Quick Reference: The bones of the fingers and toes.

Advanced Reference: The thumb and the big toe have two phalanges each, whereas the remaining digits all have three.

Pharmacodynamics   Quick reference: Indicates what effect a drug has on the body.

Advanced Reference: More specifically the effects on different systems throughout the body.

Pharmacokinetics   Quick Reference: The activity of drugs in the body.

Advanced Reference: More precisely indicates the activity over a period of time, including absorption, distribution and excretion.

Pharmacopoeia   Quick Reference: (farm-o-cap-ea) Manual containing a list of drugs.

Advanced Reference: Contains details of their formulae, preparation and dosages.

Pharynx   Quick Reference: (fa-rinx) Area continuous with the mouth and nasal cavity.

Advanced Reference: Muscular back wall of the nose, mouth and throat, extending from the base of the skull to the entrance of the oesophagus. The pharynx has three parts: the **nasopharynx**, which is concerned with breathing; the **oropharynx**, which is a passage for both air and food; and the lowest part, the laryngeal pharynx, which is involved in swallowing and situated behind the **larynx**.

Phenacetin   Quick Reference: An analgesic and antipyretic.

Advanced Reference: Little used now because of its toxicity and potential as a carcinogen affecting the bladder and kidneys.

Phenol   Quick Reference: (feen-ol) Chemical chiefly used as a disinfectant, e.g. **carbolic acid**.

Advanced Reference: Phenol is derived from coal tar and is used in many forms as a disinfectant, Dettol being one well-known preparation. It is also used for nerve block in chronic pain and for *sclerotherapy* of veins (e.g. haemorrhoids, varices).

Phenoperidine **Quick Reference:** Synthetic pethidine derivative. Also known as operidine.

Advanced Reference: Causes respiratory depression with little cardiovascular effect. Has a long duration, approximately 1 h after intravenous injection, which makes it useful for lengthy surgery, ITU use and where respiratory depression is desirable.

Pheromones **Quick Reference:** A substance secreted to the outside of the body and perceived by smell.

Advanced Reference: When detected, said to release a specific reaction of behaviour in an individual of the same species.

Phimosis **Quick Reference:** (fie-mose-is) Tightness of the foreskin so that it cannot be retracted back over the head of the penis.

Advanced Reference: Common in young children and treated by circumcision. Sometimes not solely due to tightness of the foreskin, but because the foreskin may still have attachments to underlying tissue, which can be the case with boys until 3–4 years of age.

Phlebitis **Quick Reference:** (flee-bite-is) Inflammation of a vein.

Advanced Reference: Also associated with blockage of a vein as in *thrombophlebitis*. May be found at the site of previous IV cannula insertion. Due to both inflammation and localised infection.

Phlebo **Quick Reference:** (flee-bo) Prefix indicating vein.

Advanced Reference: Phlebo, as in phlebotomy (opening of a vein in order to remove blood – venesection), thrombophlebitis. Along with veno, indicates pertaining to a vein.

Phlegm **Quick Reference:** (flem) *Mucus*.

Advanced Reference: Thick mucus secreted into the nose, throat and bronchial passages.

Phobia **Quick Reference:** Abnormal dread or morbid fear of something or situation.

Advanced Reference: A compound word is often made with phobia as the suffix in the name of the fear, e.g. agoraphobia (fear of open spaces), claustrophobia (fear of being confined). In relation to theatres could involve fear of needles or face masks.

Phosgene **Quick Reference:** Highly toxic and volatile colourless gas. Chemical formula $COCl_2$.

Advanced Reference: Rapidly fatal causing *pulmonary oedema* and *pneumonia*.

Also known as carbonic dichloride and carbonyl chloride.

Photoelectric cell Quick Reference: Piece of equipment used for the detection of light and other radiation.

Advanced Reference: An electronic device whose electrical properties are modified by the action of light. Utilised in solar cells and light meters.

Photometer Quick Reference: Device for measuring the intensity of *infrared*, *ultraviolet* and visible light.

Advanced Reference: Method used in many medical analysers, such as measuring Hb content of blood (haemoglobinometry).

Phrenic Quick Reference: Relating to the diaphragm.

Advanced Reference: The phrenic nerve supplies muscles of the diaphragm, arising on each side of the neck and passing downwards between the lungs and heart.

Physiological anaemia Quick Reference: Situation that can occur in a number of conditions, most commonly during pregnancy.

Advanced Reference: During pregnancy there can be a 50% rise in blood volume but the plasma volume increase is not proportional to the increase in red cells and so haemodilution is created leading to a physiological *anaemia*.

Physiology Quick Reference: The study of the functional processes of the body.

Advanced Reference: The science of body functions and processes of living organisms. In relation to humans, usually termed alongside anatomy (the study of the structure of the body and its parts) as Anatomy and Physiology (A&P).

Phytic acid Quick Reference: (fit-ik) Inositol hexaphosphate. Chemical formula $= C_6H_{18}P_6O_{24}$.

Advanced Reference: A compound found in the leaves of plants, and cereal grains, it interferes with the absorption of various minerals including calcium and magnesium.

Pia mater Quick Reference: Innermost of the three membranes that cover the brain and spinal cord.

Advanced Reference: A very delicate membrane separated from the arachnoid mater by a space containing the *cerebrospinal fluid (CSF)*.

Piggy-back Quick Reference: Slang term used to indicate one on top of another, hitching a ride, a piggy-back ride.

Advanced Reference: A piggy-back catheter is one in which an accessory line can be attached or joined to the main lumen. Prior to manufactured examples, it was common practice to plug an additional line into the *latex* bung of a giving-set via a *hypodermic needle*.

Pigments Quick Reference: Any colouring matter of the body.

Advanced Reference: Can be natural or synthetic. Chlorophyll is the green colouring in plants, while melanin in humans gives colouring to the skin and hair. Synthetic pigments are used to colour plastics, inks, etc.

Pilonidal (sinus) **Quick Reference:** Tract containing hair, which often becomes an irritant and infected.

Advanced Reference: Tract extending to the subcuticular level found in the midline cleft overlying the coccyx and lower sacrum. Treatment usually involves surgical excision.

Pilot balloon **Quick Reference:** External indicator on an endotracheal tube.

Advanced Reference: A balloon or 'external cuff' incorporated into the inflation tubing on an endotracheal tube designed to indicate the status of the tracheal cuff.

Pineal **Quick Reference:** Shaped like a pine cone.

Advanced Reference: The pineal gland is a pea-sized mass attached to the posterior wall of the third ventricle of the brain. Thought to play a part in development of the gonads and the secretion of the hormone *melatonin*.

Pin-index system **Quick Reference:** Safety system on anaesthetic machines for connection of medical gas cylinders.

Advanced Reference: An internationally recognised system designed to prevent cylinders from being connected to the wrong yoke on the anaesthetic machine. The yoke contains an arrangement of pins which are designed to match up with holes on the cylinder head that are numbered 1–6, each gas having its own unique configuration, e.g. oxygen $= 2 + 5$.

Piped gas supply **Quick Reference:** Form of medical gas delivery system.

Advanced Reference: Is an alternative to a cylinder supply on the anaesthetic machine. Usually involves oxygen, nitrous oxide and medical air being piped into the hospital departments from a central bank (manifold). The nitrous oxide and air are provided from a bank of large cylinders while the oxygen at such volumes is fed from a liquid tank source.

Piriton® **Quick Reference:** Proprietary antihistamine, chlorpheniramine.

Advanced Reference: Used to treat allergic reactions such as hayfever and *urticaria*.

Pituitary **Quick Reference:** An endocrine gland positioned at the base of the brain. Also called the hypophysis.

Advanced Reference: Has two lobes, the *anterior* and *posterior*. The hormones of the anterior lobe are themselves regulated by the *hypothalamus*, which is sited immediately above the pituitary. Hormones of the pituitary include adrenocorticotrophic hormone (*ACTH*), thyrotrophic, gonadotrophic, lactogenic, melanophore and growth hormones, while the posterior lobe secretes *oxytocin* and antidiuretic hormone (*ADH*).

Placebo **Quick Reference:** (plass-e-bow) A drug that is pharmacologically inert.

Advanced Reference: No longer an accepted clinical practice to prescribe placebo, but still used extensively in drug trials where a portion of the study group is given placebo and the remainder the drug being trialled. This system is referred to as a double-blind study when members of the group and the investigators are unaware of who is taking the drug and who is taking placebo.

Placenta   **Quick Reference:** (plass-enter) Organ by which the fetus receives nourishment from the mother.

Advanced Reference: The placenta is normally firmly attached to the lining of the uterus. Dissolved oxygen and nutrients diffuse from the mother's blood to the placenta and carbon dioxide and other waste travel in the opposite direction. At birth, the cord joining the fetus and placenta is divided and tied off and the placenta delivered after the baby.

Placenta accreta   **Quick Reference:** When the *placenta* invades the *myometrium*.

Advanced Reference: More likely in situations where there has been previous uterine surgery.

Placenta percreta   **Quick Reference:** When the *placenta* grows through the *uterus*.

Advanced Reference: As with *placenta accreta*, more common when there has been previous uterine surgery.

Placenta praevia   **Quick Reference:** Implantation of the placenta into the lower segment of the uterus.

Advanced Reference: As this occurs at the opening from the uterus into the vagina, it prevents vaginal delivery.

Plagiocephaly   **Quick Reference:** Misshapen head.

Advanced Reference: Indicates a lack of symmetry in the shape of the head due to irregularity in the closure of the sutures between the skull bones.

Plaque   **Quick Reference:** (plak) Term applied to the laying down or build-up of various substances throughout the body.

Advanced Reference: Dental plaque forms on the teeth and is the starting point for dental disease as it contains a mass of *micro-organisms*. Plaques also occur in areas of the central nervous system in a number of conditions such as *Alzheimer's* and *multiple sclerosis*.

Plasma   **Quick Reference:** The fluid part of the blood.

Advanced Reference: The fluid in which blood cells are suspended or the fluid remaining after blood has clotted, and is called *serum*. Total blood volume comprises 55% fluid and 45% cells.

Plasma expander   **Quick Reference:** IV fluid which increases plasma volume.

Advanced Reference: Plasma expanders, e.g. *colloids*, increase plasma volume via osmosis, i.e. drawing fluid from the extracellular and intracellular spaces. *Hypertonic* solutions have a similar but shorter-acting effect. Also referred to as volume expanders.

Plasma scalpel   **Quick Reference:** A surgical thermal knife capable of simultaneous division of tissue and coagulation of blood vessels.

Advanced Reference: Involves high-temperature argon gas plasma being passed through a direct current (DC) and so ionising the gas and raising the temperature to 3000 °C. A small plasma cutting jet is formed by a nozzle at the tip of the handpiece. Found to be most useful for liver resection, muscle division and tissue debridement.

Plasmin   **Quick Reference:** An *enzyme* that digests fibrin.

Advanced Reference: Its function is to dissolve clots.

Plasminogen   **Quick Reference:** Substance normally present in blood plasma.

Advanced Reference: Is activated to form *plasmin*.

Plaster of Paris   **Quick Reference:** (POP) *Gypsum*. Calcium sulphate (CaSO$_4$).

Advanced Reference: Treated gypsum powder impregnated into bandages which sets hard when water is applied and is used to immobilise and stabilise areas following fracture and surgical repair.

Plasticity   **Quick Reference:** Indicates that something has the capability of being moulded.

Advanced Reference: Plasticisers are a group of agents added to other organic or synthetic substances to make them soft and flexible.

Plasty   **Quick Reference:** Suffix indicating restorative or reconstructive procedures.

Advanced Reference: Most common are pyloroplasty and arthroplasty.

Platelets   **Quick Reference:** Cells that play a part in blood clotting.

Advanced Reference: Platelets or thrombocytes are produced in the bone marrow. An important constituent of blood *coagulation*, they adhere to the walls of injured vessels and help seal them off.

Plenum   **Quick Reference:** Operating ventilation (air-conditioning) system.

Advanced Reference: With the plenum system, positive-pressure air, which has been filtered, humidified and warmed/cooled, is fed into the room at ceiling level and, via downward displacement, forces air out of the lower vents, allowing for approximately 20–30 air changes per hour.

Plethysmograph   **Quick Reference:** Instrument for measuring and recording changes in the size and volume of extremities and organs resulting from fluctuations in the amount of blood or air they contain.

Advanced Reference: This is done by measuring the changes in blood volume of the structure or area. Photo-plethysmography (PPG) measures changes in light absorption as with pulse oximeter. Impedance plethysmography is a non-invasive method used to detect venous thrombosis in arms and legs.

In relation, plethysmograph is used to indicate a venous sensor that provides a waveform.

Pleura   **Quick Reference:** (plur-a) The membrane covering the lungs.

Advanced Reference: Consists of the *parietal* pleura, which covers the chest wall, and the *visceral* pleura, which covers the lungs. The space between the two membranes contains a fluid (***surfactant***) which enables the lungs to move freely within the chest.

Pleural effusion **Quick Reference:** Abnormal accumulation of fluid around the lungs.

Advanced Reference: Usually due to infection.

Plexus **Quick Reference:** A network of structures.

Advanced Reference: A network of nerves, blood or lymphatic vessels. An example is the brachial plexus, which is a system of communicating nerve branches at the root of the neck.

Pneumatics **Quick Reference:** Pertaining to air.

Advanced Reference: Pneumatics is the science that deals with the physical properties of gases.

Pneumoconiosis **Quick Reference:** Lung condition caused by inhalation of dust. Referred to as miner's lung.

Advanced Reference: Characterised by the formation of nodular fibrotic changes in the lungs due to many substances including asbestos and talc.

Pneumosilicosis is a similar condition but caused by inhalation of ***silica*** dust.

Pneumonectomy **Quick Reference:** (new-mon-ectomy) Surgical removal of the lung.

Advanced Reference: Indicates excision of the whole lung whereas ***lobectomy*** signifies removal of one lobe of a lung.

Pneumonia **Quick Reference:** (new-moan-ea) Inflammation of the lungs.

Advanced Reference: Due to infection by virus or bacteria. Unlike bronchitis, which mostly affects the upper air passages, pneumonia occurs further down the respiratory tract.

Pneumonitis **Quick Reference:** Inflammation of the lungs.

Advanced Reference: Usually caused by infectious micro-organisms but may also be due to inhalation of noxious vapours.

Pneumoperitoneum **Quick Reference:** (new-mo-perit-o-neum) Air or gas in the peritoneal cavity.

Advanced Reference: In perioperative terms, can refer to insufflation of CO_2 prior to laparoscopy to aid better viewing conditions.

Pneumothorax **Quick Reference:** (new-mo-thaw-ax) Refers to the situation when air enters the pleural cavity.

Advanced Reference: When air gets between the layers of the ***pleura*** and if the air continues to enter the cavity it could lead to a tension pneumothorax. If this develops, the pressure within the pleural space is greater than atmospheric pressure and the resultant positive pressure in the cavity displaces the ***mediastinum*** to the opposite side.

Polio (blade) **Quick Reference:** Laryngoscope (blade) with a wide-angled blade popular in obstetric anaesthesia.

Advanced Reference: Of most value when a patient has large breasts/chest and relatively short neck that could cause intubation difficulties as in late pregnancy. Originally designed for intubating patients being treated in iron-lung ventilators due to paralysis from polio.

Poliomyelitis **Quick Reference:** (polio-my-lite-is) Viral infection of the nervous system spread by poor hygiene, food and water or droplet infection.

Advanced Reference: Attacks the grey matter in the spinal cord, affecting the nerve cells responsible for stimulation and muscular contraction. If any nerve cells are damaged by the infection, the corresponding muscles can no longer function normally and eventually display signs of wasting.

Polya **Quick Reference:** A type/form of gastrectomy.

Advanced Reference: One form of partial gastrectomy, an alternative to other forms, e.g. *Billroth*.

Polyamine **Quick Reference:** Any compound containing two or more *amine* groups.

Advanced Reference: Polyamines are low *molecular weight cations* and are involved in protein *synthesis*.

Polycystic **Quick Reference:** Characterised by the presence of numerous cysts.

Advanced Reference: Examples are polycystic kidney, liver and ovary.

Polyethylene **Quick Reference:** (poly-eth-ilean) Strong, flexible synthetic resin.

Advanced Reference: Produced by the polymerisation of ethylene. Used in the production of many hospital-based products, usually single-use items.

Polyethylene terephthalate® **Quick Reference:** Trademark name of a synthetic thermoplastic resin.

Advanced Reference: In fibre form it is used as a suture material as well as in the manufacture of vascular grafts and prostheses.

Polyglactin **Quick Reference:** Suture material.

Advanced Reference: Synthetic suture material and distributed as Vicryl (coated).

Polyglycolic acid **Quick Reference:** Suture material.

Advanced Reference: Synthetic suture material manufactured under the name *Dexon*®.

Polymer **Quick Reference:** A large molecule formed from many simple molecules called monomers.

Advanced Reference: Synthetic polymers include *PVC, teflon, polythene* and nylon while naturally occurring include *starch, cellulose* and rubber.

Polymorphic **Quick Reference:** Poly = many, morph = form, structure.

Advanced Reference: Many forms or shapes. Regularly used interchangeably with *multi-formed*.

Polyp(s) Quick Reference: A growth arising from *mucous membrane*.

Advanced Reference: Usually applied to the lining of the nose and paranasal *sinuses*. They are found in many other bodily sites including the bladder and bowel. A polypectomy is the surgical removal of a polyp.

Polypeptide Quick Reference: A *molecule* that contains many *amino acids*.

Advanced Reference: Typically contains between 10 and 100 amino acids.

Polyphenols Quick Reference: Group of chemical substances found in plants.

Advanced Reference: Numerous forms have *antioxidant* properties.

Polystyrene Quick Reference: Hard transparent *thermoplastic*.

Advanced Reference: Synthetic resin produced by the polymerisation of styrene.

Polythene Quick Reference: More recently referred to as polyethylene.

Advanced Reference: A synthetic plastic material.

Polyuria Quick Reference: The production of a large volume of urine in a given period.

Advanced Reference: The urine produced is usually dilute and pale in colour and may be due to excessive fluid intake or disease such as *diabetes*.

Pons Quick Reference: Prominence on the *ventral* surface of the brainstem.

Advanced Reference: It is situated between the *medulla oblongata* and the cerebral peduncles of the midbrain.

Portal Quick Reference: Indicates the portal circulation.

Advanced Reference: The portal circulation supplies the liver, and receives all blood from the alimentary tract, pancreas and spleen via the portal vein and its branches, which pass through the liver to become the *hepatic* veins.

Portal hypertension Quick Reference: A (chronic) rise in the venous pressure in the *portal* circulation.

Advanced Reference: The condition is usually due to obstruction of blood flow through the liver, a major cause being *cirrhosis*.

Positive end-expiratory pressure (PEEP) Quick Reference: A technique used to hold the lungs in an expanded state during the expiratory phase.

Advanced Reference: Keeping the lungs in an expanded state with the pressure above atmospheric pressure by the restriction of expiration. It is used during *intermittent positive pressure ventilation (IPPV)* when certain factors affect airway resistance.

Posterior Quick Reference: Indicates behind.

Advanced Reference: Opposite to *anterior*, indicating at the back of or behind, e.g. posterior surface of something.

Post-partum (haemorrhage) Quick Reference: Post = after, partum = birth, haemorrhage = blood loss.

Advanced Reference: Indicates excessive blood loss from the genital tract after the birth of a child.

Post-perfusion syndrome Quick Reference: Also referred to as post-transfusion syndrome.

Advanced Reference: Involves *cytomegalovirus* mononucleosis occurring 3–6 weeks after *extracorporeal* circulation or multiple blood *transfusion* as with open heart surgery.

Post-traumatic stress disorder Quick Reference: (PTSD) Severe reaction to a traumatic event.

Advanced Reference: Involves re-experiencing the event through dreams, recollections and flashbacks.

Postural drainage Quick Reference: Drainage of secretions from the lungs.

Advanced Reference: Involves the patient lying down, often prone, and being encouraged to cough while the sides of the chest and back are patted with the open hand working up from the base of the lungs to upper chest level. This is intended to loosen adherent or thick secretions in the lungs.

Potassium Quick Reference: Most common positively charged particle in the body.

Advanced Reference: Symbol K. One of the important *electrolytes*. Present mainly inside cells and plays a crucial role in nerve conduction and so muscle impulse and contraction. The normal range is 3.5–5.0 mmol/l.

Pott's fracture Quick Reference: Generally indicates a fracture of the ankle.

Advanced Reference: Term originally used to indicate a variety of fractures involving the lower ends of the tibia and fibula in the region of the ankle.

Pouch of Douglas Quick Reference: The pouch is a pocket-like cavity. Commonly referred to in relation to gynaecology.

Advanced Reference: The lowest fold of the peritoneum between the uterus and rectum.

Povidone Quick Reference: A polymerised form of vinylpyrrolidone, a white powder soluble in water.

Advanced Reference: Used as a dispersing and suspending agent in drugs and other agents. It is combined with *iodine* as a topical antiseptic.

Practolol Quick Reference: *Beta-blocker* and antiarrhythmic.

Advanced Reference: Used to treat *tachycardia* and irregular heart rhythms. Works by inhibiting the contractile capacity of the heart muscle. Administration is by slow IV injection. Available as Eraldin®.

Precipitation Quick Reference: When a solution forms into solids.

Advanced Reference: Applies to drugs when sometimes mixing two together, and they solidify or react against each other.

Precursor Quick Reference: A prognostic characteristic or feature of a patient's health data.

Advanced Reference: Examples are X-ray or laboratory findings that are associated with a higher or lower risk of death than average.

Predisposing **Quick Reference:** Conferring a tendency to disease. Inclined or predisposed towards, susceptible.

Advanced Reference: A predisposing cause is anything that renders a person more liable to a specific condition without actually producing it.

Prednisolone **Quick Reference:** Synthetic corticosteroid.

Advanced Reference: Used to treat inflammation, especially in rheumatic and allergic conditions.

Pregnancy-induced hypertension **Quick Reference:** (PIH) Raised blood pressure usually in the later stages of pregnancy.

Advanced Reference: Related to *eclampsia* or toxaemia of pregnancy.

Preload **Quick Reference:** Strength of ventricular muscle fibres at each diastole.

Advanced Reference: It is reflected by ventricular pressure and volume at that part of the cardiac cycle.

Premedication **Quick Reference:** Indicates a range of drugs given prior to surgery.

Advanced Reference: Premedication, or premed as more commonly known, involves drug administration prior to anaesthesia and surgery. It is intended to be a part of the anaesthetic and can have a number of effects depending on the drugs chosen by the anaesthetist. Primarily the intention is to relieve anxiety and/or reduce secretions and diminish vagal reflexes. Can also include *prophylactic* antiemesis.

Premature **Quick Reference:** Occurring before the expected or normal time.

Advanced Reference: Examples are premature birth and premature ventricular contractions (PVCs).

Premature birth **Quick Reference:** Birth of a baby before full term.

Advanced Reference: By definition a baby that weighs less than 5.5 lbs or 2.5 kg. Causes of premature birth include: multiple pregnancy, bleeding and *pre-eclampsia*.

Presbyopia **Quick Reference:** Being unable to focus on objects up close.

Advanced Reference: Due to decreasing elasticity of the lens of the eye, there is a loss in ability to focus and further deteriorates with age.

Pressor **Quick Reference:** Substance that causes a rise in blood pressure.

Advanced Reference: A vasopressor, a drug which brings about constriction of the blood vessels and raises blood pressure.

Pressure gradient **Quick Reference:** Where fluids and gases move from an area of high pressure to an area of lower pressure.

Advanced Reference: Many bodily functions such as air exchange in the lungs are brought about by pressure gradients; in suction machines a vacuum is created to allow the passage of mucus and blood to an area of lower pressure.

Pressure head **Quick Reference:** Highest point of pressure in an irrigation or infusion.

Advanced Reference: Refers to the height of an infusion (IV or irrigation) and is the point from which the greatest pressure is exerted, i.e. within the fluid bag, giving-set.

Pressure sore   **Quick Reference:** *Bed sore*.

Advanced Reference: Caused by stagnant pressure or rubbing of the skin on the likes of bed sheets.

Priapism   **Quick Reference:** Persistent erection of the penis.

Advanced Reference: The persistent erection is the result of venous thrombosis within the organ. Treatment is usually surgical involving *embolectomy* or venous bypass.

Prilocaine   **Quick Reference:** Local anaesthetic (LA) agent.

Advanced Reference: Used as an LA for many topical applications and infiltration in minor procedures. Available as a cream and solution for injection. Proprietary versions include *Citanest*®.

Primary   **Quick Reference:** Indicates earliest or first.

Advanced Reference: Term used in relation to cancer growths and their spread. Primary is the initial site and growth of a tumour in relation to 'secondary', which indicates sites to where the disease has spread, via *metastasis*.

Primigravida   **Quick Reference:** Prim(e) = first/initial and *gravid* = pregnant.

Advanced Reference: A woman pregnant for the first time.

Prion   **Quick Reference:** Protein particles thought to be the cause of various infectious diseases mainly affecting the nervous system such as *Creutzfeldt–Jakob disease (CJD)*.

Advanced Reference: The smoke plume from *diathermy* use is thought to be one carrier of prions involving CJD.

Probe   **Quick Reference:** Surgical instrument used to explore a lumen.

Advanced Reference: Its use is intended to determine the length and direction of a cavity.

Probiotics   **Quick Reference:** Literary translates to = 'for life'. Relates to dietary supplements.

Advanced Reference: Involves the addition of beneficial bacteria or yeast to foods, *Lactic acid* Bacteria (LAB) being the most commonly used in such products as yoghurt. The bacterial *cultures* are intended to assist the naturally occurring *flora* in the *digestive tract*. There is evidence that their use strengthens the *immune system*. Prebiotics indicates foods which promote the growth of certain bacteria in the intestines.

Procainamide   **Quick Reference:** A beta-blocker used as an antiarrhythmic. Available as Pronestyl®.

Advanced Reference: Used to treat heartbeat irregularities especially after heart attack. Owing to its poor absorption properties, has lost popularity as a local anaesthetic in favour of those that are better absorbed and have a longer duration of action.

Proctocolectomy Quick Reference: Removal of the entire large bowel, rectum and anal canal.

Advanced Reference: Performed via a combined abdomino-perineal approach with creation of a permanent *ileostomy* in the right ileac *fossa*.

Proctoscope Quick Reference: Instrument for examining the *rectum* and anal canal.

Advanced Reference: Proctoscopy. Related to *sigmoidoscopy* when the rectum and sigmoid flexure are examined with a sigmoidoscope. Due to the invasive need, a proctoscope is considerably shorter than a sigmoidoscope.

Procyclidine Quick Reference: Synthetic *anticholinergic*.

Advanced Reference: Has a direct antispasmodic effect on smooth muscle.

Proflavine Quick Reference: Topical antibacterial cream.

Advanced Reference: A formulation of beeswax and liquid paraffin as as an antibacterial agent. Used as a topical application and dressing for minor skin infections, burns and abrasions.

Progesterone Quick Reference: A naturally occurring *hormone*.

Advanced Reference: Prepares the lining of the uterus for implantation of the fertilised *ovum*.

Prognosis Quick Reference: To forecast.

Advanced Reference: To forecast the probable course and outcome of an illness.

Prolactin Quick Reference: (PRL) A hormone synthesised and secreted by the anterior pituitary gland.

Advanced Reference: It is also produced in other tissues, i.e. breast and *decidua*. Secretion of prolactin is increased by stress and sexual activity, but prolactin is most notable as a stimulant of the mammary glands to produce milk (lactation) following childbirth.

Prolapse Quick Reference: The falling forward or downward of an organ.

Advanced Reference: A common area for prolapse is the uterus, which becomes displaced downwards due to weakening of the muscles of the pelvic floor. Causes include (multiple) childbirth and it is treated surgically if necessary. Postoperative problems may involve *incontinence*.

Pronation Quick Reference: To turn the hand palm downwards.

Advanced Reference: It is the movement of turning the hand palm downwards or facing backwards. *Prone* position indicates lying face downwards.

Prone Quick Reference: Patient lying face down.

Advanced Reference: The prone position is when the patient is placed on their front, face down. This is most common in spinal surgery and orthopaedics.

Propagate Quick Reference: To multiply.

Advanced Reference: To grow, culture laboratory specimens.

Prophylaxis Quick Reference: (pro-fal-axis) Treatment undertaken to prevent disease.

Advanced Reference: A prophylactic is an agent that prevents the development of a condition or disease.

Propranolol   **Quick Reference:** Beta-blocker.

Advanced Reference: Brings about a fall in heart rate and cardiac output combined with a decrease in myocardial oxygen consumption. Available as Inderal®.

Proprietary   **Quick Reference:** Refers to the brand name of a drug.

Advanced Reference: The version of a drug that is protected as a name by patent, trademark or copyright as against the *generic* name by which the drug is known or as stated in the *Pharmacopoeia*.

Prostaglandin   **Quick Reference:** A hormone-type substance produced in numerous parts of the body.

Advanced Reference: It is in fact a group of substances that regulate the actions of other hormones and are involved in many bodily functions, e.g. inflammation, gastric acid secretion, BP adjustment, clotting, renal elimination and immunity. They increase the contraction of smooth muscle, particularly in the uterus, and are used to induce abortion. May be used to induce labour. Available as synthetic versions.

Prostate   **Quick Reference:** Gland surrounding the neck of the bladder and beginning of the urethra in men.

Advanced Reference: The prostate gland produces a fluid which forms part of the semen. In later life it is susceptible to benign and malignant enlargement which may obstruct the flow of urine. Surgery is often required to remove the gland or reduce it in size.

Prosthesis   **Quick Reference:** Artificial substitute for a body part.

Advanced Reference: Theoretically involves false teeth, glass eyes and false legs, but with reference to theatres it usually indicates hips, knee and other joint replacements.

Prosthodontics   **Quick Reference:** Branch of dentistry that deals with the restoration and maintenance of oral function, appearance and health. Also termed prosthetic dentistry.

Advanced Reference: Involves the replacement of missing teeth, artificial substitutes and the care of adjacent tissues.

Protamine   **Quick Reference:** An antidote/reversal for *heparin*.

Advanced Reference: An antagonist of the anticoagulant heparin, whose action normally lasts approximately 4–6 hours, but this duration can be altered by the administration of protamine. Used regularly during *cardiopulmonary bypass* and renal *dialysis*.

Protease   **Quick Reference:** Also referred to as proteolytic *enzyme*.

Advanced Reference: A digestive enzyme that brings about the breakdown of *protein*.

Proteins Quick Reference: Large molecules composed of amino acids and essential for maintaining the structure of the body.

Advanced Reference: Proteins contain *nitrogen, carbon, hydrogen, oxygen* and in many cases *sulphur*. They are either simple or conjugated, i.e. combined with other substances as in *haemoglobin*. They can be burnt for energy but are primarily involved in growth.

Proteinuria Quick Reference: The presence of *protein* in the urine.

Advanced Reference: May indicate disease or damage in the kidney.

Protocol Quick Reference: A written or agreed plan.

Advanced Reference: A plan which specifies the procedures to be followed, e.g. an examination, research, or when providing care.

Proton pump inhibitor Quick Reference: Involves a class of drugs that inhibit gastric acid secretion.

Advanced Reference: They interfere with the movement of hydrogen ions across the cell membrane. Used in the treatment of erosive and ulcerative gastro-oesophageal reflux and excessive acid secretion.

Proximal Quick Reference: Nearer to the centre of the body.

Advanced Reference: Describes anything which is nearer to a given point of reference. In anatomy, the centre point of the body is taken as the reference point. The opposite being *distal*.

Pruritus Quick Reference: Itching.

Advanced Reference: Usually caused by local irritation of the skin or may be due to nervous disorders.

Prussic acid Quick Reference: (Hydrocyanic acid) Toxic liquid with an odour of bitter almonds.

Advanced Reference: Extremely volatile acid that can cause death if inhaled.

Pseudomembranous colitis Quick Reference: Also known as necrotising and antibiotic-associated colitis.

Advanced Reference: May result from shock and ischaemia but most commonly associated with antibiotic therapy, which alters the natural bowel *flora*. Characterised by watery diarrhoea.

Pseudomonas *Quick Reference:* (sude-a-moan-us) Gram-negative bacillus.

Advanced Reference: *Pseudomonas aeruginosa* is responsible for wound infection and can proliferate in burns, but is very common in equipment containing fluid such as humidifiers and water traps on ventilators and patient breathing circuits.

Psoas Quick Reference: Muscle (s) of the *loin*. Originating from the *lumbar* spine.

Advanced Reference: There are two, major and minor; psoas acts in conjunction with the iliacus muscle to flex the hip joint.

Psychiatry **Quick Reference:** (sigh-ki-at-ree) Branch of medicine that deals with mental illness.

Advanced Reference: Psychopathology is the study of the processes and nature of mental disorders. The branch of pharmacology that deals with the effects of drugs on the mind and behaviour is termed psychopharmacology.

Psychology **Quick Reference:** The study of normal behaviour. The workings of the normal brain.

Advanced Reference: Although referred to as behavioural medicine it is thought of as a branch of science as opposed to medicine.

Psychosis **Quick Reference:** Serious mental disorder.

Advanced Reference: Seen in schizophrenia and in manic depression. A feature is that sufferers do not recognise that there is anything wrong.

Psychosurgery **Quick Reference:** Surgery performed on the brain.

Advanced Reference: Intended to modify the behaviour in severe mental disturbances. Leucotomy was at one time the most commonly performed procedure but, mainly due to the irreversible nature of the surgery, it has been replaced by more selective operations and drug therapy.

PTFE **Quick Reference:** Teflon (Polytetrafluoroethylene).

Advanced Reference: Substance with non-stick properties invented by the Dupont company and developed via the space race (National Aeronautics and Space Administration – NASA) but more familiar in the domestic setting in non-stick kitchenware. Used in the manufacture of intravenous (IV) cannulas and catheters, which helps reduce *thrombus* formation and increase flow rate.

Puberty **Quick Reference:** The beginning of the period of life when reproduction is possible.

Advanced Reference: Marked by the development of the secondary sexual characteristics, and start of menstruation in females and production of sperm in males.

Pubis **Quick Reference:** The bone felt at the lower end of the abdomen.

Advanced Reference: The bone through which the hip bones join at the front of the pelvis forming the pubis symphysis.

Pudendal **Quick Reference:** Nerve that services the *perineum, vulva* and lower vagina.

Advanced Reference: Because of its position and route it can be damaged by the *peroneal* post on orthopaedic tables and attachments during hip and femur surgery. Pudendal nerve block is suitable for a number of obstetric situations including *forceps delivery* and *episiotomy*.

Puerperal **Quick Reference:** (purp-er-al) Indicates childbirth or the period immediately following it.

Advanced Reference: Puerperal infection involves infection of the female genital tract usually following childbirth complications.

Pulmonary artery banding   Quick Reference: An operation carried out to bring about constriction of the pulmonary artery with a band in order to reduce pulmonary blood flow and reduce *congestive heart failure*.
Advanced Reference: Carried out in children with congenital heart defects that produce right-to-left shunts between the ventricles or great veins.

Pulmonary fibrosis   Quick Reference: Disease(s) of the lungs.
Advanced Reference: Causes inflammation and subsequent scarring of the lungs and in time the resultant *fibrosis* can build up to the extent that oxygen supply to the tissues is reduced.

Pulmonary hypertension   Quick Reference: Raised blood pressure in the pulmonary circulation.
Advanced Reference: Increases pressure on the heart and leads to decreased oxygen output, causing breathlessness and exhaustion. May be of a primary cause or due to heart disease.

Pulseless electrical activity   Quick Reference: Condition related to advanced cardiac life support (ACLS).
Advanced Reference: Indicates an absence of a pulse in conjunction with a relatively normal looking ECG trace. Common causes are *hypovolaemia, hypoxia* and *hypothermia*.

Pulse pressure   Quick Reference: Is the change in blood pressure during a contraction of the heart.
Advanced Reference: Formally it is the systolic pressure minus the diastolic pressure.

Punctate   Quick Reference: Having tiny spots, points or depressions.
Advanced Reference: As with punctate haemorrhage in eye conditions such as *retinopathy*.

Purse string   Quick Reference: Suture technique used to close an opening.
Advanced Reference: Is a continuous circular closure placed around an opening to enable it to be closed when the suture ends are pulled together. Used commonly after removal of the appendix and on the urinary bladder when inserting a drainage tube or implanting the ureter.

Purulent   Quick Reference : Refers to the presence of *pus*.
Advanced Reference: Consisting of or containing pus, usually due to bacterial infection.

Pus   Quick Reference: Yellowish fluid that is a product of infection.
Advanced Reference: Tissue fluid containing dead white cells, bacteria and broken-down tissue. Has a distinctive smell but this is dependent on the type of bacteria involved.

Putrefaction   Quick Reference: The breaking down of tissue by bacteria.
Advanced Reference: Refers to the changes that take place in the bodies of animals and plants after death. Almost entirely due to bacterial action, which reduces living matter to the carbonic acid gas, ammonia, amongst

others. Usually accompanied by an offensive odour which is generated by the releasing gas.

Putti–Platt operation   Quick reference: Orthopaedic procedure for correction of persistent shoulder dislocation.

Advanced Reference: The procedure is performed to try to stabilise the shoulder following persistent dislocation.

PVC[1]   Quick Reference: Polyvinyl chloride.

Advanced Reference: Used in the manufacture of many disposable adjuncts, e.g. airways, endotracheal tubes, various catheters. Needs to be incinerated to specific guidelines of temperature and time due to the possibility of emitting *dioxins*.

PVC[2]   Quick Reference: Premature ventricular contractions or complexes.

Advanced Reference: A PVC is a depolarisation that arises in either ventricle before the next expected sinus beat, i.e. prematurely.

Pyelogram   Quick Reference: Radiological examination of the renal pelvis.

Advanced Reference: Radio-opaque dye is injected intravenously and after approximately 10 min, radiographs are taken of the kidney. Retrograde pyelogram involves inserting dye into the renal pelvis using a *cystoscope* and ureteric catheter.

Pyelonephritis   Quick Reference: (pilo-nef-ritis) Microbial infection of the kidney.

Advanced Reference: May be *acute* or *chronic* and affect the entire kidney substance. The infection may have travelled up the urinary tract from the perineum or be blood borne.

Pylorus   Quick Reference: Aperture in the stomach through which food passes into the stomach.

Advanced Reference: The pylorus is surrounded by a circular ring of muscle (pyloric *sphincter*) which controls opening and closing of the aperture.

Pyrexia   Quick Reference: Fever.

Advanced Reference: Condition in which the body temperature is above normal.

Pyrogen   Quick Reference: Any substance which causes or produces a fever.

Advanced Reference: Pyrogens can be produced during the manufacture and storage of IV fluids and although the bacteria involved have been destroyed during processing, their pyrogenic protein particles are left behind and can be the cause of reactions in patients.

Pyuria   Quick Reference: Pus in the urine.

Advanced Reference: Due to inflammation/infection in the urine.

Q

QRS complex   **Quick Reference:** Represents ventricular depolarisation.

Advanced Reference: The normal duration of this complex is approximately 0.12 seconds. The Q wave is the initial downward deflection of the QRS complex and the QT interval represents the duration of ventricular systole.

Quadrants   **Quick Reference:** Areas, regions and quarters.

Advanced Reference: The abdominal and pelvic areas of the trunk are divided into quadrants, i.e. right upper and lower quadrants and left upper and lower quadrants.

Quadriceps   **Quick Reference:** The large muscle covering the front of the thigh.

Advanced Reference: The main combination of four muscles within the lower limbs that give structure and mobility to extension and straightening of the knee.

Quadriplegia   **Quick Reference:** Paralysis of all four limbs.

Advanced Reference: Also termed tetraplegia.

Qualitative   **Quick Reference:** Pertaining to quality.

Advanced Reference: The value or nature of something. Determines the presence or absence of a substance.

Quality assurance   **Quick Reference:** Also known as Quality Management.

Advanced Reference: An aspect of general and hospital management; indicates a standard or level of excellence that assures expected quality.

Quantiflex®   **Quick Reference:** Type/make of anaesthetic machine.

Advanced Reference: The machine is common in dental anaesthesia and has a number of specific features, i.e. separated flowmeters, one common control knob that adjusts total gas flow (oxygen and nitrous oxide) and most notably that the design prevents delivery of hypoxic mixtures with the capacity to deliver no lower than 30% oxygen.

Quantitative   **Quick Reference:** Capable of being measured.

Advanced Reference: Quantitative analysis is the determination of the amounts of constituents in a sample.

Quart   **Quick Reference:** Unit of fluid volume.

Advanced Reference: Fluid measure equivalent to one-quarter of a gallon, or two pints, 32 fluid ounces, 946.24 ml.

Quartz   **Quick Reference:** A very hard crystalline form of *silica*.

Advanced Reference: Usually six-sided in shape and comes in many varieties, e.g. agate, onyx, amethyst. Used in numerous applications and industries, e.g. optical and electrical instruments.

Quadrants of abdomen

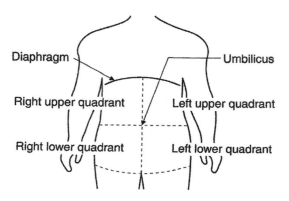

Regions of the abdominal cavity

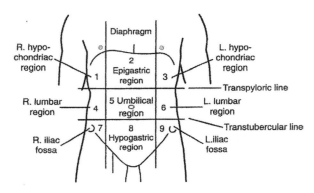

Fig. 15. Quadrants & regions of the abdomen. Reprinted with permission from Elsevier.

Quinidine   **Quick Reference:** A drug obtained from the Cinchona tree.
Advanced Reference: Used in the treatment of irregular heart action (cardiac arrhythmias), more specifically ventricular extrasystoles and ventricular tachycardia.

Quinine   **Quick Reference:** Alkaloid made from the bark of the Cinchona tree.
Advanced Reference: Used as a remedy in the treatment of malaria and can be given orally or intravenously.

Quinsy   **Quick Reference:** Abscess surrounding the tonsil.

Advanced Reference: Peritonsillar abscess, where infection has occurred in the surrounding tissue of the tonsil area. Characterised by symptoms of sore throat, fever and difficulty swallowing. Treated initially with antibiotics, however extreme cases will require surgical intervention.

Quintuplet   **Quick Reference:** Fivefold.

Advanced Reference: Five offspring born at the same *gestation* period during a single pregnancy.

Quotient   **Quick Reference:** Result obtained from dividing one quantity by another.

Advanced Reference: The respiratory quotient is the ratio between the carbon dioxide expired and the oxygen inspired during a specified time.

R

Radiation **Quick Reference:** Energy in the form of electromagnetic waves.

Advanced Reference: May be ionising or non-ionising. Examples are gamma rays, X-rays, infrared, ultraviolet and microwaves.

Radical **Quick Reference:** Relating to the root or origin. In surgery, indicates taking an extensive amount (of tissue), extensive enough to ensure all affected or diseased tissue is removed.

Advanced Reference: Also referred to as wide excision; a radical mastectomy, radical hysterectomy.

Radioactive **Quick Reference:** A chemical substance emitting radiation.

Advanced Reference: Atoms that have the same number of protons and different numbers of neutrons are commonly referred to as isotopes. A number of *isotopes* pose a threat to human life mainly due to their unstable nature, thus caused by a breakdown in their nuclei.

Radiographer **Quick Reference:** X-ray technician.

Advanced Reference: The radiographer is responsible for the production of films, images and scans, which the radiologist will diagnose.

Radiology **Quick Reference:** Medical speciality concerned with the use of electromagnetic radiation.

Advanced Reference: Radiologists can be either diagnostic or therapeutic. Work involves the diagnosis of radiographs, computerised tomography (CT) and magnetic resonance imaging (MRI) scans. Diagnostic radiologists are becoming increasingly involved in the invasive treatment of many conditions that were once treated solely with open surgery, and are now regularly referred to as interventional radiologists. The therapeutic radiologists are primarily concerned with utilising radioactive materials in the treatment of cancer.

Radio-opaque **Quick Reference:** Substance capable of obstructing X-rays.

Advanced Reference: Also referred to as contrast medium, used in X-ray procedures in the form of a dye to produce an outline or image of an area, e.g. blood vessel, biliary tree.

Radiotherapy **Quick Reference:** Treatment of disease with *radioactive* substances.

Advanced Reference: This can be achieved through the use of X-rays to identify the nature of a fracture or underlying disease. Other more direct uses of radioactive substances in radiotherapy include the insertion of a radioactive material in the form of a seed close to a tumour. The most common radioactive substance used in radiotherapy is cobalt 60 which is supplied in sealed capsules.

Radium Quick Reference: Radioactive element.

Advanced Reference: Radioactive isotopes are utilised in radiotherapy treatment for destroying cancer cells.

Radius Quick Reference: Bone of the forearm.

Advanced Reference: The outer bone of the lower arm, smaller than the *ulna* which it accompanies.

Radon Quick Reference: *Inert* gas, one of the *noble* gases. Chemical symbol = Rn.

Advanced Reference: A radioactive element produced during the decay of *radium*. Used in *radiotherapy* cancer treatment as radon seeds. Emits both alpha and gamma *radiation*.

Railroading Quick Reference: Term used in difficult intubation technique.

Advanced Reference: Indicates the situation when an endotracheal tube is fed into the larynx over an introducer, such as a '*bougie*'.

Rales Quick Reference: Abnormal sounds heard via a stethoscope when examining the chest.

Advanced Reference: Usually due to disease of the lungs involving fluid in the air passages. The sound is produced by air as it passes over or through secretions.

Ramsted's procedure Quick Reference: Operation performed to relieve stricture of the *pylorus*.

Advanced Reference: Named after the German surgeon W.C. Ramstedt. Performed for congenital stricture or stenosis of the pylorus. The condition is usually detected in a newborn who may be having difficulty retaining milk and is possibly suffering from projectile vomiting. The operation involves making a longitudinal incision into the pylorus and then resuturing it transversely, so creating a wider inner opening between the pylorus and duodenum. Otherwise known as a *pyloroplasty*.

Ranitidine Quick Reference: Antacid, H_2 receptor antagonist.

Advanced Reference: Used to reduce gastric acid production by blocking the function of H_2 receptors. Indications for use are *reflux* within the oesophagus and gastric ulcers.

Ranula Quick Reference: A *cyst* lying under the tongue.

Advanced Reference: Develops as the result of a blocked salivary or mucous gland.

Ranvier Quick Reference: More appropriately = node of Ranvier.

Advanced Reference: Small gap in the *myelin* sheath of a myelinated nerve fibre.

Rapacuronium bromide Quick Reference: Considered as a succinylcholine chloride (suxamethonium, *scoline*, Anectine®) replacement.

Advanced Reference: Has rapid onset of about 1 min, providing intubating conditions in the same time. Has a duration of approximately 20 min, which is shortened by the use of *neostigmine*.

Rash   **Quick Reference:** Temporary eruption or discoloration of the skin.

Advanced Reference: Often associated with allergy, infection and fever.

Ratchet   **Quick Reference:** A toothed bar with an interlocking system which prevents unlocking and slippage.

Advanced Reference: On artery forceps and similar surgical instruments, the toothed bar of the ratchet can be found on one side of the handle, while the other side contains the corresponding teeth that engage with the ratchet grooves. Such forceps are stored and passed to the surgeon clipped on the first ratchet. The ratchet gives added hold so the forceps remain in situ when placed on a vessel. Other surgical instruments such as mouth gags have similar ratchet design.

Raynaud's disease   **Quick Reference:** (ray-nards) Condition in which fingers and toes lose feeling and become white or blue when exposed to cold. Also referred to as Raynaud's phenomenon.

Advanced Reference: Common in young women, it produces numbness, tingling and can be painful. Also signified by redness when warmed. The cause is spasm of the arterioles supplying the digits. There is no specific or definitive treatment although vasodilator drugs help and surgery is sometimes employed for relief and involves interrupting the nerve function by severing the sympathetic nerves supplying the affected area and that have responsibility for constriction of blood vessels (*sympathectomy*).

Raytec®   **Quick Reference:** Surgical swabs often referred to as Raytec® swabs.

Advanced Reference: The Raytec® refers to the translucent lining through the middle of the swab which is intended to highlight the swab under X-ray should it be mislaid during a surgical procedure. It is a protective measure which enables swabs to be detected if they are left behind inside a body cavity. Similar measures are taken with a range of detectable materials in endotracheal tubes, ureteric stents, cannulas and catheters.

RDS   **Quick Reference:** Respiratory distress syndrome.

Advanced Reference: Involves the development of *dyspnoea* soon after birth in premature babies and is characterised by chest retraction accompanied by *cyanosis* and grunting on expiration.

Reamer   **Quick Reference:** Surgical instrument used in orthopaedics and dentistry.

Advanced Reference: Used for enlarging root canals in dentistry and clearing out the shaft of bones in orthopaedics ready for prosthesis insertion, e.g. shaft of femur for hip replacement.

Receiver   **Quick Reference:** A kidney-shaped bowl, also referred to as kidney dish.

Advanced Reference: A receiver was originally made of stainless steel but now comes in plastic and other disposable materials and is used in many settings, e.g. in surgery for holding a patient's body parts and fluids, and it is also good practice to use it to hold the surgical scalpel when being passed between scrub practitioner and surgeon. Used generally for holding many adjuncts and equipment in all areas of the operating department.

Receptor **Quick Reference:** Nerve ending adapted to a particular kind of sensation or a chemical component of a living cell.

Advanced Reference: Receptors receive stimuli in order to bring about a reaction or change.

Recipient **Quick Reference:** One who receives.

Advanced Reference: One who receives blood from another, the universal recipient is someone who can receive blood from all other blood groups. Also, a recipient receiving a donated organ for transplantation from a *donor*.

Recovery **Quick Reference:** Refers to the recovery area of a theatre suite.

Advanced Reference: Now more regularly referred to as the Post-Anaesthetic Care Unit (PACU), and in some centres it also functions as a High Dependency Unit (HDU).

Rectocele **Quick Reference:** (rec-toe-seal) Prolapse of the rectum.

Advanced Reference: Occurs commonly in women following childbirth and is due to overstretching of the vaginal wall.

Rectum **Quick Reference:** Last section of the large intestine.

Advanced Reference: The last few inches of the intestine, terminating in the anal canal, sigmoid flexure through to the anus.

Rectus sheath **Quick Reference:** Covering over the rectus abdominis muscle.

Advanced Reference: It is a thick sheath of connective tissue which covers the rectus abdominis muscle.

Recumbent **Quick Reference:** Lying down, reclining.

Advanced Reference: A recumbent position, sometimes used to describe or infer supine.

Recurarisation **Quick Reference:** Recurrence of neuromuscular block.

Advanced Reference: Happens when reversal agents wear off before the neuromuscular blocking drug is completely cleared, if at all. Happens with the longer-acting agents.

Recurrent **Quick Reference:** To recur. Happening time-after-time. Turning back so as to renew direction.

Advanced Reference: An example in anatomy is the recurrent laryngeal nerve, where one branch loops under the subclavian artery on the right side and under the arch of the aorta on the left, then returns upward to the larynx to supply all the muscles of the thyroid but excludes the cricothyroid.

Redivac®   **Quick Reference:** Pre-vacuumed surgical drain.

Advanced Reference: A pre-vacuumed, sterile, portable, closed-wound suction unit. The drain tubing is fixed into the surgical wound intraoperatively and connected once the incision is closed. The container contains measuring indicators so that blood loss can be monitored.

Reducing valve   **Quick Reference:** Pressure-regulating valve.

Advanced Reference: Device for reducing high-pressure delivery of gases to anaesthetic machines and maintaining the reduced pressure at a manageable level.

Reduction   **Quick Reference:** Relates to bone injuries, alignment, correction as well as correction of other conditions.

Advanced Reference: 1. The correction of a fracture or dislocation of a bone, may be an open or closed reduction; 2. The measures taken to reduce a hernia by surgery ensuring internal structures do not invade surrounding areas; 3. Breast reduction.

Re-fashioning   **Quick Reference:** Surgical re-suturing or re-anchoring of a structure.

Advanced Reference: Essentially this involves the re-suturing of a structure following previous surgery. Re-fashioning of a colostomy would be to re-site or correct the *stoma*.

Reflex   **Quick Reference:** Involuntary response to a stimulus.

Advanced Reference: This is the automatic reaction by the body to a stimulus, determined by impulses in nerves.

Reflux   **Quick Reference:** Backward flow. A flow of fluid in a direction opposite to the normal flow.

Advanced Reference: Term used to indicate *regurgitation* as happens in gastro-oesophageal reflux due to *hiatus hernia*. Valvular reflux is a term used to describe the backward flow past a venous valve in the lower limb due to venous insufficiency, and in relation to urine flow, vesicoureteral reflux (VUR) indicates the flow of urine from the bladder back into the ureters.

Refraction   **Quick Reference:** The turning or bending of any wave, e.g. light or sound.

Advanced Reference: In the eye it enables light to be bent so that an image is focused on the retina.

Regional anaesthesia   **Quick Reference:** Often wrongly used interchangeably with *'local' analgesia*.

Advanced Reference: Local anaesthesia tends to indicate a specific localised area, whereas regional anaesthesia has an effect over a larger area, i.e. nerve blocks, epidural/spinal techniques.

Regions of the abdomen   **Quick Reference:** Anatomical regions and quadrants of the abdomen.

Advanced Reference: Dividing the abdomen into quadrants and further subdividing into regions; makes reference much easier for surgical incisions and sites of procedures, as well as the recognition and location of pain, injury and underlying organs, etc.

Regurgitation **Quick Reference:** The back-flow of gastric contents into the mouth.

Advanced Reference: Regurgitation is a passive act whereas vomiting is active and requires muscle tone. Therefore, patients administered a muscle relaxant (non-depolariser) in their general anaesthetic regurgitate. If this occurs, the stomach contents can be aspirated into the lungs and lead to *Mendelson's syndrome.*

Rejection **Quick Reference:** Refers to the rejection of transplanted organs.

Advanced Reference: Involves the formation of antibodies against the transplanted tissue by the host, leading to eventual rejection.

Relative humidity **Quick Reference:** This is the ratio of the mass of water vapour in a given volume of the air to the mass of water vapour required to saturate the same volume of the air at the same temperature.

Advanced Reference: Relative humidity is the absolute humidity divided by the amount present when the gas (air) is fully saturated at the same temperature and pressure. Applicable to theatre environment where relative humidity should be approximately 50%–55%. Measured with a *hygrometer.*

Relaxant **Quick Reference:** Indicates muscle relaxant drugs. To paralyse the patient.

Advanced Reference: Used to provide loss of muscle tone for intubation and surgery. Includes both depolarising and non-depolarising muscle relaxants.

Relaxin **Quick Reference:** Female hormone secreted by the *corpus luteum.*

Advanced Reference: Helps to soften the cervix and relax the pelvic ligaments in childbirth.

Religion and culture **Quick Reference:** Refers to the varied treatment requirements of diverse groups.

Advanced Reference: Although theatre staff have always placed importance on attending to the needs of differing ethnic and religious groups, the issue has gained prominence so that staff must now be aware of all needs and beliefs with regard to theatre procedures. Due to this the need for further training and updating should be an on-going priority if contravention and infringements are to be avoided.

Remifentanil **Quick Reference:** Opioid analgesic.

Advanced Reference: Short-acting opioid popularly used as an infusion during anaesthesia.

Remission **Quick Reference:** The active process of surrendering, resigning or retreating.

Advanced Reference: A temporary and incomplete subsidence of the active source of pain, infection or more serious illness. Often referred to in the context of a patient's cancer going into remission. This would indicate that the symptoms have eased or the progress of the disease has slowed or halted.

Renal **Quick Reference:** Relating to the kidney.

Advanced Reference: Located or affecting the region of the kidney.

Renal failure **Quick Reference:** Inability of the kidney to carry out its normal functions.

Advanced Reference: May be acute or chronic. Acute renal failure (ARF) may be due to overdose, shock or trauma, when a lengthy drop in blood pressure may be the cause and function may/should return after a period of perfusion or dialysis. Chronic renal failure (CRF) can be due to a number of disease processes and involves long-term dialysis and eventual transplant.

Rendell-Baker **Quick Reference:** Commonly refers to a design of paediatric face mask.

Advanced Reference: Designed to minimise dead space by being anatomically moulded to fit the face.

Renin **Quick Reference:** A hormone produced in the kidneys involved in the regulation of blood pressure.

Advanced Reference: It is released into the bloodstream in response to stress and when the kidney is damaged, and stimulates the production of angiotensin, which causes vasoconstriction and so raises blood pressure.

Rennin **Quick Reference:** An enzyme present in gastric juice.

Advanced Reference: Responsible for clotting the protein casein, as the first step in the digestion of milk.

Replication **Quick Reference:** Repetition, process of duplication.

Advanced Reference: Can be applied when repeating experiments to ensure accuracy, and to the bodily process of cell reproduction.

Resect **Quick Reference:** To cut and remove a section of tissue.

Advanced Reference: Resection indicates the partial removal of tissue rather than an entire structure.

Resection **Quick Reference:** The surgical removal of an organ or structure.

Advanced Reference: Used commonly to indicate general cutting and removal in a surgical manner.

Resectoscope **Quick Reference:** Surgical instrument used in urology.

Advanced Reference: A telescope incorporating a cutting attachment passed back down the urethra and used to reduce the size of the prostate by cutting and shaving, as in *TURP* and *TURT*.

Reservoir bag **Quick Reference:** Bag incorporated into an anaesthetic circuit/breathing system.

Advanced Reference: Its function is to store gas and provide it for continued adequate ventilation. Can also be an indicator of breathing pattern and efficiency during spontaneous respiration.

Residual/residue   Quick Reference: Relating to, or being something that remains.

Advanced Reference: Can refer to the residual volume in the lungs after a maximum expiration, or residue left in the bladder following urination.

Residual volume (RV)   Quick Reference: Remainder of air.

Advanced Reference: Amount of air remaining in the lungs at the end of maximum or forced expiration.

Resistance   Quick Reference: Power or capacity to resist.

Advanced Reference: Examples are electrical resistance and resistance in breathing systems, especially in relation to paediatric anaesthesia.

Respiratory acidosis   Quick Reference: An acidosis in the blood caused by decreased ventilation of the lungs leading to a build up of carbon dioxide.

Advanced Reference: Respiratory *acidosis* may occur if the lungs are under-ventilated resulting in a heightened concentration of *carbon dioxide*. This may be due to a number of factors, e.g. obstruction, inadequate ventilation, administration of carbon dioxide, *sepsis*, severe dehydration and haemorrhagic shock, all resulting in a raised P_aCO_2 and low *pH*.

Respiratory alkalosis   Quick Reference: An alkalosis of the blood caused by hyperventilation leading to a reduction of carbon dioxide.

Advanced Reference: Occurs if the lungs are hyperventilating, resulting in an abnormal loss of carbon dioxide (hypocapnia).

Respiratory quotient   Quick Reference: The ratio of carbon dioxide produced by tissue metabolism compared to oxygen consumed.

Advanced Reference: The ratio of carbon dioxide diffusing from blood into alveoli compared to oxygen diffusion in the opposite direction.

Respiratory rate   Quick Reference: (RR) The repeated action of breathing, recorded as the number of breaths per minute.

Advanced Reference: An adult breathes approximately 12–18 breaths per minute (bpm). Breathing is controlled by the *medulla oblongata* and the *pons* areas of the *brainstem*, although there is a certain amount of voluntary control over our breathing that allows for breath-holding and hyperventilation.

Respiratory therapist   Quick Reference: A mainly USA-based health professional.

Advanced Reference: Main function involves the monitoring and therapeutic treatment of ventilated patients in ICU and HDU.

Respirometer   Quick Reference: Device for measuring expiratory gas volumes.

Advanced Reference: Available in many designs (electronic and mechanical) in anaesthetic apparatus. The Wright respirometer is a popular mechanical model. Respirometers are also used to test lung capacity and capability. Also referred to as pneumograph.

Restless leg syndrome Quick Reference: A disorder of the nerves affecting mostly the lower limbs.

Advanced Reference: The condition causes tingling, itching and aching in the lower limbs and less commonly the arms. Also known as Ekbom's syndrome.

Resusci Annie Quick Reference: A CPR resuscitation training manikin.

Advanced Reference: Slang term adopted by manufacturers for a model used in CPR training. Various models are available but primarily they respond to attempts of rescue breathing and external cardiac massage.

Resuscitaire® Quick Reference: A specially designed resuscitation trolley for the newborn.

Advanced Reference: They are a mobile combination of resuscitation trolley and incubator, equipped with oxygen, suction, heating, monitoring as well as ability to alter the position of the baby. Familiar in theatres during Caesarean section for the baby's care and transport after delivery.

Resuscitation Quick Reference: To revive, try to bring back to normal.

Advanced Reference: Term used to indicate the process of trying to revive someone who is apparently dying, as in cardiac arrest; CPR techniques. However, may be used to cover treatment of shocked and debilitated patients, to stabilise them with intravenous fluids, medication and oxygen. Often used when an extremely sick patient is being prepared for urgently needed surgery.

Retching Quick Reference: Involuntary spasm related to vomiting.

Advanced Reference: Although used in relation to vomiting, actually indicates inefficient effort and non-productive vomiting.

Retention Quick Reference: The act of keeping back.

Advanced Reference: A common example would be urinary retention which involves the inability to void urine from the bladder, usually due to obstruction.

Reticulo-endothelial system Quick Reference: Name given to a system of cells scattered throughout the body which have the function of phagocytosis.

Advanced Reference: This means that they eat up foreign material such as bacteria and the remains of dead cells. These *phagocytic* cells are called macrophages and originate in the bone marrow.

Retina Quick Reference: The innermost layer of the eyeball, involved in the receiving of images.

Advanced Reference: The light-sensitive membrane lining the back of the eye. Consists of several layers of nerve cells and fibres containing the rods and cones involved in image interpretation. The images reach the brain by way of the optic nerve. Retinal detachment involves the separation of the retina from the underlying layer of blood vessels.

Retinitis pigmentosa **Quick Reference:** An inherited *retinal* disorder that produces night blindness and constriction of the visual field.

Advanced Reference: Leads to progressive deterioration of the retina, which eventually causes blindness.

Retinopathy **Quick Reference:** Any disorder of the *retina*.

Advanced Reference: Usually indicates conditions that result in impairment of vision through damage to the blood vessels, such as occurs in *diabetes* and *hypertension*.

Retinoscope **Quick Reference:** Optical instrument used for examining and assessing refraction in the eye.

Advanced Reference: Hand-held, it utilises a beam of light to view shadows produced on the subject's pupil. Also referred to as a skiascope.

Retract **Quick Reference:** To pull or hold back tissues so to expose a structure or other tissues.

Advanced Reference: Retraction is mostly carried out by the surgeon's assistant with the use of specific retractors or the hands and fingers, although there are many self-retaining types of instruments that sit within the wound or are fixed to an external point such as the operating table.

Retractors **Quick Reference:** Instruments used during surgery to hold back organs.

Advanced Reference: A retractor is used to hold open a wound or cavity or pull tissue aside so as to give the surgeon an improved view and increased room to work. Retractors come in many shapes and sizes, depending on what they are designed for. Some of the most common used in surgery are: Devers, Czerny, Volkman, Waltons malleable version, Traverse, Balfour and Roux; even skin hooks are classified as retractors. There are self-retaining versions, hand-held ones and models which attach to the operating table or towel rail.

Retrognathia **Quick Reference:** Better known as receding jaw. It is an abnormal positioning of one or both jaws, particularly the mandible.

Advanced Reference: A congenitally acquired condition in which the lower jaw is set back from the upper jaw. One of the anatomical conditions associated with *difficult intubation*.

Retrograde **Quick Reference:** Going against the normal direction. The prefix retro indicates going backwards.

Advanced Reference: Occurring or performed in a direction opposite to the usual direction of conduction or flow. Retrograde priming is carried out when preparing IV infusions. Retrograde prostatectomy is another term for TURP, i.e. going back down the urethra to resect the prostate. A retropubic prostatectomy is an open technique that involves going behind the pubic bone to access the prostate for removal.

Retrograde amnesia Quick Reference: Loss of memory for a period of time preceding a particular incident.

Advanced Reference: Type of memory loss that follows a severe blow to the head resulting in unconsciousness.

Retrograde ejaculation Quick Reference: Abnormal ejaculation of sperm, usually into the bladder.

Advanced Reference: In this condition the *sperm* travels up the *urethra* instead of down and exiting the body. Occurs commonly after *TURP* but may also be due to spinal cord injuries, diabetes or following major abdominal/pelvic surgery.

Retrograde intubation Quick Reference: Technique used with difficult intubation.

Advanced Reference: Involves passing a retrograde guide (often an epidural or CVP catheter) through the cricothyroid membrane, then feeding it upwards into the mouth or nose and the endotracheal tube is guided over it via the larynx and trachea.

Retropubic Quick Reference: Retro = backwards or behind, pubic = pubis bone.

Advanced Reference: Indicates behind the pubic bone. A retropubic prostatectomy is removal of the gland by incising the prostate capsule following a *suprapubic* incision.

Retroversion Quick Reference: Backward displacement of an organ.

Advanced Reference: When related to the uterus, a normal uterus slopes downwards and backwards while a retroverted one may lie vertically or slope downwards and forwards.

Retrovirus Quick Reference: A group of highly active and resilient viruses.

Advanced Reference: These viruses infect and destroy helper T-cells of the immune system. Human immunodeficiency virus (HIV), the virus responsible for human acquired immunodeficiency syndrome (AIDS), is a member of this group.

Reynolds Risk Score Quick Reference: Heart attack risk factor assessment system used mainly for women.

Advanced Reference: It takes in such factors as age, blood pressure, cholesterol levels and smoking plus parental history in relation to cardiac condition.

Rhabdomyolysis Quick Reference: Disintegration of muscle.

Advanced Reference: Associated with excretion of *myoglobin* in the urine.

Rhesus factor Quick Reference: (re-sus) Rh factor. Rhesus blood group system.

Advanced Reference: A group of antigens that may or may not be present on the surface of a person's red blood cells. People with this factor are Rh-positive and those who lack the factor are Rh-negative. Incompatibility between the two is a cause of transfusion reactions and of haemolytic disease of the newborn.

Rheumatic fever   **Quick Reference:** Condition that is due to infection by a haemolytic group A *Streptococcus*.

Advanced Reference: Most commonly affects children causing painful joints but more importantly it weakens the heart muscle and damages the mitral valve resulting in incompetence, which often requires replacement surgery. The aortic and tricuspid are less commonly affected.

Rheumatoid   **Quick Reference:** (ru-mat-oid) Disorder affecting the joints causing inflammation and degeneration.

Advanced Reference: Relates to such conditions as *arthritis*. The patient has a rheumatoid condition. Rheumatism is a term loosely applied to pain and inflammation of the joints and muscles which causes stiffness and difficulty in moving. It includes many diseases, principally *osteoarthritis* and rheumatoid arthritis.

Rhinitis   **Quick Reference:** Inflammation of the *mucous membrane* of the nose.

Advanced Reference: May have an *allergic* origin or due to such things as the common cold. In chronic situations may lead to *inflammation* of the *sinuses* and the formation of nasal *polyps*.

Rhinoplasty   **Quick Reference:** Rhino = nose and plasty = corrective surgery. Corrective nasal surgery.

Advanced Reference: Surgical procedure performed to alter/correct the shape and size of the nose, usually for cosmetic reasons, but can be done if misalignment is affecting normal breathing.

Rhinovirus   **Quick Reference:** Group of viruses that cause respiratory tract infection.

Advanced Reference: Responsible for the common cold and strike more commonly in Spring and Autumn. Also called coryza virus.

Rhizotomy   **Quick Reference:** Interruption of a cranial or spinal nerve root.

Advanced Reference: The surgical procedure involves the cutting of selected nerve roots at the point where they exit the spinal cord. Carried out to relieve pain or hypertension.

Rhys-Davies exsanguinator   **Quick Reference:** A limb exsanguinator used prior to the application of a tourniquet in orthopaedic surgery.

Advanced Reference: A black-rubber (sausage) device that has a central hole through which a patient's arm/leg can be inserted, followed by rolling it up the limb (to the level of the tourniquet), which has the effect of squeezing blood (venous) out of the limb. Once at this level, the tourniquet is inflated to stem arterial flow into the limb, so creating a bloodless flow. The exsanguinator is an alternative to the *Esmarch* bandage.

Rib   **Quick Reference:** A curved bone that forms part of the thoracic cage.

Advanced Reference: There are 12 pairs of ribs within the thoracic cage. Each rib is flat and curved and joined at the spinal vertebrae by cartilage. The top seven pairs of ribs are directly connected to the sternum while the remaining five pairs are classified as false ribs connected to each other by cartilage. The last two pairs of false ribs are often referred to as floating ribs because they are attached to the vertebrae at the back but are not connected at the front. Ribs are useful landmarks for identifying key insertion points for intercostal chest drains, CVP catheters, etc.

RIDDOR Quick Reference: Reporting of Injuries Diseases and Dangerous Occurrences.

Advanced Reference: A section of the Health and Safety regulations which deals with the reporting and recording of relevant details of accidents and incidents in the workplace. Incorporated in the regulation are timeframes for when events should be reported.

Rigor Quick Reference: Intense shivering.

Advanced Reference: Involves shivering and a sensation of coldness accompanied by a rise in temperature. Often indicates fever if in combination with sweating. Rigor mortis is the stiffening of the body that occurs within approximately 8 h of death (dependent on temperature) and is due to changes in muscle tissue after death.

Ring block Quick Reference: Subcuticular infiltration of local anaesthetic.

Advanced Reference: Used to anaesthetise extremities such as fingers and toes. Involves infiltrating local anaesthetic around the full circumference of the extremity proximal to the site. Useful for emergency situations when a full anaesthetic is both unsuitable and the required period of fasting has not taken place.

Ringer's lactate Quick Reference: IV maintenance and replacement fluid.

Advanced Reference: Consists mainly of normal saline with small amounts of calcium and potassium.

Risk management Quick Reference: Process initially involved with managing health and safety within an organisation but can be applied to a range of activities.

Advanced Reference: Involves highlighting an activity and assessing the risks in comparison to need and then implementing changes and/or alternatives or substitutes.

RNA Quick Reference: Ribonucleic acid.

Advanced Reference: A substance included in all living cells by which information contained in the inherited *DNA* is used in the formation of protein molecules. DNA is found in the cell nucleus whereas RNA is in the ribosome (granules in the substance of living cells and where the synthesis of proteins takes place). It is through this mechanism that *hereditary* characteristics are handed down through generations.

Robertshaw tube   Quick Reference: A double-lumen endotracheal tube with an angled (left or right) end.

Advanced Reference: Used and designed for one-lung anaesthesia. Originally available in red rubber but now disposable plastics are more popular; also in a range of sizes and left/right design to facilitate insertion into either bronchi. Has two channels and is used with either a single or double catheter mount connection in order to facilitate one- or two-lung ventilation. Both have a tracheal and bronchial cuff and the right-sided model has an eye to facilitate right upper lobe ventilation.

Robinul®   Quick Reference: A proprietary *anticholinergic* drug.

Advanced Reference: It is a preparation of glycopyrronium bromide (glycopyrrolate). Used in combination with neostigmine as an alternative to *atropine* for reversal of the actions of non-depolarising muscle relaxants.

Rocuronium   Quick Reference: Non-depolarising muscle relaxant.

Advanced Reference: Has rapid onset and therefore often used in place of suxamethonium with an intermediate duration of action. Trade names include Esmeron™ and Zemuron™.

Rodent ulcer   Quick Reference: A malignant tumour of the skin.

Advanced Reference: Arises from the basal cells and is usually found on the face, particularly in those who have been exposed to sunlight. Has the appearance of a raised ulcer that will not heal. Rodent ulcers do not give rise to secondary growths in other parts of the body but if left untreated are capable of spreading into underlying bone.

Rogitine®   Quick Reference: Proprietary antihypertensive drug. Phentolamine.

Advanced Reference: An alpha-blocker used in the treatment of hypertension and heart failure.

Roller-ball   Quick Reference: A control clamp/switch on an IV administration set.

Advanced Reference: The roller-ball is a controlling clamp fitted to an IV infusion set downstream of the chambers, on the tubing. Designed to control the flow of fluid in graduations through the giving-set.

Ronguer   Quick Reference: (ron-jure) A surgical instrument used for nibbling bone.

Advanced Reference: Derived from the French word meaning to nibble. Most often used to take small bites of bone in orthopaedic and neurosurgery.

Ropivacaine   Quick Reference: Local anaesthetic.

Advanced Reference: Similar in action to *bupivacaine* but less cardiotoxic.

Rotameter®   Quick Reference: Trade name of a design of *flowmeter*.

Advanced Reference: Used in anaesthetic machines, it consists of a tapered-glass tube (wider at the top) mounted vertically, and inside is a rotating bobbin that is free to move up and down the tube as gas flows up and past it, recording flow rates by the markings (litres per minute) on the tube. The tapered shape of the glass tube creates an annular orifice between the bobbin and the walls of the tube and as this orifice increases in diameter the bobbin moves upwards, controlled by a needle valve.

Rotary clamp Quick Reference: Operating table fixation device.

Advanced Reference: Type of fixation clamp for table attachments. Its design (rotary) allows for a range of adjustments not possible with fixed clamps, e.g. low lithotomy, but extra vigilance is required as the nature of the clamp can allow slippage and lead to a less stable fixation.

Rotavirus Quick Reference: Genus of *virus* that has a wheel-like appearance.

Advanced Reference: Normally transmitted via the faecal–oral route causing infantile *gastroenteritis* signified by vomiting, *diarrhoea*, fever, abdominal pain and dehydration. In severe cases may be fatal.

Round-bodied needles Quick Reference: Refers to a suture needle which has a rounded shaft but a sharp tapered point for passing through delicate tissue.

Advanced Reference: Round-bodied needles are used for *approximation* of soft tissues and are intended to separate tissue rather than cut through them. An example is when suturing bowel tissue.

Roux-en-Y Quick Reference: (ru-en-why) A type of *anastomosis*.

Advanced Reference: An anastomosis of the small intestine in the shape of the letter Y. The proximal end of the divided intestine is anastomosed end-to-side to the distal loop and part of the distal loop is anastomosed to another part of the digestive tract, e.g. the oesophagus.

Rowbotham connector Quick Reference: (row-bottom) A metal endotracheal tube connector.

Advanced Reference: It is of a right-angled design and was originally used in both oral and nasal tubes. Now superseded by preformed tubes and plastic connectors.

RTA Quick Reference: Road traffic accident.

Advanced Reference: A term used throughout critical care areas of hospitals but gradually being replaced by motor vehicle collision (MVC).

Rubber shod Quick Reference: Indicates a protective cover placed over the ends of artery forceps, e.g. Halsteads.

Advanced Reference: Usually made of rubber, PVC or silicone. When placed over the ends of the artery forceps it creates a more atraumatic hold.

Ruben valve Quick Reference: A one-way or non-re-breathing valve.

Advanced Reference: A one-way valve similar in design and function to the Ambu valve. Allows for a constant flow of fresh gas as there is no mixing of fresh and expired gases. Seldom used in anaesthetic circuitry but still found in resuscitation-type circuits, e.g. the bag-valve-mask (*BVM*).

Ruga Quick Reference: A crease or fold. Plural is rugae.

Advanced Reference: Particularly applies to folds of mucous membrane which line the stomach.

Rule of nines **Quick Reference:** Assessment measuring system used in relation to patients with burns.

Advanced Reference: Used for assessing external burns by percentage of overall body surface area. For an adult each of the following areas is assessed as: front of thorax and abdomen 18%, back of thorax and abdomen 18%, each leg 18%, each arm 9%, head 9%. The area of the perineum is about 1%. In children the head is assessed as 15%–20% because it is proportionally much greater. Another useful measure is the front of the patient's hand, which represents approximately 1% of the surface area.

Ryles tube **Quick Reference:** A plastic-weighted tube inserted into the gastric system via the nasopharynx.

Advanced Reference: Also termed nasogastric tube. Available in a range of gauges and contains a radio-opaque line for X-ray purposes and metal ball in the tip for weighting. Used during gastric, hepatic and bowel surgery to allow escape of gas and gastric fluid. In theatres they are often stored in a fridge to give a degree of rigidity to aid insertion.

S

Sacral hiatus **Quick Reference:** Anatomical landmark formed by the failure of fusion of the fifth sacral *vertebrae*.

Advanced Reference: The *coccyx* lies below the sacral *hiatus*. Used as a landmark in *caudal* anaesthesia.

Sacrohysteropexy **Quick Reference:** Surgical procedure for correction of uterine prolapse.

Advanced Reference: Involves the insertion of a permanent supportive mesh.

Sacrum **Quick Reference:** (say-crumb) Bone at the base of the spinal column.

Advanced Reference: Triangular in shape formed by the fusion of five vertebrae. It unites above with the lumbar vertebrae and below with the coccyx.

SADS **Quick Reference:** Sudden arrhythmic death syndrome.

Advanced Reference: Genetic cardiac disease. Can affect all ages, be of sudden onset and be the cause of death where no cardiac irregularities have been previously identified. This is not to be confused with the regularly used SADs abbreviation (seasonal affected disorder).

Sagittal **Quick Reference:** An imaginary line extending from front to back.

Advanced Reference: With reference to the human body, it indicates the midline of the body, dividing right and left.

Saliva **Quick Reference:** Commonly referred to as spittle.

Advanced Reference: Secretion of the salivary glands which contains water, mucus, ptyalin and starts the process of digestion.

Salmonella **Quick Reference:** The main cause of food poisoning.

Advanced Reference: Genus of Gram-negative bacteria. Parasites of the gastrointestinal tract responsible for common types of food poisoning as well as typhoid and paratyphoid fevers.

Saphenous **Quick Reference:** (saf-een-us) Refers to veins in the leg.

Advanced Reference: The long saphenous vein runs up the inside of the leg from the ankle to the groin and the short saphenous from the outside of the ankle to the back of the knee. The long saphenous is the longest vein in the body. Both are used regularly as grafts, the short saphenous being very popular for coronary bypass grafting.

Sarcoma **Quick Reference:** A tumour of connective tissue often highly malignant.

Advanced Reference: May occur in any part of the body and tends to grow rapidly and metastasise early to distant sites.

SARS   Quick Reference: Severe acute respiratory syndrome.

Advanced Reference: Viral infection first detected in China in 2002 and has now spread to many more countries, particularly in Asia and the Orient.

Saturation   Quick Reference: Refers to oxygen saturation. SpO_2.

Advanced Reference: Most commonly encountered as the reading from an oxygen analyser or saturation monitor. It is the relative measure of the amount of oxygen dissolved in the blood.

Saviour sibling   Quick Reference: Term used in relation to producing babies for stem cell harvesting.

Advanced Reference: A planned pregnancy with the intention of extracting stem cells for the treatment of disease in a brother or sister.

Savlodil   Quick Reference: An antiseptic agent.

Advanced Reference: Produced in the form of sterile sachets and is a compound preparation of the disinfectants/antiseptics, *chlorhexidine* gluconate and cetrimide (Savlon®).

Scabies   Quick Reference: Skin infection.

Advanced Reference: Caused by a *mite*, the female of which burrows under the skin to lay eggs which then become adult in approximately 10 days. Is passed on via contact and causes rash and itching on the hands, under the arms, genitals and buttocks.

Scalene   Quick Reference: Muscles of the neck/shoulder. Also referred to as scalenus.

Advanced Reference: There are four scalene muscles: anterior, medius, minimus and posterior. They extend from the cervical area to the first and second ribs and are responsible for raising these during inspiration and bending the neck forward and to the sides.

Scavenging system   Quick Reference: Method of removing waste gases from theatre and related areas.

Advanced Reference: More specifically, removes waste gases via the expiratory ports of anaesthetic and ventilator circuits. Can be either a passive or active system; the passive system is rarely used now and involved directing the gases through a carbon-filled container (*Cardiff Aldasorber*), which absorbed some vapours. Other systems just simply fed the gases away to a remote ventilation system. Active systems are standard in all designs of theatre suites now, using an active vacuum (suction) system to remove expired gases.

Schimmelbusch mask   Quick Reference: (shim-em-bush) Early design of anaesthetic mask for delivering volatile anaesthetic gases.

Advanced Reference: Although referred to as a mask, it is also classified as a vaporiser. Was in fact a wire mask-shaped frame covered with gauze which fitted over the patient's face. The anaesthetic agent was then sprinkled onto the gauze which became impregnated and consequently the patient inhaled the vapours. No measurement of dosage or strength was involved and those in the vicinity also inhaled a certain amount of the vapour.

Schizophrenia   Quick Reference: A group of severe mental disorders.

Advanced Reference: Characterised by detachment from reality, delusions, hearing of voices and the feeling of being externally controlled.

Schrader   Quick Reference: Design of anaesthetic gas pipeline fitting/valve.

Advanced Reference: Classed as a valve or simply a fitting. It refers to the wall- or ceiling-mounted outlet coupling for piped oxygen, nitrous oxide, air and the vacuum. The valve ensures that the gas is shut off when no probe is in place and each is colour-coded and unique to each gas.

Schwann cells   Quick Reference: The *myelin*-secreting cell surrounding a myelinated nerve fibre.

Advanced Reference: Situated between two nodes of ***Ranvier***.

Scissors   Quick Reference: Refers to those designs used in surgery and related areas.

Advanced Reference: They are available in numerous shapes, sizes and forms designed usually for a specific use or purpose, e.g. curved, single-edged, off-set angle, combined scissor/forceps. Besides surgical scissors, such as McIndoe, Mayo, Potts and Metzenbaum, there are others manufactured for specific use, i.e. bandage and Plaster of Paris scissors. Scissors intended for cutting tissues should never be used for general surgical use to cut sutures and dressings as this will blunt and alter the cutting edge.

Scirrhous   Quick Reference: A type of cancer.

Advanced Reference: Pertaining to a hard tumour, or scirrhus, a growth of connective tissue, such as hard carcinoma of the breast.

Sclerosis   Quick Reference: Hardening of tissue.

Advanced Reference: Due to inflammation and the formation of fibrous interstitial tissue, as with atherosclerosis (hardening of the arteries).

Sclerotherapy   Quick Reference: Injecting of sclerosing agents to produce fibrosis.

Advanced Reference: Treatment used for ***haemorrhoids, varicose veins*** and oesophageal ***varices***. Preparation of suxamethonium chloride. It has a duration of up to 5 min and is commonly used for intubating in general anaesthesia. ***Fasciculation*** occurs before paralysis is achieved.

Scoline apnoea   Quick Reference: *Apnoea* caused by prolonged muscle paralysis due to depolarising muscle relaxant.

Advanced Reference: Occurs when the patient is administered a depolarising muscle relaxant, e.g. suxamethonium chloride. If the patient is low on the enzyme cholinesterase, which naturally breaks down the suxamethonium, the result is prolonged muscle paralysis. Treatment is to keep the patient sedated and ventilated until spontaneous reversal occurs.

Scopolamine   **Quick Reference:** Hyoscine.

Advanced Reference: A central nervous system (CNS) depressant. Has sedative, hypnotic and antiemetic effects. Used as a premedication, usually in combination with a narcotic. It is a more powerful drying agent (*antisialogogue)* than atropine.

Screen   **Quick Reference:** Refers to the barrier device between the surgical and anaesthetic areas of the operating table.

Advanced Reference: Also termed towel rail. Has the intention of separating the sterile surgical field from the socially clean area of the anaesthetist as well as preventing drapes, etc. from falling on the patient's face. A number of designs are available that either clamp to the table or slide under the mattress.

Scrub area   **Quick Reference:** Area or room where theatre staff scrub up prior to surgery.

Advanced Reference: Usually a room adjoined to theatre, it should be easily accessible but separate from general and patient entrances and exits.

Sebum   **Quick Reference:** Oily substance secreted by the sebaceous glands of the skin. A semi-fluid composed of fat, keratin and epithelial debris.

Advanced Reference: Sebum lubricates the skin and hair. It coats the skin, slowing evaporation of water, as well as having an antibacterial action, and reaches the skin through small ducts.

Secretion   **Quick Reference:** The process by which a gland expels the particular substance for which it is responsible.

Advanced Reference: The secretions of exocrine glands are carried away in ducts or poured straight into the place where they are to be utilised. The secretions of endocrine glands (hormones) are released into the blood to be carried to their site of action.

Sedation   **Quick Reference:** The state of calming.

Advanced Reference: Involves the use of a sedative or tranquilliser, drugs which lessen excitement. Barbiturates and hypnotics are also used to produce sedation.

Sedation assessment scales   **Quick Reference:** Various scales used to assess the adequacy of sedation, comfort, agitation, consciousness, medication requirements, ventilator synchrony and tolerance.

Advanced Reference: There are many that cover both ventilated and non-ventilated patients but no one is considered suitable for all criteria and patient groups. Examples are: Ramsay scale, motor activity sedation scale, sedation agitation scale, Richmond agitation sedation scale.

See-saw breathing   **Quick Reference:** Also known as paradoxical breathing.

Advanced Reference: Seen in patients with airway obstruction. Upon observation, the chest falls as the abdomen rises when the patient attempts to breathe.

Seldinger wire Quick Reference: Device used to assist blood vessel cannulation/catheterisation.

Advanced Reference: A sprung wire originally used by radiologists and later adapted for venous/arterial cannulation. After venous access has been established, the wire is fed through the cannula followed by the indwelling catheter, threaded over the wire. Upon successful catheterisation, the wire is withdrawn. Wires now have at least one end in the shape of a J (J-wire) which eases passage through tortuous routes and causes less trauma to vessel walls.

Selectatec Quick Reference: Vaporiser locking/securing mechanism.

Advanced Reference: With this system, only when the vaporiser is locked in position can gas flow. The system is also designed to prevent two vaporisers being used simultaneously.

Selective abortion Quick reference: Term used to indicate the aborting of one gender in preference to another.

Advanced Reference: A practice carried out in certain countries in order to control numbers and genders of children. Mostly involves the aborting of female fetuses for cultural and financial reasons.

Sellick's manoeuvre Quick Reference: Manoeuvre carried out to prevent aspiration of stomach contents into the lungs.

Advanced Reference: Involves pressure being externally exerted on the cricoid cartilage during induction of anaesthesia, in an attempt to prevent regurgitation of stomach contents entering the lungs. This manoeuvre is effective because the cricoid cartilage is a circular structure and when depressed occludes the oesophagus which lies behind. Utilised during emergency inductions when a patient may not have been fasted, although certain groups, such as those undergoing *Caesarean section*, are always in danger of regurgitation and always require Sellick's during induction. Others include patients with *hiatus hernia*. The manoeuvre is named after the anaesthetist who first described its use. Also termed crash induction and rapid sequence induction.

Semen Quick Reference: (sea-men) The male testicular fluid.

Advanced Reference: Semen contains spermatozoa plus secretions of the prostate gland and seminal vesicles.

Semiconductors Quick Reference: Materials that can act as a conductor or insulator of electricity.

Advanced Reference: Solid crystalline substances whose electrical conductivity is intermediate between that of a conductor and an insulator.

Seminoma Quick Reference: Testicular cancer.

Advanced Reference: A germ cell tumour.

Sengstaken-Blakemore tube Quick Reference: (seng-stark-en) Multilumen tube used for applying pressure to oesophageal *varices*.

Advanced Reference: The tube has both gastric and oesophageal balloons which, after oral insertion, are inflated with saline to compress against the bleeding area. Traction is also applied to the external end of the tube as a further means of suppressing bleeding. The Minnesota tube is similar but has an extra lumen for oesophageal drainage.

Sensitive larynx Quick Reference: Anaesthetic term sometimes used to indicate that anaesthetic agents (*volatiles*) may cause irritation during induction and recovery.

Advanced Reference: Applies mainly to smokers whose larynx may be more prone to irritation with resultant coughing and mucus production.

Sepsis (septic) Quick Reference: An infection by *pus*-forming bacteria, i.e. septic.

Advanced Reference: Destruction of the tissues by disease-causing bacteria or their *toxins*.

Septicaemia Quick Reference: The presence of bacterial toxins in the bloodstream. Blood poisoning.

Advanced Reference: Can lead to widespread tissue injury as the toxins are dispersed throughout the body in the blood.

Septic arthritis Quick Reference: Also referred to as infective *arthritis*.

Advanced Reference: Involves infection in the fluid and tissues of a joint, usually caused by bacteria but can be due to certain viruses and fungi.

Septum Quick Reference: A partition between two sides of a structure.

Advanced Reference: An example is the nasal septum, a sheet of cartilage between the nostrils and the interventricular septum dividing the two sides of the heart.

Serotherapy Quick Reference: Also referred to as serum therapy and plasma therapy.

Advanced Reference: The treatment of a disease by the injection of immune *serum* or *antitoxin*.

Serotonin Quick Reference: A *monoamine* vasoconstrictor found in many body tissues.

Advanced Reference: Has numerous physiological properties including: inhibition of gastric secretions, stimulation of smooth muscle, it is a central *neurotransmitter* and a precursor of *melatonin*.

Serous membrane Quick Reference: Often referred to as the serosa. Smooth transparent membrane.

Advanced Reference: Consists of a single cell layer (mesothelium) and underlying fibrous connective tissue and lines many large cavities of the body such as the *peritoneum*, *pleura* and the membrane surrounding the heart, the pericardium.

Serum Quick Reference: The clear fluid that separates from whole blood when it clots.

Advanced Reference: It is plasma with fibrinogen removed and also contains antibodies and antitoxins.

Servo **Quick Reference:** Feedback. Servomechanism, a self-regulating feed-back system.

Advanced Reference: Term applied to patient ventilators or the system they utilise. Indicates that feedback is provided on the patient's condition and needs, and the ventilator is able to make suitable adjustments.

Servo-vent **Quick Reference:** Name given to a type and design of patient ventilator.

Advanced Reference: The servomechanism is a control system applied to many ventilators but used to indicate others, i.e. Manley Servo-vent and Siemens Servo-vent.

Sesamoid **Quick Reference:** Bony mass said to resemble a sesame seed.

Advanced Reference: A small bony mass formed in tendons. The patella is the largest of the sesamoid bones.

Set-up room **Quick Reference:** A specific area in theatres for laying out sterile instruments before surgery.

Advanced Reference: Some theatres have a separate designated room for this function, usually adjacent to theatre, and it allows for the scrub practitioner to prepare sterile instrument trolleys separate from other activities and prior to the start of a procedure.

Sevoflurane **Quick Reference:** Volatile anaesthetic agent.

Advanced Reference: One of the more recently introduced drugs. Delivered via a vaporiser, and is relatively soluble so it has a rapid induction and recovery. Also suitable for gas induction in children due to its lack of irritating odour as with other agents.

Sharps **Quick Reference:** Refers to sharp items in hospitals that have the potential to puncture and cause injury.

Advanced Reference: Items such as hypodermic needles, cannulas, suture needles, scalpels or even large drain introducers and laparoscopic trocars, plus glass. Under *COSHH* regulations, these must be disposed of in a designated container. These items pose many hazards with *needle-stick injury* being common.

Shelf-life **Quick Reference:** Indicates the time within which an item should be used.

Advanced Reference: Corresponds to a sell-by date. In relation to theatres, involves sterilised items such as instrument packs, although pre-packed manufactured sundries and pharmaceuticals all have expiry dates which must be adhered to. As within any organisation, stock rotation should be standard practice.

Shock Quick Reference: Term used generally to indicate distress, but in medical terms refers to specific situations, each with their own causes and treatment protocols.

Advanced Reference: Shock is in fact a *syndrome* in which, irrespective of cause, tissue perfusion is inadequate, causing a number of signs and symptoms, e.g tachycardia, sweating, hypotension and rapid shallow breathing. Can be due to many causes and take many forms, i.e. anaphylactic shock, cardiogenic shock, septic shock, toxic shock, hypovolaemic shock, neurogenic shock, obstructive shock and distributive shock. Obstetric shock is also now recognised as a specific type but requires changes in treatment regimes due to the two-lives situation and the undesirable actions of *vasopressors* on mother and baby as well as the *placenta*.

Shod Quick Reference: Artery forceps with rubber fitted over the gripping ends.

Advanced Reference: Designed and used to hold fine sutures.

Shunt Quick Reference: Diversion of flow, as with circulation of blood. To push or send in a certain direction.

Advanced Reference: In relation to *haemodialysis*, involves the insertion of connecting tubing into an adjacent artery and vein (common sites are wrist and ankle). This is then used as access to the arterial and venous systems for connecting to the dialysis machine.

Sickle-cell anaemia Quick Reference: A genetically transmitted form of anaemia involving abnormal haemoglobin (Hb).

Advanced Reference: Under certain conditions, including hypoxia, hyper-carbia, hypothermia and acidosis, the affected Hb may distort (sickle) and rupture, leading to blockage of small blood vessels and reduced oxygen-carrying capacity (haemolytic anaemia). Normal Hb is referred to as A with abnormal termed S. When the disease is inherited from both parents and a majority of the Hb is abnormal the condition is referred to as HbSS. However, when inherited from only one parent and there is a presence of both normal and abnormal Hb, this is referred to as HbAS.

Known to originally affect mainly certain races (of African decent) and those from certain areas but can now be found in a broad range of any population.

Sievert Quick Reference: (Sv) SI unit of radiation.

Advanced Reference: Others include the Roentgen (R) and the Gray (Gy). All relate to the amount of energy deposited.

Sigmoidoscope Quick Reference: Device used to examine the lower bowel.

Advanced Reference: Originally a rigid metal scope with a detachable light source, long enough to view the sigmoid colon and rectum. These have been supplemented and replaced by flexible versions with integral fibre-optic light illumination systems.

Signs and symptoms Quick Reference: Observation and assessment of a patient's condition.

Advanced Reference: Sign = an observation by a physician that the patient may not be aware of. Symptom = an indication of a disorder from the patient themselves.

Silica Quick Reference: Crystalline compound occurring abundantly as *quartz*, sand and many other minerals. In the form of silicon dioxide the formula is SiO_2.

Advanced Reference: Used in the manufacture of such products as glass and concrete.

Silicon(e) Quick Reference: A rubber-like material used in many medical sundries and devices.

Advanced Reference: An organic polymeric compound (polysiloxane) that has many useful properties, i.e. water resistant, *inert*. The latter allows for devices made from silicone to remain in the body for much longer periods than those made of plastics. These include: IV catheters and cannulas, dialysis and oncology catheters, *TPN* lines as well as endotracheal tubes intended for use on ICU and extended placement.

Silver nitrate Quick Reference: Substance used as an antimicrobial, *astringent* and corrosive agent. Chemical formula $AgNO_3$.

Advanced Reference: Seen primarily in the form of a stick used in the treatment of warts. Also used as an antiseptic in eye drops and in laboratories as a bacterial staining agent.

Sinoatrial node Quick Reference: The natural pacemaker of the heart.

Advanced Reference: Situated in the atrium of the heart and instigates the heart beat.

Sinus Quick Reference: Indicates a pathway.

Advanced Reference: A hollow or cavity. There are a number of anatomical sinuses, brain, coronary, nasal and bone, but it also refers to a blind-ended opening or tract which usually starts from the body surface and heads inwards, often becoming inflamed and/or infected.

Sinus arrhythmia Quick Reference: Variation in the heart rate.

Advanced Reference: Common in young healthy people it is signified by a variation in rate often associated with the respiratory cycle (accelerates on inspiration and slows on expiration). Otherwise meets all the criteria for normal *sinus rhythm*.

Sinus rhythm Quick Reference: Refers to the (normal) rhythm of the heart.

Advanced Reference: Sometimes referred to as normal sinus rhythm(each P wave being followed by a QRS complex). Indicates that the rhythm is initiated by the *sinoatrial node*.

Skin clips/staples Quick Reference: An alternative skin closure method to suturing and/or steri-strips.

Advanced Reference: Made of non-corrosive metal and often supplied with an applicator. They are quickly and easily applied and removed, and reduce postoperative scarring.

Sleep apnoea   **Quick Reference:** Condition brought on during sleep involving obstruction of the airway.

Advanced Reference: Can be due to a number of reasons that cause the cessation of breathing, and so the waking and arousal of the patient.

Sliding scale   **Quick Reference:** Refers to an insulin regime used to regulate blood glucose levels with diabetic patients.

Advanced Reference: Aimed at tightly regulating blood sugar levels depending on need. Often used throughout the perioperative period as an intravenous infusion. An alternative to the *Alberti regime*.

Slipped disc   **Quick Reference:** Everyday term for a prolapsed intervertebral disc.

Advanced Reference: Involves the disc between two vertebrae bulging out, usually under strain, and pressing on a nerve root causing pain that is both local as well as in areas supplied by the nerve. Most often occurs in the lower back. In severe cases is treated with surgery, i.e. laminectomy.

Sloops   **Quick Reference:** Used during surgery to identify various structures.

Advanced Reference: Available in various colours, i.e. red, blue, white and yellow, they are used to identify structures, e.g white for nerves, yellow for ureters, blue for veins and red for arteries. The red and blue are regularly used during vascular surgery to occlude veins and arteries.

Slough   **Quick Reference:** (sluf) Necrotic tissue.

Advanced Reference: Sloughing is the process of the slough separating from viable tissue.

Smith's fracture   **Quick Reference:** Fracture of the *distal* portion of the **radius**.

Advanced Reference: Otherwise known as a reverse *Colles* fracture.

Sniffing the (morning) air   **Quick Reference:** Refers to the head position in anaesthesia.

Advanced Reference: Describes when the head is flexed/extended for intubation. Variations are employed for differing age groups, size, physical condition and any current injuries.

Soda lime   **Quick Reference:** Compound used to absorb carbon dioxide in anaesthetic circuits.

Advanced Reference: Used to absorb the patient's exhaled carbon dioxide. Composed of 94% calcium hydroxide, 5% sodium hydroxide and a trace of potassium hydroxide. Silica is added to prevent powdering of the granules and a dye to indicate when the soda lime is exhausted and cannot absorb any further chemical. Depending on which variety is in use, colour changes vary, e.g. pink to white or white to violet.

Sodium   Quick Reference: Soft white element normally found in combination with other elements, i.e. sodium chloride = common (table) salt. Chemical symbol = Na.

Advanced Reference: Essential for normal health and life and forms the principal *cation* in the extracellular fluids. Commonly taken in the form of sodium chloride (common salt). Helps maintain electrical potential in the nervous system. An excess leads to hypernatraemia which can result in *oedema*.

Sodium bicarbonate   Quick Reference: Chemical symbol – $NaHCO_3$. An alkali.

Advanced Reference: Has varying uses as an alkali and antacid. Most commonly seen during the *CPR* setting when used to correct *acidosis*.

Bicarbonate itself is utilised as a buffer in the blood, a crucial component of the acid/base process maintaining *homeostasis*. Approximately 85%–90% of carbon dioxide is converted into bicarbonate (H_2CO_3); i.e. $CO_2 + H_2O \rightleftharpoons H_2CO_3 \rightleftharpoons HCO_3^- + H^+$.

Sodium chloride   Quick Reference: NaCl, common salt.

Advanced Reference: Widely used as normal saline (0.9%) for IV infusion as a replacement and maintenance fluid. Also used for irrigation during cystoscopy but not *TURP*/TURT, when diathermy is used as it is conductive; *glycine* is used in this situation.

Sodium citrate   Quick Reference: Alkaline compound used to treat infections of the urinary tract.

Advanced Reference: Also used to assist in the secretion of *uric acid*.

Sodium hydroxide   Quick Reference: Caustic soda (NaOH).

Advanced Reference: A strong alkaline compound or solution used externally.

Sodium hypochlorite   Quick Reference: Compound used as a disinfectant.

Advanced Reference: Mainly used for cleaning abrasions. Available in 1% and 8% concentrations.

Sodium lactate   Quick Reference: Hartmann's solution.

Advanced Reference: Crystalloid IV solution used as a replacement and maintenance fluid.

Soft palate   Quick Reference: Posterior portion of the roof of the mouth.

Advanced Reference: The soft palate extends from the palatine bones to the *uvula*.

Solar cell   Quick Reference: Is an electric cell that produces electrical energy from light.

Advanced Reference: It is based upon a *semiconductor* device called a *photoelectric cell* which creates a small current because of the movement of electrons.

Solubility   Quick Reference: Susceptible to being dissolved.

Advanced Reference: The amount of a substance that can be dissolved in a given amount of *solvent*. *Bile* salts increase the solubility of fat-soluble *vitamins* to aid their absorption. Insoluble indicates that something is incapable of being dissolved.

Solu-Cortef® **Quick Reference:** Proprietary corticosteroid.

Advanced Reference: Used to replace steroid deficiency, suppress inflammation or allergic symptoms and in the treatment of shock. Supplied in powder form for reconstitution.

Solu-Medrone® **Quick Reference:** Proprietary corticosteroid. Methylprednisolone.

Advanced Reference: Used to treat shock and suppress allergic and inflammatory symptoms.

Solution **Quick Reference:** Liquid in which a substance is dissolved.

Advanced Reference: A fluid which contains a dissolved substance (solute).

Solvent **Quick Reference:** A substance in which another substance is dissolved, forming a *solution*. Capable of dissolving a substance.

Advanced Reference: Solvent abuse involves the deliberate inhalation of fumes from glues and polishes to become intoxicated.

Somatic **Quick Reference:** Of or relating to the body (non-reproductive parts).

Advanced Reference: As opposed to the mind. Somato is a prefix indicating the body.

Sonor **Quick Reference:** Son = sound.

Advanced Reference: Sonograph, ultrasound. A sonographer is trained in the use of ultrasound for diagnostic and therapeutic purposes.

Sotalol **Quick Reference:** *Beta-blocker* and antihypertensive.

Advanced Reference: Used to treat hypertension, arrhythmias and angina.

Spatula **Quick Reference:** A flat blunt-edged instrument.

Advanced Reference: Seen commonly as a tongue depressor; normally made of wood, metal or plastic.

Specimens **Quick Reference:** Indicates a sample (tissue, fluid) taken from a body part or area during surgery/examination.

Advanced Reference: Specimens are taken to determine their nature and/or the presence of disease. Depending on the tissue involved and the examination required, specimens are placed in various containers and mediums. Examples include blood, cells, tissue, fluids and pus.

Speculum **Quick Reference:** An instrument for inspecting the interior of natural body passages.

Advanced Reference: Often fitted with illumination or mirrors, suitable for viewing peripheral areas. There are various models designed for viewing the vagina, rectum, nose and outer ear.

Sperm **Quick Reference:** Spermatozoon. Spermatozoa.

Advanced Reference: A mature male sex cell produced in the testis.

Spermatocele **Quick Reference:** (sperm-at-o-seal) A *cyst* of the *epididymis*.

Advanced Reference: Aspiration reveals a milky fluid. Treatment is by surgical removal.

Spermaturia **Quick Reference:** The presence of *sperm* in the *urine*.

Advanced Reference: Their presence is not abnormal but in large numbers can discolour the urine making it cloudy.

Spermicidal **Quick Reference:** Substances that destroy/inactivate sperm.

Advanced Reference: Not a contraceptive in themselves but are used in barrier methods such as creams and to coat condoms.

Sphenoid **Quick Reference:** Wedge shaped.

Advanced Reference: Relates to the sphenoid bone.

Sphincter **Quick Reference:** A ring of muscle.

Advanced Reference: Has the ability to constrict and close a natural passage or orifice, e.g. anal sphincter, gastro-oesophageal sphincter.

Sphygmomanometer **Quick Reference:** (sfig-mo-man-ometer) Instrument for non-invasively measuring blood pressure.

Advanced Reference. A cuff and graduated glass tube containing mercury used in conjunction with a stethoscope to record BP. The cuff is inflated (mercury column rises in tandem) and then allowed to deflate slowly and as the blood pressure cuts in the reading causes the mercury to jump, so indicating systolic pressure. The pressure continues to drop, and as the mercury stops pulsing this is taken as diastolic pressure.

Spina bifida **Quick Reference:** A developmental defect where part of the spinal cord is exposed through a gap in the lower back.

Advanced Reference: Affects the posterior part of the spinal column so that the arches of the vertebrae fail to meet and fuse. Often signified by a tuft of hair or *naevus* in the overlying skin leading to interference with the nervous system and developing leg weakness and *incontinence*.

Spinal **Quick Reference:** Term used to describe *spinal* anaesthesia. Intradural.

Advanced Reference: Involves the passage of a fine needle into the *subarachnoid* space which contains cerebrospinal fluid (*CSF*), followed by the injection of a local anaesthetic drug to bring about loss of pain. Spinal needle sizes are in the range of 22 G to 29 G and approximately 10 cm in length with a 15-cm version available for obese patients and a 5-cm one for paediatric use. The two most common designs are the Whitacre, which has a pencil-point tip, and the bullet-shaped Sprotte design. Needles in the range of 24 G are the most popular as the finer versions have a tendency to bend and give problems with identifying back-flow of CSF.

Spinal column **Quick Reference:** The back bone. Also termed the vertebral column.

Advanced Reference: A bony and flexible column which reaches from the base of the skull to the small of the back, made up of individual bones (*vertebrae*). It protects the *spinal cord* and articulates with the hips, ribs and skull while providing attachments for the muscles of the back.

Spinal cord **Quick Reference:** The section of the central nervous system enclosed within the vertebral column.

Advanced Reference: It extends from the *brain* as far as the second *lumbar vertebra* where it is continues as the filum terminale.

Spirochetes **Quick Reference:** (spiro-keets) Spiral bacterium.

Advanced Reference: Bacterial group responsible for, e.g. *syphilis*, leptospirosis.

Spirometer **Quick Reference:** Device used to measure lung volumes.

Advanced Reference: Various types are in use which involve moving a cylinder up a column or dial. Incorporated into ventilators and for investigative purposes in assessment clinics. Example is the vitalograph.

Splanchnic **Quick Reference:** Denotes the *viscera*.

Advanced Reference: System of neurones conducting impulses from the splanchnic (visceral) receptors.

Spleen **Quick Reference:** It forms part of the *reticulo-endothelial* and *immune* system.

Advanced Reference: It produces *antibodies*, *lymphocytes* and plasma cells and breaks down worn out red blood cells. In the *fetus*, it is the origin of red blood cells although it later gives up this activity. It lies in the upper left portion of the abdominal cavity behind the *stomach*.

Spondylolisthesis **Quick Reference:** The slipping of one *vertebra* (commonly lumbar) in front of another.

Advanced Reference: Spondylo = vertebrae; listhesis = slippage.

Sponge holder **Quick Reference:** Surgical instrument for holding small swabs.

Advanced Reference: Involves wrapping a small (e.g. 4 × 4) swab around the end of the instrument (Rampleys) and is used for prepping with antiseptic and swabbing. Also referred to as swab on a stick.

Staging **Quick Reference:** The determination of distinct phases in the course of a disease.

Advanced Reference: Utilised chiefly in the classification of *neoplasms* according to the extent of the *tumour*.

Stainless steel **Quick Reference:** Alloy of steel and chromium and sometimes with an additional metal such as nickel or molybdenum.

Advanced Reference: Practically incapable of rusting and ordinary corrosion. Used for a number of implants.

Staphylococcus **Quick Reference:** A round *(coccus) micro-organism*.

Advanced Reference: A Gram-positive organism that grows in clumps. Superficially it can infect cuts leading to boils but if it gains access to the interior of the body it can cause *pneumonia*, *septicaemia* and other *septic* conditions.

Starch　Quick Reference: A polysaccharide found in green plants.

Advanced Reference: Polysaccharides are a group of natural carbohydrates in which the molecules are made from simple sugars (monosaccharides).

Stasis　Quick Reference: To stop. Stagnation of natural movement.

Advanced Reference: Could be applied to an interruption of flow or natural movement of *blood*, lymph, *urine* and the onward peristaltic motion of the *intestines*.

Stasis dermatitis　Quick Reference: Inflammation and scaling on the lower legs. Due to impaired and/or insufficient venous return.

Advanced Reference: Characterised by *oedema*, pigmentation and often ulcers, which may lead to infection of the affected area. A common cause is varicose veins, when insufficient venous return results in pressure in the capillaries resulting in both fluid and cell leakage followed by the breakdown of red cells which is responsible for the discoloration of the skin, often referred to as venous flaring. Other related terms are varicose eczema and acroangiodermatitis.

Static　Quick Reference: With reference to theatres indicates static electricity.

Advanced Reference: Involves the build-up of an electrical charge in a non-conductor. This may occur in two unlike surfaces rubbing together, as with patient's clothing and the operating table covers. Can lead to sparking which has the potential of the clothing becoming ignited with support from oxygen. It was standard at one time for carbon to be impregnated into patient circuit tubing and table mattresses to act as a conductor.

Statins　Quick Reference: Cholesterol-lowering drugs.

Advanced Reference: Statins work by inhibiting the enzyme involved in *cholesterol* synthesis and so lower low-density lipoprotein (LDL) cholesterol.

Status　Quick Reference: In medicine, a continuing state or condition.

Advanced Reference: Examples include: status asthmaticus, in which the *asthma* continues with increasing breathlessness, as opposed to an attack which abates or recovers; also status epilepticus, in which the patient suffers repeated epileptic *convulsions* without regaining full consciousness.

Stem cell　Quick Reference: A generic cell that can make exact copies of itself indefinitely.

Advanced Reference: An unspecified cell that gives rise to a specific specialised cell via daughter cells.

Stemetil®　Quick Reference: Proprietary antiemetic. Prochlorperazine.

Advanced Reference: Used as a postoperative antiemetic and for nausea caused by vertigo, inner ear infections, etc.

Stenosis　Quick Reference: Abnormal narrowing of a natural orifice or passage.

Advanced Reference: Narrowing of the *mitral* and *aortic* valves of the heart; pyloric stenosis is narrowing of the passage from the stomach to duodenum.

Stent Quick Reference: Device used as a support or splint.

Advanced Reference: Stents are used in urology, cardiac surgery, vascular surgery, ophthalmic surgery as well as in the bile ducts and oesophagus, and in many other specialities to maintain the patency of vessels and orifices. Placed across an obstruction to maintain an open or continuous lumen. Also used as a support after creation of an anastomosis. Many absorbable types are now being introduced and trialled.

Stereotaxy Quick Reference: An intracranial approach using accurate geometric calculations to set a target in order to obtain biopsy samples or perform a specialised neurosurgical procedure.

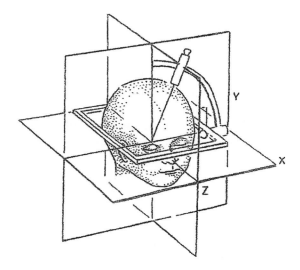

Principles of stereotactic apparatus used to locate (and treat) the target area.

Fig. 16. Principles of stereotactic apparatus. Reprinted with permission from Elsevier

Advanced Reference: Predetermined anatomical landmarks are used as a guide. Special head fixation devices have been developed for use with radiography, fluoroscopy, computerised tomography scans and magnetic resonance imaging to permit accurate placement of a probe directed at the target area inside the skull.

Sterile field Quick Reference: Indicates an area that has been made free from contamination.

Advanced Reference: The surgical sterile field refers to the area designated aseptic, surrounding the operative site. Covered, screened and isolated with sterile drapes and the domain of only those prepared by washing and gloving, who are gowned appropriately.

Sterilisation   Quick Reference: Actually indicates the inability for living things to reproduce.

Advanced Reference: Can be used to mean operative procedures such as vasectomy and tubal ligation/clipping, but generally indicates the process of ridding articles of bacteria and infection, which can be done via a number of methods, i.e. steam, heat, chemical, gas or irradiation.

Sternal notch   Quick Reference: Anatomical landmark located at the upper end of the sternum.

Advanced Reference: The notch where the sternum reaches the cricoid area of the neck.

Sternomastoid   Quick Reference: Large muscle at the side of the neck.

Advanced Reference: The muscle extends from the top of the sternum and clavicle to the skull behind the ear. It facilitates flexing of the head and rotation of the neck. Also a common landmark during *CVP* cannula/catheter insertion.

Sternum   Quick Reference: The breast bone.

Advanced Reference: The flat bone at the front and centre of the chest to which the upper ribs are attached. The upper part, or manubrium, slopes downwards and forwards making an angle with the vertical body section. A joint at the manubrium allows the sternum to straighten when the ribs rise during inspiration.

Steroids   Quick Reference: Naturally occurring and synthetic agents based on sterone.

Advanced Reference: In the body they include *hormones* of the adrenal cortex and sex glands (oestrogen, testosterone).

Stethoscope   Quick Reference: Instrument used to listen to internal body sounds.

Advanced Reference: Used mainly for listening to heart and lungs. Invented by a French physician, traditionally consists of listening ear pieces fitted to tubing that ends in a pick-up for placing on the body surface. There are variations for listening to fetal heartbeat in the uterus as well as oesophageal stethoscopes, all available in manual and electronic models.

Stoma   Quick Reference: A mouth-like opening.

Advanced Reference: Usually refers to an artificial opening made in the skin surface as a collection point/conduit for various internal anatomy, e.g. *colostomy, ileostomy*.

Stomach   Quick Reference: That part of the digestive tract between the lower end of the oesophagus and the beginning of the intestine.

Advanced Reference: The first part of the stomach is the *fundus*, which forms a dome under the left side of the *diaphragm*. The second part, the body, broadens and runs down from the fundus to the third part, the *antrum*, which is funnel-shaped and travels upwards to the right and ends in the midline of the body at the pylorus, which is a muscular tube that acts as a valve between the stomach and the ***duodenum***.

Strabismus   Quick Reference: Squint. Also known as heterotropia.

Advanced Reference: A mostly congenital condition in which the two eyes point in different directions. May be divergent with the eyes deviated out, or convergent where they point inwards, or vertical when the faulty eye points up or down. Due to an imbalance of the eye muscles so that there is poor correlation between focusing and convergence of the axes of the eyes.

Streptococcus   Quick Reference: A round Gram-positive ***micro-organism*** that grows in chains.

Advanced Reference: Various strains are responsible for causing ***pneumonia, endocarditis*** and scarlet fever.

Streptokinase   Quick Reference: Enzyme used therapeutically as a fibrinolytic agent, i.e. ***thrombolytic***, clot buster.

Advanced Reference: One of a number of agents used to break down clots in the treatment of thrombosis and embolism.

Streptomycin   Quick Reference: An **antibiotic**.

Advanced Reference: Mostly used now in the treatment of tuberculosis (TB) and usually in combination with other antibiotics.

Stress ulcer   Quick Reference: Gastrointestinal mucosa injury related to critical illness. Common to ICU patients, especially those on long-term ventilation. Also referred to as Curling's ulcer.

Advanced Reference: Regularly witnessed in patients suffering burns, shock or trauma. Due to a number of factors including reduced blood flow, imbalance in oxygen supply, loss of the ability to neutralise acid and a reduction in the production of ***prostaglandin***. The condition is not related to a history of peptic ulcer disorder.

Stricture   Quick Reference: A narrowing in cavity.

Advanced Reference: Can be of congenital origin or due to disease. Many urethral strictures are due to gonococcal infection.

Stridor   Quick Reference: Noise/sound of the respiratory tract.

Advanced Reference: Sound made by the breath passing an obstruction in the larynx or trachea.

Stripper   Quick Reference: A surgical instrument used for removal of varicose veins, usually of the leg.

Advanced Reference: Made of flexible, sprung metal with a removable cone end (choc). The wire is threaded down the vein then the choc is attached and pulled back up the vessel, so stripping out the vein from the surrounding tissue.

Stroke   Quick Reference: A CVA – cerebrovascular accident. Sudden interference with the blood supply to a part of the brain.

Advanced Reference: Caused by a haemorrhage, thrombosis or embolism occurring in a blood vessel which supplies any part of the brain, resulting in unconsciousness and paralysis and can be fatal.

Stroma   **Quick Reference:** Connective tissue framework of an organ.

Advanced Reference: As distinct from tissues that perform specialised functions of the organ.

Stupefy   **Quick Reference:** To render insensible. To be groggy.

Advanced Reference: Could be used to describe the effect of many drugs used in anaesthesia, narcotics, or induction agents.

Stylette   **Quick Reference:** (sti-let) Endotracheal tube (ETT) introducer.

Advanced Reference: A malleable introducer designed to assist re-shaping of the ETT in the event of *difficult intubation*. Made from various materials including metal, copper, plastic and plastic-coated metal.

Subarachnoid   **Quick Reference:** Fluid-filled space between the coverings of the brain and spinal cord.

Advanced Reference: The subarachnoid space lies beneath the arachnoid membrane and pia mater of the brain and contains cerebrospinal fluid (CSF).

Subclavian   **Quick Reference:** Under the collar bone (clavicle).

Advanced Reference: The subclavian artery and vein accompany each other below the clavicle. The vein is regularly used for *CVP* insertion.

Sublimaze®   **Quick Reference:** Fentanyl. Narcotic analgesic.

Advanced Reference: Synthetic drug derived from pethidine and commonly used for intraoperative analgesia. In small doses lasts approximately 30 min but given in larger boluses can have a duration of 2–3 h. A powerful respiratory depressant but has virtually no cardiovascular effects.

Suction   **Quick Reference:** Indicates a suction machine or the act of suctioning.

Advanced Reference: General term to indicate a suction machine for use in all patient areas of theatre. Hospital suction machines tend to be electrically powered, mechanically driven or function via a central vacuum system. They all utilise a vacuum process where 0 (zero) is equal to atmospheric pressure and a suction increase is indicated by a rise in vacuum pressure. Across the range of paediatrics through to adults airway suction is in the range of 50 mmHg to 150 mmHg, with lower readings utilised for wound drainage and cell salvage machines, as high suction in this setting is thought to cause *haemolysis*.

Sufentanil   **Quick Reference:** Synthetic opioid.

Advanced Reference: A relative of fentanyl with similar effects but less potent and has a shorter elimination period.

Sugam(m)adex   **Quick Reference:** A reversal agent specific to the muscle relaxant *rocuronium*.

Advanced Reference: Because of its mode of action it does not rely on the inhibition of *acetylcholinesterases* therefore avoiding the instability potential of neostigmine (*anticholinesterase*) and atropine (*antimuscarinic*).

Sulphonamide   **Quick Reference:** (sul-fon-a-mide) Literally a sulphur drug.

Advanced Reference: Drugs that prevent the growth of bacteria. Often confused with antibiotics but are in fact a distinct group and in some cases may be used as an alternative where there may be sensitivity to antibiotics.

Sulphonic Acid   **Quick Reference:** (RSO_3H) A group of strong organic acids.

Advanced Reference: Used in the manufacture of detergents, dyes and drugs such as antibacterial sulphur drugs.

Sulphur   **Quick Reference:** Yellow non-metallic element.

Advanced Reference: It is widely distributed in both the free state and in compounds forming sulphates, sulphides and oxides.

Summer smog   **Quick Reference:** Occurs when sunlight reacts with pollutants in the air of mainly urban areas producing a low level ozone.

Advanced Reference: The main pollutants are nitrogen dioxide, sulphur dioxide and *carbon monoxide*, with motor vehicles being the major contributor. Those with *asthma*, heart and lung disease are the most affected.

Sump drain   **Quick Reference:** A double-lumen surgical wound drain.

Advanced Reference: Made of plastic or rubber and used to drain accumulated fluids from cavities. Can be used with or without positive suction.

Supination   **Quick Reference:** Indicates turning the hand so that the palm is uppermost.

Advanced Reference: The opposite is *pronation*. The supinator muscle of the forearm acts to turn the hand upwards.

Supine   **Quick Reference:** Positioned face up.

Advanced Reference: A patient flat on their back, possibly the most common surgical position.

Supine hypotension syndrome   **Quick Reference:** Most commonly associated with late-stage pregnancy and during labour when a woman is lying flat on her back.

Advanced Reference: The fall in blood pressure is due to compression of the large pelvic veins and inferior *vena cava* by the pregnant uterus leading to a diminished return of blood to the right side of the heart and a low-output hypotension. Also referred to as veno or *aortocaval compression*.

Suppository   **Quick Reference:** A solid medicated capsule designed to dissolve at body temperature.

Advanced Reference: Prepared for rectal and vaginal use. Rectal versions are used to deliver both locally acting medications and those designed to be absorbed and act on other sites, whereas those given vaginally are used to treat gynaecological disorders.

Suppuration   Quick Reference: The formation of *pus*.

Advanced Reference: A suppurating wound is one discharging pus.

Supranuclear palsy   Quick Reference: Disorder characterised by muscle stiffness.

Advanced Reference: Also includes the inability to move the eyes and weakness of the throat muscles.

Suprapubic   Quick Reference: Indicates above the pubic bone.

Advanced Reference: Used in relation to a number of procedures. Suprapubic cystotomy involves making an incision or opening into the urinary bladder. Suprapubic prostatectomy indicates the removal of the prostate gland by an approach from above the pubic bone, as opposed to transurethral.

Supraventricular   Quick Reference: Situated or occurring superior to the ventricles.

Advanced Reference: Any cardiac rhythm originating above the ventricles either normally in the *SA node* or abnormally elsewhere in the *atria* or in the *AV node*, i.e. supraventricular *arrhythmia*.

Surfactant   Quick Reference: Lubricating agent.

Advanced Reference: Pulmonary surfactant is secreted by the alveoli, lowering surface tension and so allowing free expansion of the lungs and chest wall. An absence of surfactant can lead to respiratory distress syndrome.

Surgical assistant   Quick Reference: Non-medical specialist working alongside the surgeon carrying out a number of extended roles under supervision.

Advanced Reference: Originally a USA-based role, developed initially in the cardiac surgery speciality to harvest the *saphenous* vein during bypass procedures. Has become established within the UK working in several specialities.

Often mistakenly confused with scrub assistant who supervises and accounts for instrumentation and surgical adjuncts, while first and second assistants literally provide extra hands to the surgeon rather than performing autonomously.

Surgical instrument mechanics and structure   Quick Reference: The unique and varying workings of basic instruments.

Advanced Reference: Grasping instruments and scissors especially have many individual and unique aspects, i.e. joints, teeth, serrated jaws, locking ratchets, to suit the mechanical need, type of tissue and the access that certain procedures can present.

Surgical technologist   Quick Reference: USA-based health professional.

Advanced Reference: Opposite number to UK-based scrub assistant (scrub-nurse or ODP). Direct-entry specialist who works alongside and interchangeably with nurses.

Surgicel   Quick Reference: Surgical haemostatic agent.

Advanced Reference: Oxidised cellulose, reacts with body tissues and swells to form a seal over the area of bleeding.

Surrogate **Quick Reference:** Substitute.

Advanced Reference: One put into the place of another, e.g. surrogate mother.

Sus **Quick Reference:** Form of tobacco preparation.

Advanced reference: It is placed under the lip allowing for absorption of *nicotine* into the bloodstream. Although it reduces the likelihood of diseases associated with conventional smoking of tobacco, there is evidence that it can cause cancers of the *pancreas* and oral cavity as well as increasing the risk of *hypotension* and *heart attack*.

Suture **Quick Reference:** A stitch used to close a wound; or in relation to anatomy, a junction between two bones as in the cranium and occipital regions.

Advanced Reference: Sutures of all sizes and materials are used to close and repair during surgery. May be natural or synthetic, absorbable or non-absorbable, mono- or multifilament. Suturing describes the act of sewing; methods and styles vary according to need and tissue involved. Attached needles are also specific to need and can be blunt, cutting, round-bodied as well as straight, or curved.

Suxamethonium **Quick Reference:** A depolarising muscle relaxant also known as Scoline, Anectine®, succinylcholine and colloquially as Sux.

Advanced Reference: A depolarising neuromuscular blocker used to induce short duration muscle relaxation. It imitates the action of *acetylcholine* at the neuromuscular junction and is then degraded by pseudocholinesterase, which is a slower process than that of acetylcholinesterase breaking down acetylcholine. Following injection there is a period of stimulation of the acetylcholine receptor, which results in disorganised muscle contractions (*fasciculation*).

Swab **Quick Reference:** An item used to absorb blood.

Advanced Reference: Besides being used as an absorbent, swabs can be used to pack cavities during surgery and aid blunt dissection. Usually made of cotton gauze, they are available in a range of sizes and designs. There are also pledglets and *patties* (small swabs) for finer work. All swabs that are to enter the body should have some form of detection system in case they are mislaid, usually an X-ray-detectable strip. The swab count is a safety monitoring measure to reduce the possibility of loss and, if so, at what stage their loss occurred.

Swage **Quick Reference:** Needle that is permanently attached to a suture.

Advanced Reference: More accurately refers to the area of a needle where the suture is attached rather than the entire product.

Swan-Ganz catheter **Quick Reference:** Balloon-tipped multi-lumen catheter used to measure pulmonary artery pressures.

Advanced Reference: Also termed pulmonary artery and floatation catheter. Via venous access, the catheter is inserted and guided (floated) into the right

Pulmonary Artery Catheterisation

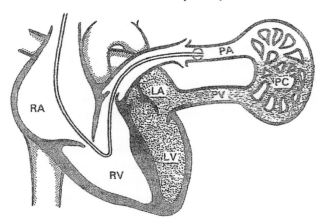

Pulmonary artery wedge pressure. Flow-guided balloon-tipped pulmonary artery catheter. RV, right ventricle; RA, right atrium; LV, left ventricle; LA, left atrium; PA, pulmonary artery; PV, pulmonary vein; PC, pulmonary capillary bed.

Fig. 17. Pulmonary artery catheter. Reprinted with permission from Elsevier

atrium, on to the right ventricle and eventually the pulmonary artery in order to obtain diagnostic pressure readings of ventricular function and output performance indirectly via the pulmonary artery (pulmonary wedge pressure – PWP).

Symbiosis **Quick Reference:** An association between two organisms.

Advanced Reference: Living together or close association of two dissimilar organisms.

Symmetry **Quick Reference:** (sim-et-ree) Equal on both sides.

Advanced Reference: Where body parts are arranged regularly around a central axis. *Asymmetry* is a lack of symmetry in corresponding parts or sides of the body. Dissymmetry indicates an absence of symmetry.

Sympathectomy **Quick Reference:** Surgical division of sympathetic nerve fibres.

Advanced Reference: Carried out to improve circulation to a part of the body by reducing sympathetic activity.

Sympathetic **Quick Reference:** Refers to part of the *autonomic nervous system*.

Advanced Reference: Responsible for regulating the subconscious autonomic processes.

Sympathomimetic **Quick Reference:** Mimicking the effects of the *sympathetic* nervous system.

Advanced Reference: Includes *amines* that have the same action as *catecholamines* such as epinephrine (*adrenaline*), norepinephrine (*noradrenaline*) and *dopamine*.

Symphysis pubis Quick Reference: The cartilaginous junction of the two pubic bones.

Advanced Reference: A symphysis is a joint separated by cartilage which has the effect of limiting movement and makes the structure rigid.

Synapse Quick Reference: Point where processes of different nerve cells meet.

Advanced Reference: Where nerve impulses are transmitted by the release of chemical substances.

Synchronised intermittent mandatory ventilation Quick Reference: (SIMV) A breathing mode that allows the mechanical ventilator to synchronise with the patient's respiratory cycle.

Advanced Reference: SIMV allows the patient to breathe whilst the ventilator guarantees a mandatory number of breaths and the synchronisation of the ventilator detects the patient's respiratory cycle preventing machine inspiration coinciding with the patient's expiration.

Syncope Quick Reference: Sudden loss of consciousness, a faint.

Advanced Reference: Commonly due to a fall in blood pressure which interrupts circulation to the brain.

Syndrome Quick Reference: A set or combination of *signs and symptoms*.

Advanced Reference: As a syndrome, these signs and symptoms occur together in a definite pattern.

Synergistically Quick Reference: Acting together.

Advanced Reference: Organs that act in concert with one another.

Synovial Quick Reference: Indicates the area incorporating a joint.

Advanced Reference: Synovial fluid is secreted by the synovial membranes, and acts as a lubricant. *Synovitis* is inflammation of the membrane.

Synovitis Quick Reference: Inflammation of the *synovial* membrane.

Advanced Reference: The synovial membrane lines the joints, *tendon* sheaths and *bursae* and secretes a lubricating fluid.

Synthesis Quick Reference: The process of combining separate elements.

Advanced Reference: The production of a compound by a chemical reaction.

Synthetic Quick Reference: Artificial, not naturally created.

Advanced Reference: Produced by chemical *synthesis*.

Synthetic absorbable suture materials Quick Reference: Many are available, made from synthetic polymers.

Advanced Reference: Examples are polydioxanone (PDO), polyglycolide (PGA), polylactic acid (PLA), polycaprolactone (PCL). All have differing degradation durations and are *biocompatible* and *biodegradable*.

Syntocinon® **Quick Reference:** Proprietary preparation of the hormone *oxytocin*.

Advanced Reference: Brings about increased contraction of the uterus during labour. Administered therapeutically to induce or assist labour and control postnatal bleeding. Used in similar circumstances to *ergometrine*.

Syntometrine® **Quick Reference:** A proprietary preparation of the alkaloid ergometrine together with oxytocin. Produces similar effects to *ergometrine* and *Syntocinon®*.

Advanced Reference: Used during the final stages of labour to contract the uterus and control postnatal bleeding.

Syphilis **Quick Reference:** Sexually transmitted disease.

Advanced Reference: A chronic disease caused by bacteria entering the body during sexual intercourse. Treatment is with *penicillin*, or, in those sensitive, *tetracycline* and *erythromycin*. The disease passes through stages ranging from the early infection stage followed by a latent period of many years. The later, non-infectious stage, involves disorders of the nervous and vascular systems.

Systemic **Quick Reference:** Affecting the entire body (system).

Advanced Reference: Rather than a single organ or body part. The systemic circulation (circulatory system, minus pulmonary circulation). Systemic disease is one where the effects are present throughout the body, as opposed to a localised condition or disease.

Systole **Quick Reference:** Contraction period of the heart muscle.

Advanced Reference: Atrial systole is the phase when blood is pumped from the atria to the ventricles, while ventricular systole involves the pumping of blood into the aorta and pulmonary arteries.

T

Tachycardia **Quick Reference:** (tacky-cardia) Rapid heartbeat. Tachy indicates fast or rapid.

Advanced Reference: May be due to many causes: fever, emotional change, exercise, infection, pain, anaemia, haemorrhage, drugs or disorders of cardiac rhythm. Can also be of atrial, *supraventricular* or ventricular origin.

Tamiflu® **Quick Reference:** An anti-viral drug.

Advanced Reference: Recognised internationally as the drug of choice in the event of pandemic flu.

Tamoxifen® **Quick Reference:** An oral non-steroidal medication used in the treatment of breast cancer.

Advanced Reference: Has anti-oestrogen action and is used as an antineoplastic in the prophylaxis and treatment of breast cancer.

Tamponade **Quick Reference:** Abnormal pressure on a part of the body which affects its function.

Advanced Reference: An example is cardiac tamponade, when the presence of fluid, e.g. blood, between the *pericardium* and the heart itself exerts excessive pressure which interferes with normal function.

Tannin **Quick Reference:** Tannic acid. An *astringent* found in plants.

Advanced Reference: Used as a suppository in the treatment of haemorrhoids and to treat burns. Its use is mostly discontinued now as it is suspected of causing liver damage.

Tare weight **Quick Reference:** Empty weight.

Advanced Reference: Marking on a nitrous oxide cylinder to indicate the weight of the empty cylinder. Contents can be assessed by weight because the contents are liquid and not a gas.

Tarsus **Quick Reference:** Base of the foot. Of the seven tarsal bones only one, the talus, articulates with the leg to form the ankle joint.

Advanced Reference: Also, it is the flat firm plate of connective tissue which supports the eyelid.

TED stockings **Quick Reference:** Thromboembolism deterrent.

Advanced Reference: Worn by the patient throughout the perioperative period with the intention of preventing venous stasis and pooling in the legs (calves) and so reducing the potential for thrombus formation.

Temazepam **Quick Reference:** Short-acting *benzodiazepine*.

Advanced Reference: Often used to treat insomnia and regularly as a premedication.

Temgesic® **Quick Reference:** Narcotic analgesic.

Advanced Reference: Used in many forms of pain relief, it is a preparation of the opiate buprenorphine hydrochloride.

Temporomandibular joint **Quick Reference:** Joint between the temporal bone of the skull and the lower jaw.

Advanced Reference: The joint lies just in front of the ear and is of a sliding-hinge design which allows movement of the mandible from side to side. The two bones are separated by a plate of cartilage inside the joint. Stiffness, deformity and/or injury to this joint may lead to difficult intubation.

Tendon **Quick Reference:** Sinew.

Advanced Reference: Cord structure comprised of fibrous tissue which attaches muscle to bone.

Tenesmus **Quick Reference:** A painful condition of either bladder or bowel.

Advanced Reference: An uncomfortable and painful condition enhanced by straining on attempting to empty bladder or bowel.

Tenosynovitis **Quick Reference:** Inflammation of mucous membranes around tendons.

Advanced Reference: The resultant swelling associated with the inflammation compresses the nerve.

Tenotomy **Quick Reference:** Surgical division of a tendon.

Advanced Reference: An operative procedure on the tendon carried out to correct a deformity caused by shortening. Also an ophthalmic procedure to correct a squint (*strabismus*).

TENS **Quick Reference:** Transcutaneous electrical nerve stimulation. Method of pain relief.

Advanced Reference: The power unit (pulse generator and transformer) is attached to the skin via electrodes and uses electric signals to stimulate nerves through unbroken skin. Used in palliative care, to treat neuropathic (damaged nerves) pain and in obstetrics during labour.

Other forms of neurostimulation include: percutaneous tibial nerve stimulation (PTNS), where the post tibial nerve at the ankle is stimulated in the treatment of a variety of urological conditions such as overactive bladder (OAB); microcurrent electrical neuromuscular stimulation (MENS) is another and is utilised to treat macular degeneration, wound healing, tendon repair and ligament rupture.

Tensile **Quick Reference:** Tensile strength is the greatest longitudinal stress a substance can withstand without tearing apart.

Advanced Reference: Alternatively, a measure of the resistance that a material offers to stress before breaking. Term related to the strength of suture material.

Teratogenicity **Quick Reference:** Process leading to developmental abnormalities in the *fetus*.

Advanced Reference: A teratogen indicates any substance or process that causes the formation of developmental abnormalities in a fetus.

Termination   **Quick Reference:** Commonly used to indicate a termination of pregnancy.

Advanced Reference: Abortion, usually surgical, but can include alternative methods using drugs.

Test dose   **Quick Reference:** Administration of a small amount of a drug to test reaction.

Advanced Reference: Term applied to injection of local anaesthetic in epidural procedures and intravenous antibiotics. With epidural, a small dose of drug is injected before the main dose in order to identify accidental subarachnoid or intravenous injection. With antibiotics it is done to determine sensitivity to the drug.

Testis   **Quick Reference:** The male sex organs contained within the *scrotum*. Testicles.

Advanced Reference: They produce spermatozoa and the male sex hormones. In the fetus they are housed within the abdomen but in normal circumstances descend after birth; if not, they may become non-functional and even malignant and need to be removed. Removal of a testicle is termed *orchidectomy*.

Testosterone   **Quick Reference:** Male sex hormone, being the principal hormone of the testis.

Advanced Reference: Testosterone is necessary for the development of the secondary sexual characteristics, i.e. beard growth, pubic hair, enlargement of the genital organs, lowering of the voice at puberty together with a change in body shape. Also involved in the production of semen.

Tetanus   **Quick Reference:** An acute disease affecting the nervous system.

Advanced Reference: Caused by the micro-organism *Clostridium tetani*. Contamination is commonly from soil. Initially, muscle stiffness occurs around the site of the wound, then followed by rigidity of the face and neck muscles and the mouth becomes difficult to open fully (lock-jaw). Prevention is by active immunisation with tetanus toxoid. Booster doses are given at recommended intervals.

Tetracaine   **Quick Reference:** Local anaesthetic. Also available as amethocaine.

Advanced Reference: Available mainly as a topical 4% gel and in eye drops.

Tetracyclines   **Quick Reference:** Antibiotic class of drugs.

Advanced Reference: They have broad-spectrum activity but many organisms have developed resistance but they are still used to treat *Chlamydia* and *Rickettsia*. Tetracyclines are deposited in growing bones and teeth, staining the latter yellow, and are therefore not given to pregnant women, those breast-feeding or children under 12 years of age.

Tetrahydrocannabinol Quick Reference: (THC) The active ingredient of marijuana, cannabis and hashish.

Advanced Reference: Although used for its relaxing properties, the use of THC-derived drugs can also lead to *paranoia* and anxiety.

Tetraplegia Quick Reference: Also referred to as quadriplegia.

Advanced Reference: Paralysis of all four limbs.

Thalamonal® Quick Reference: A proprietary preparation of *fentanyl* and *droperidol*.

Advanced Reference: This preparation of a narcotic and tranquilliser/anti-emetic may be used for patients undergoing diagnostic or minor surgical procedures.

Thalamus Quick Reference: Two masses of nerve cells positioned at the base of the *cerebrum*.

Advanced Reference: Sensations of all kind are carried to the thalamus and then relayed to the cerebral cortex where they are perceived. If the thalamus is damaged, the perception of pain sensation can be affected.

Thalassaemia Quick Reference: (thal-a-seem-ea) An inherited defect in the formation of *haemoglobin*. Widespread in the Mediterranean, Asia and Africa.

Advanced Reference: The initial problem is anaemia but further symptoms include enlargement of the spleen and abnormalities of the bone marrow. Can be inherited from either one or both parents, so deciding severity. Treatment is with repeated blood transfusions.

Thalidomide Quick Reference: Morning sickness medication.

Advanced Reference: Withdrawn in 1961 after thousands of children were born with limb deformities after it had been taken as a morning sickness remedy during pregnancy. Now being used in the treatment of cancer, it prevents the creation of new blood vessels and so inhibits tumour growth. It was this property that caused the original limb development problems, as the drug prevented blood vessel growth to supply the arms and legs.

Thallium Quick Reference: Soft white poisonous metallic element. Utilised as a radioactive *isotope* – thallium 201.

Advanced Reference: Used in the treatment of many types of tumour including testicular cancer and has a half-life of 3.05 days. Its poisonous effects are cumulative and lead to liver damage, bone destruction and permanent hair loss.

Theophylline Quick Reference: A drug which dilates the bronchi.

Advanced Reference: Derived from tea leaves or made synthetically, theophylline is used in the treatment of *asthma* and *bronchospasm*.

Therapeutics Quick Reference: The study of the science of treating disease.

Advanced Reference: Therapy is the treatment of disease.

Therm Quick Reference: Unit of heat.

Advanced Reference: Thermal indicates a relationship to heat.

Thermistor   **Quick Reference:** Device involved in temperature measurement.

Advanced Reference: Found in temperature probes and pulmonary artery (PA) catheters for assisting in measuring cardiac output. A semiconductor whose resistance decreases as the *ambient* temperature increases. Used to measure extremely small temperature changes.

Thermocouple   **Quick Reference:** Device involved in identifying and reacting to temperature change.

Advanced Reference: Involves two strips of dissimilar metals which expand at different rates. The metals expand and contract in response to temperature changes and produce an electrical potential that then makes reference to pre-settings. Found in autoclaves.

Thermodilution   **Quick Reference:** Method of measuring blood flow.

Advanced Reference: Involves the injection of a known quantity of cool or cold indicator such as saline solution or distilled water into the cardiovascular system. Measurements are then taken using a *thermistor* over time and at a specific point in the system.

Thermogenic   **Quick Reference:** Relating to heat or the production of heat.

Advanced Reference: Fat (*adipose*) is the thermogenic tissue of the body.

Thermoplastics   **Quick Reference:** Plastic that softens under heat.

Advanced Reference: Are capable of being moulded into shape with pressure, then harden on cooling without undergoing a chemical change.

Thermoregulation   **Quick Reference:** Regulation of temperature such as the body heat of warm-blooded animals. Thermostasis.

Advanced Reference: In humans this involves *homeostasis*.

Thermostat   **Quick Reference:** Apparatus for regulating temperature.

Advanced Reference: Automatically maintains temperature between certain set levels.

Thiazides   **Quick Reference:** Diuretic group of drugs.

Advanced Reference: They act on the first part of the convoluted tubule in the kidney, blocking the re-absorption of sodium. Used in the treatment of high blood pressure and heart failure.

Thiopentone   **Quick Reference:** IV anaesthetic agent. Pentothal sodium or intraval sodium.

Advanced Reference: Short-acting barbiturate used in a 2.5% solution in the UK and 5% in the USA. Also referred to as the truth drug in the USA as it is used in small increments to question suspected criminals. Stored as a yellow powder for reconstitution with sterile water. Gives off a smell and taste of garlic due to the sulphur content. Although active as a sleep-inducing agent for only minutes, remains in the circulation for up to 24 h. Also used as an anticonvulsive agent.

Thomas splint   **Quick Reference:** Splint used to immobilise leg (knee, femur).

Advanced Reference: The Thomas splint is a cylindrical frame which fits over the limb right up to the groin. Slings are fitted to rest the leg on, adhesive tape is affixed to the lower leg, and secure the splint to the leg, and downward traction and weights are applied to assist reduction of the fracture. Mostly superseded now by external fixation (scaffolding) devices.

Thoracic   Quick Reference: In relation to the chest cavity (*thorax*).

Advanced Reference: Thoracic surgery indicates procedures carried out on or within the chest cavity.

Thoracic duct   Quick Reference: The large *lymph* vessel that begins at the cisterna chyli, which is a sac lying adjacent to the aorta at the opening of the *diaphragm*.

Advanced Reference: Into this area drains the right and left lumbar lymph trunks, which serve the lower limbs and intestinal trunk. From here the thoracic duct runs up through the thorax to the neck and comes to lie on the right side of the oesophagus. The lymph carried by the thoracic duct runs into the subclavian vein. Also, the right lymphatic duct, which is about 1 cm in length, lies at the root of the neck and opens into the right subclavian vein. This duct also receives lymph from the right half of the thorax, head and neck and right arm.

Thoracocentesis   Quick Reference: Thoraco = chest, centesis = puncture.

Advanced Reference: Involves removal of fluid from the pleura via needle biopsy.

Thoracoscopy   Quick Reference: Inspection of the interior chest through an endoscope.

Advanced Reference: More specifically involves examination of the pleural cavity as well as the thoracic cavity.

Thorax   Quick Reference: The chest compartment.

Advanced Reference: The thorax is enclosed by the ribs, reaching from the first rib to the diaphragm.

Throat spray   Quick Reference: Refers to a local anaesthetic spray used in anaesthesia.

Advanced Reference: Used after induction to spray the laryngeal and tracheal mucosa with a topical lignocaine (4%) preparation, which is intended to decrease the stimulus and presence of the endotracheal tube. Originally the sprays were reusable/refillable models (Macintosh, Forrester) but more recently replaced with sealed, pre-loaded disposable versions.

Throb   Quick Reference: To beat or pulse.

Advanced Reference: Felt in the area of injury or infection when the pain is likened to a throbbing sensation.

Thrombin   Quick Reference: An enzyme involved in the coagulation of blood.

Advanced Reference: Thrombin converts fibrinogen to fibrin during the blood-clotting process.

Thrombocytopenia   **Quick Reference:** (thrombo-sigh-toe-peen-ea) Deficiency in the number of platelets circulating in the blood.

Advanced Reference: May lead to multiple small haemorrhages especially under the skin (purpura) in addition to prolonged bleeding after injury and spontaneous bruising. Due to disturbances in the bone marrow where platelets are produced and to a lesser degree via inheritance.

Thrombocytosis   **Quick Reference:** An increase in the number of platelets in the blood.

Advanced Reference: May be due to chronic infection, cancers and blood diseases. Can lead to intravascular clotting.

Thromboembolic   **Quick Reference:** Indicates a potential for the development of thrombi.

Advanced Reference: Could indicate an individual, procedure, or material.

Thrombogenic   **Quick Reference:** Producing a *thrombus* or clot.

Advanced Reference: Thrombogenic indicates a lower or reduced tendency to form a thrombus. Many medical and surgical sundries such as vascular catheters and cannulas or vascular grafts are coated or impregnated with anticoagulant substances to reduce clotting potential.

Thrombolysis   **Quick Reference:** The breakdown of a thrombus.

Advanced Reference: Usually by infusion of an enzyme such as *streptokinase*. Thrombolytic indicates an agent with the ability to dissolve thrombi.

Thrombolytics   **Quick Reference:** Clot busters.

Advanced Reference: Group of drugs, injected intravenously, used to break down clots following coronary thrombosis, stroke, etc. Work by adjusting plasminogen action. *Streptokinase* was an early version, others in use include *urokinase*, alteplase (tPH), tenecteplase (TNK).

Thrombophilia   **Quick Reference:** (thrombo-fill-ea) A disorder in which blood clots easily or excessively.

Advanced Reference: Those with thrombophilia need to have their thrombin levels tested, *anticoagulant* therapy and to be screened for clotting (*DVT*) potential.

Thrombophlebitis   **Quick Reference:** Inflammation of a vein with consequent thrombosis.

Advanced Reference: With reference to theatre patients, it is commonly associated with postoperative effects of IV cannulation sites. Following removal of the cannula, the site often forms a hard clot and inflammation of the vessel lining occluding the lumen.

Thrombo-prophylactic   **Quick Reference:** (thrombo-pro-fil-actic) Blood thinning or antithrombus actions and activity.

Advanced Reference: Refers to drugs or procedures that are designed to prevent the creation of thrombi. In relation to surgery this includes preoperative **heparin** and the use of **TED stockings** and mechanical devices that massage the lower limbs in order to prevent pooling of blood.

Thrombosis   **Quick Reference:** Formation of a clot or thrombus in a blood vessel.

Advanced Reference: May occur in arteries when the walls have been roughened by atherosclerosis or in veins when the circulation becomes sluggish or stagnant. A thrombus indicates a blood clot that formed within the vessel (usually a vein) and is stationary. Once it moves from its original site, it is termed an **embolus**.

Thymol   **Quick Reference:** A mild antiseptic derived from oil of thyme.

Advanced Reference: A hydrocarbon also used as an antioxidant in some volatile agents. Other uses are as a disinfectant, mouthwash and deodorant.

Thymus   **Quick Reference:** Gland which lies at the root of the neck behind the breastbone in the upper mediastinum.

Advanced Reference: The gland grows from birth to puberty and thereafter diminishes in size but remains active. It is an important part of the lymphatic system, being responsible for the formation of lymphocytes (T-cells) which are essential in the immune reaction.

Thyroid   **Quick Reference:** A ductless gland lying in the neck.

Advanced Reference: The thyroid lies at the front of the neck in front of the trachea and just below the larynx. It has two lobes and secretes two hormones, of which thyroxine is the most prominent. Swelling of the gland is known as a goitre and normal function of the gland depends on an adequate intake of **iodine** in the diet.

Thyrotoxicosis   **Quick Reference:** Overactivity of the **thyroid** gland.

Advanced Reference: Also termed hyperthyroidism. Involves enlargement of the gland and a speeding up of metabolism, resulting in nervousness, sweating, emotional overactivity and loss of weight.

Thyroxine   **Quick Reference:** *Hormone* synthesised and secreted by the **thyroid** gland.

Advanced Reference: Absence of thyroxine leads to underactivity (**hypothyroidism**) of the thyroid. Can be administered orally.

TIA   **Quick Reference:** Transient ischaemic attack. Minor stroke.

Advanced Reference: Involves numbness in the affected part, face, arm, etc., sometimes with speech disturbance, nausea, double vision but not usually loss of consciousness. It is due to small clots partially blocking arteries in the brain and connected nerves lose function temporarily; unlike a major stroke, where there is no return of function. However, TIAs may indicate future stroke.

Tibia   **Quick Reference:** The shin bone.

Advanced Reference: One of the two parallel bones in the lower leg which extend from the knee to the ankle. Corresponding with the radius in the forearm. The tibia is much more heavily built as it carries all the body weight.

Tidal volume   Quick Reference: Volume of air that moves into the lungs with each inspiration.

Advanced Reference: Tidal volume (TV) is used in relation to minute volume (MV) and respiratory rate (RR).

$MV = TV \times RR$.

Time   Quick Reference: Refers to seconds, minutes and hours.

Advanced Reference: Seconds (abbreviation and symbol, s) is the SI base unit of time. A millisecond = one-thousandth of a second, kilosecond = 1000 seconds.

Minute (symbol and abbreviation, min) is not recognised as an official SI unit; 1/60th of an hour.

Hour (symbol, h), also not an official SI unit of time; 1/24th of a median (day).

Tincture   Quick Reference: An alcoholic solution of a medication.

Advanced Reference: Commonly seen in theatres as in relation to antiseptics, e.g. tincture of iodine, alcoholic chlorhexidine (hibitane), more than actual drug preparations.

Tinea   Quick Reference: Superficial fungal infection of the skin.

Advanced Reference: Tinea pedis is athlete's foot, which produces moist lesions between the toes. Other infections of this group involve the nails, groin, scalp and ringworm.

Tinnitus   Quick Reference: Noises in the ear.

Advanced Reference: May be buzzing, ringing, hissing, or whistling and may follow disease of the *auditory* nerve or *cochlea*.

Tissue fluid   Quick Reference: Also termed extracellular fluid.

Advanced Reference: Watery fluid percolating through all the minute spaces of/between the body cells.

Tissue forceps   Quick Reference: An instrument used for grasping tissue during surgery.

Advanced Reference: There are numerous types and designs, among the most commonly used are Allis, Lanes, Babcock and Duvals.

Titanium   Quick Reference: Grey metallic element.

Advanced Reference: Used in many implants and prostheses such as for hips and knees. Has many desirable properties, i.e. low solubility, strong, non-toxic, non-carcinogenic, non-irritant, relatively inert.

TIVA   Quick Reference: Total intravenous (IV) anaesthesia.

Advanced Reference: Aimed at avoiding the use of inhalation (vapours) agents and usually given via infusion. Has the benefits of avoiding pollution and the unwanted effects of nitrous oxide, volatile agents.

TLC   Quick Reference: Ventilation terminology for: trigger, limit, cycling.

Advanced Reference: Trigger is the signal that opens the inspiratory valve allowing air/gas to the patient; limit is the factor which limits the rate at which gas/air flows into the lungs; cycling indicates the signal which stops inspiration and opens the expiratory valve.

TMJ syndrome **Quick Reference:** (Temporomandibular joint). TMJ connects the lower jaw to the skull (temporal bone) and with this syndrome can be painful, stiff and difficult to open.

Advanced Reference: This situation presents difficulty during airway control and intubation. People affected by Pierre Robin and Treacher-Collins syndromes present similar problems as they have a small and/or receding jaw (micrognathia) usually combined with *cleft palate* and a tendency for the tongue to fall back into the *pharynx*. Both create the scenario for potential *difficult intubation*.

Tobramycin **Quick Reference:** Antibiotic, Tobralex.

Advanced Reference: Effective against many forms of bacteria as well as a range of other micro-organisms.

Tomography **Quick Reference:** X-ray intended to show structures lying in a selected plane.

Advanced Reference: Can involve the use of X-rays or ultrasound waves in order to view a layer of body tissue irrespective of depth.

Tonic **Quick Reference:** Refers to tension or pressure.

Advanced Reference: Tonicity is the status of tissue tone or tension. With reference to body fluid physiology, it is the effective osmotic pressure equivalent. Also muscles, when they are in a state of continuous contraction as opposed to the normal situation of contraction and relaxation.

Tonometry **Quick Reference:** Procedure that measures the pressure inside the eye (*intraocular*).

Advanced Reference: Test used to screen for *glaucoma* and carried out with a tonometer.

Tonsils **Quick Reference:** A mass of lymphoid tissue.

Advanced Reference: Two lymph glands situated at the back of the throat between the pillars of fauces which form part of *Waldeyer's ring*.

Topical anaesthesia **Quick Reference:** Surface application of local anaesthetic.

Advanced Reference: Applied to skin, mucous membrane (pharynx, nasal passages, urethra, conjunctiva) via direct application with sprays, pastes and swabs.

Torecan® **Quick Reference:** Proprietary antiemetic.

Advanced Reference: Used to relieve nausea and vomiting, Torecan® is a preparation of thiethylperazine.

Toronto frame **Quick Reference:** Piece of patient positioning equipment.

Advanced Reference: Also referred to as the Montreal frame among other descriptions. Used as a support and positioning device during spinal surgery with the patient placed over it lying face down.

Torr **Quick Reference:** Non SI unit of pressure.

Advanced Reference: Torr = mmHg.

Torsade de Pointes **Quick Reference:** (TdP) (Turning of the points). Abnormal heart rhythm.

Advanced Reference: A condition signified by rapid ventricular tachycardia with variations in the *amplitude* of the *QRS complex* and rotation of the complex about the *isoelectric line*. Can progress to ventricular *fibrillation*.

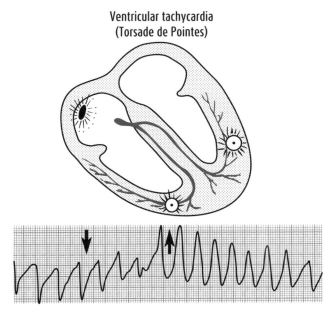

Fig. 18. Ventricular tachycardia (Torsade de Pointes).

Torsion **Quick Reference:** The act of twisting.

Advanced Reference: Torsion of testis is twisting of the spermatic cord which carries blood vessels and nerves and if left untreated leads to loss of blood supply to the testicle and consequent removal. Similarly, twisting of the bowel can happen, cutting off blood supply leading to ischaemia in the affected area and the need for resection.

Tortuous **Quick Reference:** Crooked, curved, indirect, winding, circuitous.

Advanced Reference: Term sometimes applied to the veins, usually of the hand and arm.

Total spinal **Quick Reference:** Inadvertent effects when local analgesic solutions reach the level of the cranium.

Advanced Reference: Can occur if/when patient is placed head down following intrathecal injection of local analgesic agents or if an epidural needle inadvertently pierces the dura mater and the larger drug volumes involved reach higher levels, and so affect cranial nerves producing respiratory paralysis, hypotension and unconsciousness.

Tourniquet Quick Reference: (turn-i-kay) A constrictive band placed around a limb to stem the flow of blood. However, with reference to first-aid, tourniquets are no longer recommended and have been replaced by elevation wherever possible and/or digital pressure of the artery supplying the bleeding area.

Advanced Reference: The objective of a tourniquet is to compress both an artery and a vein with the intention of stemming blood flow, to prevent the spread of a poison, or, as is the common purpose when used in theatres, to create a bloodless field for the surgeon. Numerous designs are available but all with the same intention. The limb is drained of venous blood and then the tourniquet is inflated to prevent entry of arterial blood. Local policy will dictate pressures and times for inflation as well as methods of recording these criteria.

Toxaemia Quick Reference: Blood poisoning.

Advanced Reference: This occurs due to an underlying bacterial infection within the body.

Toxic shock syndrome Quick Reference: Form of blood poisoning.

Advanced Reference: Caused by bacterial invasion and displays all the usual signs of *shock*. In females can be caused by *menstrual* tampon use.

Toxin Quick Reference: A poison. Toxic indicates poisonous.

Advanced Reference: Toxicology is the study of poisons and their actions. The source of the toxin may be varied but the term is used commonly to indicate those of bacterial or animal origin. Toxoid refers to modified bacterial toxins that have lost their poisonous properties but can still act as antigens to provoke the formation of *antibodies* but the toxoid does not produce symptoms of the disease. *Tetanus* toxoid is used to induce immunity to tetanus.

TPN Quick Reference: Total parenteral nutrition.

Advanced Reference: Involves providing nutrition via a vein when the patient cannot take or absorb food by the enteral route. May be due to coma, obstruction in the intestines, bowel removal, or for a temporary period following intestinal surgery or when a patient is on long-term ventilation.

Trabecula Quick Reference: Dividing band of tissue passing from the outer part of an organ to its interior.

Advanced Reference: As it extends into the interior it divides the organ into chambers.

Trace elements Quick Reference: An element essential to nutrition and physiological processes.

Advanced Reference: Found in minute quantities, a minor presence, hence the term trace.

Trachea **Quick Reference:** The windpipe.

Advanced Reference: The trachea runs from the larynx downwards into the upper mediastinum and divides into the right and left main bronchi.

Trachelectomy **Quick Reference:** Procedure for removal of the cervix in early stage cancer.

Advanced Reference: Performed vaginally in combination with an abdominal laparoscope, to remove the cervix, parametrial tissue and pelvic lymph nodes while preserving the uterus and ovaries.

Tracheostomy **Quick Reference:** (track-e-ostomy) Creating an artificial opening in the trachea.

Advanced Reference: Involves entering the trachea through a hole in the front of the neck at approximately the level of the third tracheal ring. Carried out for numerous reasons, i.e. obstruction, long-term ventilation, or laryngectomy, followed by insertion of a tracheostomy tube which can be permanent or temporary depending on the cause and need. At one time it was classified as a surgical procedure but various models for emergency and direct insertion are now available, e.g. percutaneous tracheostomy, which is usually carried out with the patient in their bed in the likes of an intensive care unit and involves the use of a trochar, guide wire and dilators for insertion rather than being a full surgical procedure.

Trachlite **Quick Reference:** A lighted intubation *stylette*.

Advanced Reference: An intubating device used as an alternative to conventional direct laryngoscopy. The endotracheal tube is fed over the stylette before intubation in the normal way and then introduced; following successful placement of the tube, the stylette is withdrawn. Can be used via the nasal or oral route and is useful in cases of suspected or discovered difficult intubation while also quoted as being suitable for awake as well as asleep intubation. Is similar in design and use to earlier intubation wands and the Surch-lite device.

Trachoma **Quick Reference:** Chronic eye disease.

Advanced Reference: A form of conjunctivitis caused by the bacteria *Chlamydia* trachomatis.

Tracrium® **Quick Reference:** Non-depolarising muscle relaxant.

Advanced Reference: Tracrium® is the trade name for atracurium, which has a short duration of action and is useful with renal and liver failure patients as it does not require their function for total degradation and elimination.

Tractotomy **Quick Reference:** Surgical severing or incising of a nerve tract.

Advanced Reference: Can be in the brainstem or spinal cord. Carried out for the relief of pain.

Train of four **Quick Reference:** (ToF). Refers to using nerve stimulation to assess muscular blockade with a muscle relaxant drug.

Advanced Reference: In relation to peripheral nerve stimulators, ToF is a method used to monitor the degree of neuromuscular block. The ToF ratio compares the strength of the fourth to first twitch produced by the stimulator.

Tramadol   **Quick Reference:** Opioid analgaesic, e.g. Zydol®.

Advanced Reference: Reported to have fewer of the typical opioid side-effects, notably less respiratory depression, reduced constipation action and it is less likely to cause addiction.

Tranquillisers   **Quick Reference:** Group of drugs used to sedate and allay anxiety.

Advanced Reference: Intended to have a general calming effect in many situations and conditions. The group has been divided into a number of classes: the major are used to treat psychotic states, and at the lesser end, they are used to treat and as aids for sleep problems. Minor tranquillisers are also known as anxiolytics, while those used to treat more major conditions are antipsychotics and neuroleptics.

Trans-cranial Doppler   **Quick Reference:** Form of Doppler ultrasonography in which pulses are directed at vascular formations in the base of the skull.

Advanced Reference: This allows measurement of blood flow velocity in the major intracranial arteries.

Transcutaneous   **Quick Reference:** Through the skin or unbroken skin. Transdermal, *percutaneous*.

Advanced Reference: Pertains to any procedure where internal access is achieved via puncture of the skin, as opposed to cutting of the skin as in open surgery. Transdermal usually refers to medications applied to the skin for absorption, as with creams, lotions and slow-release skin patches.

Transducer   **Quick Reference:** Device (receptor) that translates one form of energy to another.

Advanced Reference: Includes temperature, pressure. Commonly seen in theatres when used in the invasive monitoring of blood pressure. Transducers convert one form of energy (mechanical pressure) into another (electric impulse) and a pulse to an electrical signal.

Transect   **Quick Reference:** To cut across an organ or section of tissue.

Advanced Reference: Cutting across a blood vessel or piece of bowel perpendicular to the length is transecting the structure.

Trans-fatty acids   **Quick Reference:** Solid fats. Also known as trans-fats.

Advanced Reference: Found in dairy products and processed foods due mainly to the process of hydrogenation, which is used to extend the shelf-life of products.

They boost harmful cholesterol and therefore increasing the risk of heart disease.

Transformer   **Quick Reference:** A device for changing the voltage of an alternating current.

Advanced Reference: Transformers can be made to step-up or step-down a voltage.

Transfusion   **Quick Reference:** The transfer of blood.

Advanced Reference: Used to replace lost volume or a blood product. May be from one human to another or autotransfusion (own pre-harvested blood). Exchange or replacement transfusion is the removal or replacement of all or the majority of a recipient's blood. Direct transfusion involves immediate transfer from one to another without a period of storage.

Translucent   **Quick Reference:** Allowing light to pass through.

Advanced Reference: Although not necessarily transparent.

Transluminal   **Quick Reference:** Passing or occurring across a lumen.

Advanced Reference: As of blood vessels.

Transmission   **Quick Reference:** A passage or transfer.

Advanced Reference: As with a disease passing from person to person or an impulse within the nervous system passing from neurone to neurone.

Transplantation   **Quick Reference:** Transfer of tissue or entire organ from one place to another.

Advanced Reference: Usually indicates one person to another whereas grafting implies moving tissue from one place to another on the same person. Can involve hearts, kidneys, livers, lungs, or the cornea. Donor is the source, and recipient is the one receiving.

Transponder   **Quick Reference:** A wireless communication device that receives and transmits audio signals at a prescribed frequency range and, after receiving the signal, will broadcast it at a different frequency.

Advanced Reference: Used in satellite communications, and location identification navigation systems. Transponder is a combination of the words transmitter and responder.

Transposition   **Quick Reference:** A developmental fault in relation to the heart.

Advanced Reference: Involves the aorta arising from the right side of the heart instead of the left and the pulmonary artery (PA) from the left instead of the right. Dextrocardia indicates a mirror image to normal, with the apex of the heart being towards the right.

Transverse   **Quick Reference:** To go across, at right angles to the long axis of the body.

Advanced Reference: A transverse incision is across the abdomen as opposed to an 'up and down' midline incision.

Trauma   **Quick Reference:** An injury or wound.

Advanced Reference: Can be applied to both physical and mental situations. A traumatic event as well as a traumatic injury to body tissues.

Trendelenburg   **Quick Reference:** Title of both an operation and patient position.

Advanced Reference: Indicates head-down with the body sloping downwards and backwards. Used now for a number of procedures but originally for the operation of varicose veins and named after the German surgeon, Fredrich Trendelenburg. In the original position, the knees were bent and hanging down at about 40°.

Trephine   **Quick Reference:** (tref-ine) Surgical instrument used in neurosurgical operations.

Advanced Reference: Used for removing a circle or disc of bone in the skull. A trepan is a cylindrical saw used for the same purpose. A similar instrument is used in ophthalmic surgery to cut out a piece of cornea.

Triage   **Quick Reference:** To sort, sift or filter.

Advanced Reference: Classifying and prioritising patients or casualties at the scene of an accident or in A&E departments according to severity of their injuries.

Trichiasis   **Quick Reference:** A condition in which the eye-lashes invert and rub against the eyeball.

Advanced Reference: Can lead to ulceration of the cornea. Can also happen in conditions of **trachoma** when the eyelid shrinks and turns inwards.

Tricuspid   **Quick Reference:** Having three cusps or flaps.

Advanced Reference: The tricuspid valve is situated between the right atrium and right ventricle of the heart.

Tricyclic antidepressants   **Quick Reference:** Class of antidepressant drugs.

Advanced Reference: They are used in more serious cases of depression. Side-effects include **convulsions, heart block** and **arrhythmias**.

Tridil   **Quick Reference:** Vasodilator drug.

Advanced Reference: Used to treat **angina pectoris**. Available for injection/infusion as glyceryl trinitrate (GTN).

Trigeminal nerve   **Quick Reference:** Fifth cranial nerve.

Advanced Reference: Sensory nerve of the face. It has three divisions, i.e. ophthalmic, maxillary and mandibular or first, second and third, as well as a motor branch which supplies the muscles involved in chewing.

Trigeminy   **Quick Reference:** Irregular pulse or heartbeat.

Advanced Reference: Can be seen on an ECG trace when there are three beats followed by a missed beat. Refers to heartbeats in groups of three, e.g. premature ectopics.

Triglycerides   **Quick Reference:** Compound consisting of three individual **fatty acids**.

Advanced Reference: A neutral fat synthesied from **carbohydrate**; an energy source that is the chief constituent of fats and oils. It forms most of the fat stored by the body.

Trilene   **Quick Reference:** Trichloroethylene. Volatile anaesthetic agent.

Advanced Reference: No longer available. It had analgesic properties and was popular for use in labour combined with oxygen. Could not be used in a closed circuit with soda lime as it produced toxic metabolites which caused cranial nerve damage. Used in industry as a dry-cleaning agent and solvent.

Trimester   **Quick Reference:** A 3-month period.

Advanced Reference: The three trimesters of pregnancy.

Trimetaphan   **Quick Reference:** (tri-met-a-fan) Drug used to lower blood pressure. Arfonad®.

Advanced Reference: Technically a hypotensive agent with a short duration of action. Popular for lowering BP in many types of surgery.

Triple-A   **Quick Reference:** Refers to vascular surgical operation.

Advanced Reference: Indicates abdominal aortic aneurysm.

Triple-testing   **Quick Reference:** Term used in the diagnosis and treatment of breast cancer.

Advanced Reference: Indicates: (1) breast examination, (2) imaging (*mammography, ultrasonography*), (3) biopsy utilised to identify tumours.

Triptans   **Quick Reference:** A specific drug group that targets the receptors that stimulate the nerves supplying the cerebral blood vessels.

Advanced Reference: Used to treat *migraine* during onset (rather than the symptoms). Also used to treat depression.

Trismus   **Quick Reference:** Spasm of the jaw muscles.

Advanced Reference: May be due to inflammation from a tooth abscess, throat infection or irritation of the nerves controlling the muscles of the jaw (lock-jaw).

Trocar   **Quick Reference:** Sharp instrument used for piercing a body tissue/cavity.

Advanced Reference: Used in combination with a cannula (trocar and cannula), which is a slightly shorter hollow tube enclosing the trocar so that the sharp tip protrudes. When they are both assembled and introduced, the trocar is withdrawn and fluid and air are allowed to escape through the cannula, or anything necessary can be inserted. Used for such procedures as *hydrocele, pneumothorax, cystostomy*, or *gastrostomy*.

Trochanter   **Quick Reference:** The protuberance below the neck of the femur in each hip joint.

Advanced Reference: The lesser and greater trochanter, to which are attached various muscles acting on the hip.

Trochlea(r)   **Quick Reference:** (troc-lia) Pulley shaped.

Advanced Reference: The trochlear nerve, which is the fourth cranial nerve, supplies the superior oblique eye muscle. Also indicates the frontal bone through which the tendon of the superior oblique eye muscle passes.

Trouser graft   **Quick Reference:** Synthetic vascular graft.

Advanced Reference: Y-shaped (inverted) synthetic vascular graft used to replace a portion of the abdominal aorta and femoral arteries.

Trypsin   **Quick Reference:** A digestive enzyme.

Advanced Reference: Trypsin converts protein into amino acids and is secreted in the pancreas and converted into active trypsin in the intestine.

Tubal ligation   **Quick Reference:** Surgical female sterilisation.

Advanced Reference: Involves interruption of Fallopian tube continuity by excision and tying off or clipping. May be done laparoscopically or as an open procedure.

Tubercle   **Quick Reference:** A small lump.

Advanced Reference: Most often refers to a prominence on a bone but also indicates the lesion produced by the *tuberculosis (TB)* micro-organism.

Tuberculosis   **Quick Reference:** TB. Infectious disease caused by *Mycobacterium tuberculosis*.

Advanced Reference: The disease process destroys the tissue involved, lungs being the most recognised, but can manifest in numerous parts of the body, bladder being common. Treatment was revolutionised by the discovery of streptomycin but after falling figures for many decades it is now increasing again. Immunisation is with Bacilli Calmette Guerin (BCG) vaccine, which is an attenuated strain of *Mycobacterium bovis*. Due to developing resistance other names and descriptions are involved when discussing TB, i.e. MDR-TB (multi-drug-resistant TB) and XDR-TB (extensive drug resistant TB).

Tuberosity   **Quick Reference:** A protuberance on a bone.

Advanced Reference: The tibial tuberosity is a raised surface on the tibia and the radial tuberosity has the same on the shaft into which the tendon of the *biceps* muscle inserts.

Tube support   **Quick Reference:** Device used to support the anaesthetic tubing at the table end/head of the patient during surgery.

Advanced Reference: Designed to keep the tubing away from the patient's face and to prevent drag and kinking as well as helping to give necessary direction. Various models are available which either fit to the table or slide under the table mattress.

Tubigrip   **Quick Reference:** Type of cylindrical support bandage.

Advanced Reference: Provides extra support to wound dressings and bandages as well as being popular in the treatment of sprains and strains.

Tubocurarine   **Quick Reference:** Non-depolarising muscle relaxant.

Advanced Reference: The first in fact of this class of muscle relaxant. It is the active part of curare, a South American arrow poison. A pure alkaloid D-tubocurarine (DTC) was first isolated in 1935. Also referred to as tubarine.

Tubule   **Quick Reference:** Small tube.

Advanced Reference: The collecting and conveying tubules in the kidney medulla which carry urine to the pelvis of the kidney.

Tudor Edwards   **Quick Reference:** Name given to a piece of patient positioning equipment, i.e. back support.

Advanced Reference: Used primarily in orthopaedics when the patient is in the *lateral* position. Traditionally said to be named after a surgeon who designed or first used the device.

Tulle gras **Quick Reference:** (tule-grar) A net of pliant material impregnated with soft paraffin.

Advanced Reference: May also be mixed with ointment containing antiseptic and/or antibiotic. Used as a dressing for raw surfaces such as abrasions, burns, scalds and ulcers.

Tumour **Quick Reference:** A growth, swelling.

Advanced Reference: Usually used to indicate a *benign* or *malignant* growth of cancer. A new growth is called a *neoplasm*.

Tungsten **Quick Reference:** A heavy, hard and corrosion resistant metal. Also known as wolfram (symbol – W).

Advanced Reference: Greyish in colour, it has a very high melting point and is utilised in electrical components as well as X-ray tubes and alloys.

Tunnelling **Quick Reference:** Refers to the technique of fixing catheters under the skin with the likes of IV *feeding tubes*.

Advanced Reference: The catheter is tunnelled in the subcutaneous tissue to emerge at a remote site a few centimetres away and so reducing the possibility of sepsis spreading down the tract via the catheter and into the vein. Used when catheters are to be left in place for an extended period as with IV nutrition.

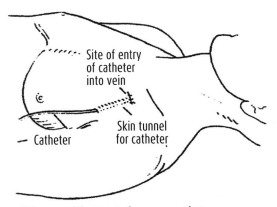

Skin tunnel for central venous catheter.

Fig. 19. Skin tunnelling. Reprinted with permission from Elsevier.

Tuohy **Quick Reference:** (tu-ee) Epidural needle.

Advanced Reference: An epidural needle with an oblique bevelled tip and 1-cm markings (Alfred-Lee type), designed to indicate the depth of insertion.

The needle tip (Huber) is of a blunt and bevelled design intended to push through the tissues, rather than a long cutting type as with hypodermic and lumbar-puncture needles such as the Quincke. The Weiss needle was the original winged-type design. Needle gauges for epidural are in the range 16–18 G and approximately 8–10 cm in length. There is a 15-cm version available for obese patients with a 19-G/5-cm model for paediatric use.

Turbinates **Quick Reference:** Bones of the nasal cavity.

Advanced Reference: Three scroll-shaped bones, superior, middle and inferior, that help form the walls of the nasal cavity.

Turgor **Quick Reference:** Fullness.

Advanced Reference: Skin turgor is one way to estimate the status of hydration and, to a lesser extent, nutritional state.

TUR hook **Quick Reference:** Piece of equipment used in endoscopic genitourinary procedures.

Advanced Reference: Intended to be a support for light cables, irrigating tubing, during TUR procedures. Commonly suspended from the ceiling or operating lights but there are also models which attach to the operating table.

TURP **Quick Reference:** Transurethral resection of prostate. Reduction or removal of the gland via an endoscope.

Advanced Reference: Also termed transurethral retrograde prostatectomy. Involves excision of the prostate using a resectoscope attached to a cystoscope passed via the urethra into the bladder. May also indicate the similar use of laser probes. An alternative operation is open prostatectomy (retropubic and transvesical), the approach being via a lower abdominal incision. TURT = Transurethral resection of tumour; TURBN = Transurethral resection of the bladder neck.

TUR syndrome **Quick Reference:** Condition/syndrome associated with transurethral prostatectomy.

Advanced Reference: Due to absorption of irrigating fluid (glycine) via the open vessels of the prostatic bed during prostatectomy. Causes overload and hyponatraemia due to the diluting effect on the circulation. Signs and symptoms include bradycardia, hypotension, convulsions, confusion and dyspnoea.

Twelve-Lead ECG **Quick Reference:** Diagnostic ECG.

Advanced Reference: Takes a much broader view than the usual three-lead standard version as used during surgery, which basically provides information on rhythm and rate. There are six limb leads (1, 11, 111, AVR, AVL, AVF) and six chest leads ($V_1, V_2, V_3, V_4, V_5, V_6$), which provide for a much more specific diagnosis.

Two-lives syndrome **Quick Reference:** Refers to mother and baby (fetus).

Advanced Reference: More specifically term used to denote the risk and related hazards during *labour* when an anaesthetic may be required for the likes of *Caesarean section*.

Tympanic membrane **Quick Reference:** (tim-panic) The eardrum.

Advanced Reference: A greyish membrane which detects sound vibrations.

Tympanoplasty **Quick Reference:** Repair of the eardrum.

Advanced Reference: Generally involves any reconstructive operation on the middle ear with the intention of improving hearing.

Typhus **Quick Reference:** An infection spread by lice.

Advanced Reference: Primarily a disease of dirt caused by Rickettsiae.

Typology **Quick Reference:** The study or systematic classification of types that have common characteristic or traits.

Advanced Reference: An example is, as with bacteria, according to type.

U

Ulcer **Quick Reference:** A chronic defect in the surface of skin or mucous membrane.

Advanced Reference: Can be due to many causes and occur in numerous sites, i.e. *gastric* and *duodenal ulcers* of the stomach, leg ulcers involved with *varicose veins; rodent ulcers* associated with cancers.

Ulceration **Quick Reference:** The formation of an ulcer.

Advanced Reference: Ulceration defines the break in continuity with the tissue surface. This can occur due to pressure on the surface, causing restricted blood flow and potential **necrosis** of the tissue. Ulceration can occur on the skin, mucous membrane and even within the trachea due to direct pressure of the over-inflated or extended inflation of the endotracheal tube cuff.

Ulcerative colitis **Quick Reference:** Disease of the colon and rectum.

Advanced Reference: The condition involves inflammation of the large bowel and possible *ulceration*. Cause is unclear but theories range from infection, allergy to autoimmune reaction.

Ulna **Quick Reference:** The bone on the underside of the forearm connecting the wrist and humerus.

Advanced Reference: The ulna is one of the essential structures of the forearm along with the radius. Both bones give protection to the radial and ulnar arteries that run parallel to the bone surface. The ulnar nerve is a branch of the *brachial plexus*, which descends on the medial side of the upper arm to the elbow. The ulnar is one of the most prominent nerves in terms of injury and damage in relation to positioning of the patient on the operating table.

Ultrasonic **Quick Reference:** Sound waves which are beyond the upper range audible to humans.

Advanced Reference: Utilised in various forms for medical and diagnostic equipment, i.e. extracorporeal shock-wave lithotripsy (ESWL), ultrasound.

Ultrasonic washer **Quick Reference:** A device used to clean debris from the surface of surgical instruments and anaesthetic equipment.

Advanced Reference: The device emits ultrasonic waves, which create high-frequency rippling that strikes the object shaking off any debris.

Ultrasonography **Quick Reference:** The use of ultrasound to produce images of internal body structures. Ultrasonics involves sound waves that are of a frequency above the range of audible sound.

Advanced Reference: The echoes of reflected sound waves form an electronic image. Based on the principle of SONAR (sound navigation and ranging), it was first applied medically to monitor fetal growth and development in the uterus but now has a wide range of diagnostic uses. Three-dimensional ultrasound shows images in three planes, i.e. transverse, longitudinal and horizontal; four-dimensional involves the further dimension of time.

Ultrasound **Quick Reference:** The utilisation of ultrasonic waves to examine the interior of the body.

Advanced Reference: Also used therapeutically in the treatment of soft-tissue pain and **lithotripsy** shock-wave therapy to break up renal and other stones.

Ultraviolet **Quick Reference:** Relates to *electromagnetic* light waves.

Advanced Reference: The waves are shorter than those visible to the eye but longer than X-rays. Emitted by the Sun and referred to as UVA, UVB, UVC, which signifies the level of radiation and penetrative powers. They act on the skin to promote the formation of *vitamin* D but overexposure can lead to skin *cancer*. Ultraviolet light is also produced by various artificial means such as arc-welding machines, which can cause eye-flash damage.

Umbilical cord **Quick Reference:** Cord which connects an unborn fetus to the placenta.

Advanced Reference: The cord which supplies nourishment to the fetus and is composed mainly of two arteries and a vein plus vestigial structures surrounded by a membrane.

Umbilicus **Quick Reference:** The naval, belly-button.

Advanced Reference: Depression in the middle of the abdomen where the umbilical cord enters.

Undecylenic acid **Quick Reference:** Unsaturated fatty acid. Also termed undecenoic acid.

Advanced Reference: Used as a topical agent in the treatment of fungal infections.

Underwater seal drainage **Quick Reference:** Type of chest drain.

Advanced Reference: Used after chest surgery, the drain is inserted into the pleura as a way of equalising pressure with the external atmosphere. Allowing air to remain in and enter the pleura would cause collapse of the lung. The tubing from the pleura connects to further tubing whose end is placed below the surface of a level of sterile water in a jar and so allows air to exit but none to return.

Unilateral block **Quick Reference:** Unilateral = one-side, block = spinal or epidural analgesia.

Advanced Reference: Indicates the block affecting only the nerves on one side of the body. May be intentional or unintentional on the part of the anaesthetist, depending on requirements.

Unipolar Quick Reference: Having a single pole or process.

Advanced Reference: A psychiatric disorder characterised by episodes of *mania*.

Unit Quick Reference: A single item. One.

Advanced Reference: Designates quantity, a standard of measurement.

Univent tube Quick Reference: A bronchial-blocker tube. Introduced as an alternative to double-lumen tube.

Advanced Reference: Used for one-lung anaesthesia, it is a single-lumen endotracheal tube with a moveable bronchial-blocker incorporated into a second lumen on the tube's concave surface. Also proven to be useful in difficult intubation settings where the blocker is advanced as a guide (in the manner of a bougie) and also allowing for the delivery of oxygen and monitoring of carbon dioxide.

Universal Quick Reference: Refers to blood – primarily the universal donor (O−).

Advanced Reference: This is possible because group O blood will not react with the serum of the other groups as it has no *antigens*, and if no anti-D, therefore Rh-negative. Conversely group AB (+) is the universal recipient.

Universal precautions Quick Reference: Infection control guidelines designed to protect health workers from exposure to diseases spread by blood and certain body fluids.

Advanced Reference: Universal precautions apply to tissue, blood and other body fluids, e.g. semen and vaginal secretions. Formulated in America in 1987 by the Center for Disease Control and Prevention, the guidelines indicate and advise that all patients should be treated as a positive risk until proven otherwise.

Upsher Quick Reference: Rigid fibre-optic laryngoscope.

Advanced Reference: As with alternative rigid scopes, intention and use are similar, i.e. is useful when conventional laryngoscopy does not allow alignment of the oral, pharyngeal and laryngeal axes as well as in difficult intubation settings, cases of anterior larynx and those with immobility of the temporomandibular joint (TMJ). Requires less head manipulation so has a value when the patient has an unstable cervical spine, but does require a minimum mouth opening to be used as intended. The Airtraq single-use disposable is a similar device.

Uraemia Quick Reference: (your-eem-ea) Excess of urea in the blood.

Advanced Reference: Results from defective function of the kidneys.

Urea Quick Reference: (your-ear) End-product of protein breakdown.

Advanced Reference: Urea is excreted in the urine and an excess in the blood is termed *uraemia*.

Ureter Quick Reference: (your-et-er) Tube leading from the kidney to the bladder.

Advanced Reference: There are two ureters, one from each kidney. They are muscular tubes and convey urine from the kidney to the bladder. The term ureteric is used when making reference to the ureters, e.g. ureteric catheter.

Ureterolithotomy **Quick Reference:** (your-et-ero-lith-ot-omy) Surgical removal of a ureteric *calculus*.

Advanced Reference: Carried out if the stone is causing recurrent pain, obstruction or infection. Involves exposure and excision of the ureter for direct removal of the stone.

Urethra **Quick Reference:** Tube carrying urine away from the bladder.

Advanced Reference: The urethra is longer in the male than the female, one consequence being that males have increased protection against infections such as *cystitis* compared to females. Urethritis is inflammation of the urethra.

Urethropexy **Quick Reference:** Bladder neck suspension.

Advanced Reference: Surgical procedure carried out to suspend the bladder in an effort to correct urinary incontinence in women. Also termed colpo-suspension, cystourethropexy and referred to as Burch procedure.

Uric acid **Quick Reference:** A normal constituent of urine. Lithic acid.

Advanced Reference: Uricaemia is the accumulation of uric acid in the blood. A build-up can lead to renal *calculi* formation.

Urinalysis **Quick Reference:** (UA) Laboratory analysis of urine.

Advanced Reference: Physical, chemical, microscopic examination of urine usually for the determination of infection, tumour, diabetes or the detection of a specific substance.

Urinary diversion **Quick Reference:** Surgical procedure carried out to divert the ureters, usually following bladder removal, contracted bladder or irreparable vesico-vaginal *fistula*.

Advanced Reference: Two of the most common procedures are utero-sigmoidostomy and uretero-ileostomy. In the former the ureters are trans-planted into the sigmoid colon but this procedure creates the disadvantage of ascending infection. The latter, also termed ileal conduit, involves isolating a section of ileum and bringing it to the abdominal wall then implanting the ureters into this *conduit* and so creating an ileostomy for urine collection.

Urine **Quick Reference:** Fluid secreted by the kidneys, stored in the bladder and expelled via the *urethra*.

Advanced Reference: It is composed of 96% water and 4% solids, the most important being *urea* and *uric acid*. Urinalysis involves the bacteriological and chemical examination of urine.

Urodynamics **Quick Reference:** The investigation of disorders of the lower urinary tract.

Advanced Reference: Involves the urinary bladder and urethra, and investigations to confirm symptoms related to urinary flow and pressure.

Urography Quick Reference: X-ray examination of the urinary tract. Also referred to as *retrograde* urography.

Advanced Reference: The examination is carried out with the use of contrast media (Urograffin). Urogram involves a radiograph of the urinary tract. Related procedures include cystography (bladder) and pyelography (kidney).

Urokinase Quick Reference: An enzyme produced in the kidney.

Advanced Reference: Is capable of breaking down blood clots by activating plasminogen to plasmin, which dissolves the clots.

Urology Quick Reference: Branch of medicine dealing with the urinary tract and related structures.

Advanced Reference: Involves disease and disorders of the urinary tract in both sexes and especially those of the genital organs in males.

Urostomy Quick reference: Surgical construction of an artificial excretory opening from the urinary tract.

Advanced Reference: May be temporary or permanent but generally relates to such procedures as urinary diversion or ileal conduit.

Urticaria Quick Reference: (hurt-te-care-ea) Allergy reaction signified by redness of the skin, especially around the neck and upper chest. Also referred to as nettle-rash.

Advanced Reference: The redness is due mainly to *histamine,* which is released when tissue is injured and causes capillaries to leak. Signs and symptoms generally include redness, itching and burning sensations, sometimes combined with blistering.

Uterotonics Quick Reference: Agents which cause contraction of the uterus.

Advanced Reference: Also termed oxytoxics, include *ergometrine, Syntocinon*® *Syntometrine*® as well as the *prostaglandin*-based preparations, i.e. Hemabate.

Uterus Quick Reference: Refers to the female womb.

Advanced Reference: Triangular-shaped, hollow, muscular organ sited in the pelvis between the rectum and bladder.

Uvula Quick Reference: Fleshy prolongation at the back of the mouth.

Advanced Reference: The uvula hangs down in the middle of the throat over the base of the tongue.

U-wave Quick Reference: A positive deflection seen on an ECG recording.

Advanced Reference: A positive deflection but of low amplitude. Not always present and thought to represent slow repolarisation of minor muscle in the cardiac anatomy.

V

Vaccine   **Quick Reference:** (vax-seen) Vaccination. To introduce a substance into the body, usually by injection, in order to confer immunity.

Advanced Reference: Involves the introduction of a modified virus or bacterium, which provokes immunity but does not produce the disease itself. Vaccination is now used synonymously with immunisation and *inoculation.*

Vacuum   **Quick Reference:** A space in which there is no matter.

Advanced Reference: Generally consists of a double-walled glass bottle between which a vacuum is created and the surfaces are silvered so that together the transfer of heat by *convection* and *radiation* is reduced to a minimum.

Vagal tone   **Quick Reference:** Indicates a level of activity in the *parasympathetic* nervous system.

Advanced Reference: The inhibitory control exerted by the vagus nerve over heart rate and atrioventricular (AV) conduction.

Vagina   **Quick Reference:** Lower part of the female reproductive tract.

Advanced Reference: A muscular passage lined with mucous membrane extending from the cervix to the exterior.

Vaginal cuff   **Quick Reference:** Anatomical closure created following hysterectomy.

Advanced Reference: Structure created by the surgeon at the end of the top of the *vagina* where the *cervix* used to be.

Vaginismus   **Quick reference:** Physical and psychological condition affecting vaginal penetration.

Advanced Reference: Generally a condition of unknown or specific cause which causes the muscles surrounding the vagina to go into spasm and so preventing penetration.

Vagotomy   **Quick Reference:** Surgical division (entire or partial) of the vagus nerve in the abdomen.

Advanced Reference: The object of removing the influence of the *vagus nerve* from the stomach is to reduce the secretion of gastric acid. Selective (highly) vagotomy diminishes the gastric secretion but leaves the emptying mechanism of the stomach intact, whereas complete (truncal) vagotomy may be accompanied by a pyloroplasty or gastro-enterostomy, which ensures continued emptying of the stomach.

Vagus nerve   **Quick Reference:** Component of the *parasympathetic* nervous system.

Advanced Reference: The tenth cranial nerve, also called vagus. It carries autonomic fibres to the organs of the abdomen and thorax, supplies motor fibres to the oesophagus, larynx and pharynx, and sensory fibres to the larynx, pharynx, tongue and ear.

Valency   **Quick Reference:** The bonding potential of atoms.

Advanced Reference: Measured by the number of hydrogen ions (H^+) that the atom could combine with or replace.

Valgus   **Quick Reference:** Bent, twisted outwards.

Advanced Reference: Abnormal position of a limb. Indicating away from the midline.

Valium®   **Quick Reference:** A tranquilliser with mild muscle-relaxant properties.

Advanced Reference: A proprietary preparation of the benzodiazepine group which may be used as a general sedative, for *premedication* and is also a skeletal-muscle relaxant.

Vallecula   **Quick Reference:** (val-ek-you-la) Any crevice or depression on the surface of an organ or structure.

Advanced Reference: A groove between the base of the tongue and the *epiglottis*.

Valsalva manoeuvre   **Quick Reference:** A test of the *baroreceptor* reflex.

Advanced Reference: Involves the patient exhaling forcefully against a closed larynx, resulting in an increased intrathoracic pressure which leads to decreased venous return and in turn a reduction in cardiac output coupled with a fall in blood pressure. The reduced baroreceptor discharge to the vasomotor centre then brings about vasoconstriction and an increase in heart rate.

Valve   **Quick Reference:** Refers to a number of valves in the body which allow passage of fluid or air in one direction. A fold of membrane, e.g. heart valve.

Advanced Reference: A valve may consist of two or three flaps or folds attached to a structure or vessel such as those in the veins of the legs intended to prevent back flow of blood.

Valvotomy   **Quick Reference:** A surgical procedure involving entering and opening into a valve.

Advanced Reference: Usually performed to correct a defect and to allow effective opening and function. Mitral valvotomy performed to relieve mitral stenosis removes fibrosed tissue that is affecting function.

Vancomycin   **Quick Reference:** An antibiotic.

Advanced Reference: Can be taken orally in the treatment of such conditions as colitis or via the intravenous route for endocarditis.

Vaporiser   **Quick Reference:** A piece of anaesthetic equipment which converts a liquid into a vaporised anaesthetic agent.

Advanced Reference: A device that allows controlled vaporisation of liquid anaesthetic gases. Although working on the same principle, there are many available because each is specific to a particular agent, unlike the early multi-use models. The early custom-made vaporisers even carried the name of the agent, i.e. Fluotec for Fluothane (halothane) and Tritec for Trilene, but all are now specific to and colour-coded with the agent to be used.

Varices **Quick Reference:** (var-is-seas) Dilated *friable* veins, e.g. as those around the gastro-oesophageal junction.

Advanced Reference: Normally associated with life-threatening bleeding due to back-pressure from an enlarged and obstructed liver as common with conditions related to alcoholism.

Varicocele **Quick Reference:** Varicose swelling of the testicular veins.

Advanced Reference: If symptomatic, treated by surgery which involves excision of the affected veins.

Varicose veins **Quick Reference:** Swollen or dilated veins.

Advanced Reference: Particularly those of the legs, which show as swollen and tortuous beneath the skin. Due to weakness and failure of the venous valves, they allow back-flow and pooling of blood. Haemorrhoids are a form of varicose veins, also *varicocele* of the testes, *varices* of the oesophagus.

Vas deferens **Quick Reference:** The duct of the testis.

Advanced Reference: It carries spermatozoa via the *prostate* to the urethra.

VAS scores **Quick Reference:** Visual analogue scale. Measures the intensity and magnitude of sensations.

Advanced Reference: Primarily a pain measurement scale but also used to measure a variety of stimuli such as emotional distress and nausea. The most common method utilises a horizontal line of 100 mm in length and, with reference to pain, 0 is stated as no pain and 100 as worst pain. The patient then identifies severity in relation to distance along the scale in response to questioning.

Vasa praevia **Quick Reference:** Critical condition in which blood vessels of the placenta and *umbilical cord* are trapped between the *fetus* and the opening of the birth canal leading to oxygen depletion.

Advanced Reference: Occurs in low-lying or unusually formed *placenta* as sometimes found with **in-vitro** fertilisation pregnancies, twins/triplets, etc. When diagnosed, *Caesarean section* is indicated.

Vascular **Quick Reference:** Relating to blood vessels. Also a surgical speciality.

Advanced Reference: May also relate to blocked, injured or diseased arteries and veins. The most common vascular surgery procedures are: aorto-bifurcation graft (*Trousers* graft), aorto-femoral bypass graft, femero-femero graft, axillary-femoral graft, *femoro-popliteal bypass graft* and carotid *endarterectomy*.

Vascular graft materials Quick Reference: Besides *autografts*, many synthetic materials are used for various blood vessel replacements.

Advanced Reference: *PTFE, Dacron* and Gortex (a waterproof and re-breathable fabric) are the three most commonly used materials, available in a number of forms, i.e. knitted or woven, and coated/impregnated with various substances to enhance their performance, e.g. antimicrobial, heparinised, collagen coated. Some are also biodegradable and break down over time allowing tissue to build up around and replace/reinforce the graft. The basic compounds for some of these materials are similar to those used in synthetic absorbable suture manufacture, i.e. Dacron and polydioxanone (PDO), which is combined with *elastin* for additional strength and flexibility.

Vasculature Quick Reference: The circulatory system.

Advanced Reference: Arrangement of blood vessels in the body or in an organ or body part. Vascularisation is the formation of blood vessels.

Vasectomy Quick Reference: Male sterilisation.

Advanced Reference: Division and tying off of the *vas deferens*, usually carried out via an incision in the *scrotum.*

Vas-occlusive contraception Quick Reference: (VOC) Contraceptive method for men.

Advanced Reference: All devices and methods available involve preventing the *sperm* from travelling down the *vas*.

Vasoconstriction Quick Reference: Reflex widening (relaxing) or narrowing of blood vessels.

Advanced Reference: Selective constriction or dilatation of blood vessels that can change or compensate blood pressure.

Vasomotor Quick Reference: Indicates the vasomotor centre in the medulla oblongata.

Advanced Reference: Responsible for the regulation of blood pressure and cardiac function via the *autonomic nervous system*.

Vasopressin Quick Reference: A natural body hormone secreted by the posterior lobe of the pituitary gland. Involved in the reabsorption of water by the kidney.

Advanced Reference: Also known as antidiuretic hormone or ADH. Available as a drug used to raise blood pressure as it constricts the blood vessels.

Vasopressor drugs Quick Reference: Drugs that bring about *vasoconstriction.*

Advanced Reference: These drugs are used to increase vasoconstriction and/or raise blood pressure. One example is *adrenaline* (epinephrine) which is used during resuscitation, and is added to local anaesthetics such as *lignocaine* to bring about localised vasoconstriction and therefore slow absorption.

Vasovagal attack   **Quick Reference:** Fainting. Also referred to as vagovagal, which is a reflex response.

Advanced Reference: Involves stimulation of the vagus nerve. A reflex action, e.g. irritation of the larynx or trachea, which results in bradycardia. The vasovagal response generally causes a drop in blood pressure, *bradycardia* and fainting.

Vasoxine   **Quick Reference:** A vasoconstrictor drug.

Advanced Reference: Used to raise blood pressure. A preparation of methoxamine hydrochloride.

Vector   **Quick Reference:** An insect or any living creature that carries an infective organism or parasite and passes it on to another, e.g. the mosquito in malaria.

Advanced Reference: This transport of infection can be to either the same or different species, i.e. with malaria from mosquito to human.

Vecuronium   **Quick Reference:** (vec-you-rone-eum) A non-depolarising muscle relaxant, Norcuron®.

Advanced Reference: Has a duration of action of 20–30 min with little effect on the cardiovascular system and does not trigger *histamine* release. Secreted in the bile and only to a minor degree through the kidneys so is suitable for use with renal failure patients.

Vegetative state   **Quick Reference:** (VS) Condition of patients with severe brain damage. Often follows *coma*. Sufferers are considered to be unconscious and unaware. Also referred to as persistent and permanent vegetative state (PVS).

Advanced Reference: Involves loss of cognitive function and awareness and develops when coma has progressed to a state of wakefulness without detectable awareness.

Veins   **Quick Reference:** Blood vessels that carry deoxygenated blood, many of which contain one-way *valves*.

Advanced Reference: Veins are relatively thin-walled and act as transport for the blood after it has given up its oxygen, i.e. from the capillaries back to the right side of the heart.

Velocity   **Quick Reference:** The rate of change of an object's position.

Advanced Reference: The speed at which an object travels, e.g. a bullet.

Velosef®   **Quick Reference:** Proprietary antibiotic.

Advanced Reference: One of the cephalosporin group of antibiotics available as a syrup, in tablet form or as a powder for reconstitution with water.

Vena cava   **Quick Reference:** The two largest veins in the body.

Advanced Reference: Comprise: (1) the superior vena cava (SVC) into which blood drains from the head, neck, arms and chest; (2) the inferior vena cava (IVC), which receives blood from the legs and abdomen. Both connect to and empty into the right atrium of the heart.

Venepuncture   **Quick Reference:** Transcutaneous access to a vein.

Advanced Reference: Cannulation. Puncture of a vein with a cannula or needle in order to give drugs, take blood or set up an intravenous drip.

Venereal   **Quick Reference:** Pertaining to a sexually transmitted disease (STD).

Advanced Reference: A disease transmitted via sexual activity, e.g. gonorrhoea, which affects the mucous membranes of the genital tract.

Venflon™   **Quick Reference:** Type of and trade name of an IV cannula.

Advanced Reference: A name that has become a term synonymous with cannula generally although it is actually a brand name. Available in a full range of adult and paediatric gauges and has a top-mounted injection port.

Venography   **Quick Reference:** X-ray study of a vein.

Advanced Reference: Usually carried out to detect a blockage.

Venous pump   **Quick Reference:** Process of blood returning to the heart.

Advanced Reference: Involves the combination of muscular contraction, venous valves in the leg and positive/negative pressure fluctuations of the thorax due to respiration (thoracic pump).

Ventilator   **Quick Reference:** A machine intended to breathe for a patient. In lay terms often referred to as a life-support machine.

Advanced Reference: There are numerous designs and types – gas driven, electrically powered, those that work on time cycles and those that utilise breathing volumes and rates – but all generally use positive pressure to inflate a patient's lungs. The models used in theatres tend to be simpler versions of those designed specifically for intensive care use, which have more intricate facilities in order to deal with a patient on long-term support and the varying needs they develop.

Ventilation-associated pneumonia   **Quick Reference:** (VAP) Type of *nosocomial pneumonia* seen in patients breathing with a ventilator.

Advanced Reference: Usually caused by *aspiration* of contaminated secretions or stomach contents. May be viral, bacterial or fungal.

Ventolin®   **Quick Reference:** A bronchodilator drug.

Advanced Reference: Used in the treatment of asthma and other conditions where the alveoli need to be opened up in order to absorb adequate oxygen. Available for injection and inhalation (inhaler) use.

Ventouse   **Quick Reference:** (von-toos) Vacuum extractor.

Advanced Reference: Device used in *obstetrics* to assist vaginal delivery. Involves the attachment of a suction cap to the head of the fetus and application of backward pull to assist removal from the *uterus*.

Ventral   **Quick Reference:** Refers to the front surface of the body.

Advanced Reference: Relating to or situated at or close to the front of the body or anterior part of an organ.

Ventricle   **Quick Reference:** A small pouch or cavity.

Advanced Reference: Includes the ventricles of the heart and brain.

Ventricular assist device   **Quick Reference:** (VAD) Implantable mechanical pump.

Advanced Reference: There are both left- and right-sided devices and they are intended to replace the function of a failing heart, quite often prior to heart transplant.

Ventro   **Quick Reference:** Prefix indicating in front of.

Advanced Reference: A ventro-fixation involves stitching a retroverted uterus to the abdominal wall and a ventro-suspension is carried out to correct displacement of the uterus.

Venturi mask   **Quick Reference:** Oxygen delivery system.

Advanced Reference: Type of oxygen mask that utilises the Venturi principle. The concentration of oxygen can be varied and set from 24% to 50% using a selection of detachable pre-set connectors, which, along with set delivery rates of oxygen, provides a fixed percentage.

Venturi principle   **Quick reference:** Physics-based principle involving pressure and flow.

Advanced Reference: The Venturi principle relates to the Bernoulli effect involving the effect on pressure of flow through a constriction, in that the inclusion of a side-arm to a pipe or tubing will involve the entrainment of fluid or gas causing the mixing of the two. This principle is utilised in the *Venturi* or Mix-O-Mask oxygen delivery system, which allows for precise percentage oxygen settings by use of the detachable connectors which have been pre-set by boring out differing diameters for oxygen flow.

Venule   **Quick Reference:** A small vein.

Advanced Reference: Venules drain blood from capillaries and then unite to form veins.

Verapamil   **Quick Reference:** A calcium-antagonist antiarrhythmic drug.

Advanced Reference: Used to treat high blood pressure, angina and arrhythmias. Available as Cordilox®.

Veriform   **Quick Reference:** Worm-shaped structure.

Advanced Reference: Pertaining to the worm-shaped structure, as with the appendix.

Verruca   **Quick Reference:** Type of *wart*. A watery skin *lesion*.

Advanced Reference: Caused by papilloma virus and occurs commonly on the underside of the foot.

Vertebra   **Quick Reference:** The bone(s) of the spinal column (backbone). Pleural = vertebrae.

Advanced Reference: The vertebra is one of 33 irregular bones forming the spinal column, divided into: 7 *cervical*, 12 thoracic, 5 *lumbar*, 5 sacral, 4 coccygeal. They are bound together by ligaments and intravertebral discs.

Vertebroplasty   Quick Reference: Repair of a collapsed *vertebra.*

Advanced Reference: An acrylic bone *cement*, polymethylmethacrylate (PMMA) is injected into the collapsed vertebra. Kyphoplasty is a similar procedure in which an orthopaedic balloon is used to expand the vertebra back to its normal state prior to injection of acrylic bone cement.

Vertex   Quick Reference: The crown of the head.

Advanced Reference: Position of the fetus when the crown of the head appears first in the vagina.

Vesicle   Quick Reference: A small bladder.

Advanced Reference: Usually containing fluid.

Vesico-vaginal fistula   Quick Reference: Pertaining to bladder and vagina.

Advanced Reference: An abnormal passage between the bladder and the vagina.

Vestibule   Quick Reference: An entrance, space, going into, entering.

Advanced Reference: The oral vestibule is the area of the mouth between the teeth and cheeks, i.e. entrance to the oral cavity.

Viable   Quick Reference: Capable of independent life.

Advanced Reference: The term applied to a *fetus* capable of living outside the *womb* after the 28th week of pregnancy.

Viagra   Quick Reference: Anti-impotence medication. Also known as silde-nafil. A powerful vasodilator.

Advanced Reference: Commonly used to treat erectile dysfunction but originally developed for use in general hypertension, pulmonary artery hypertension and angina.

Vibrio   Quick Reference: A *Gram-negative* bacterium.

Advanced Reference: Includes the organism that causes *cholera* and others responsible for gastric upsets and diarrhoea.

Villi   Quick Reference: Small finger-like projections.

Advanced Reference: A small protrusion from the surface of a mucous membrane, e.g. the small intestine.

Virilism   Quick Reference: The appearance of masculine characteristics in the female.

Advanced Reference: This includes body hair, baldness at the temples, deepening of the voice, increased muscular growth and loss of periods. The cause is excess of *androgenic* male hormones such as *testosterone.*

Virology   Quick Reference: The study of *viruses* and viral diseases.

Advanced Reference: Specifically their growth and the diseases that viruses cause.

Virulence   Quick Reference: The ability of *micro-organisms* to produce *toxins.*

Advanced Reference: This is dependent on the number and power of invading organisms. To be virulent indicates that something is dangerously poisonous.

Virus   **Quick Reference:** A micro-organism so small that many cannot be seen even under a light microscope. Responsible for numerous diseases.

Advanced Reference: A microbe that lives inside a host cell and uses it to multiply. Viruses are unaffected by antibiotics.

Viscera   **Quick Reference:** (vis-sera) Organs within the body cavities.

Advanced Reference: Usually applies to the large internal organs of the abdomen, pelvis and thorax, i.e. liver, lungs, intestines.

Viscosity   **Quick Reference:** Resistance to flow of a fluid.

Advanced Reference: Indicates the thickness of a fluid and so its ability to flow freely.

Vital capacity   **Quick Reference:** The maximum volume of air that can be exhaled after maximum inhalation.

Advanced Reference: The volume exhaled can be measured with a *spirometer* or respirometer.

Vitamins   **Quick Reference:** Group of substances which are essential for the normal functioning of the metabolic processes of the body.

Advanced Reference: Vitamin A is also known as retinol. Vitamin B involves a number of sub-varieties: B_1(thiamine), B_2 (riboflavin), B_3 (niacin), B_5 (pantothenic acid), B_6 (pyridoxine), B_{12} (cyanocobalamin), folic acid (pteroylglutamic acid). Vitamin C (ascorbic acid); vitamin D is a number of substances (D2 – calciferol, and D3 – cholecalciferol); vitamin E (tocopherol); vitamin K (phytomenadione and menaquinone).

Vitreous humour   **Quick Reference:** Transparent fluid that fills the eye.

Advanced Reference: It is in fact jelly-like and fills the posterior chamber of the eye between the *retina* and the lens.

Vitro (in)   **Quick Reference:** Interprets literally to 'in glass'.

Advanced Reference: Term related to artificial insemination, i.e. test-tube baby or fertilisation in a laboratory, outside of a womb, whereas in vivo indicates within the living animal.

Vocal cords   **Quick Reference:** Two folds of mucous membrane that lie in the *larynx.*

Advanced Reference: They can be relaxed or made tense by the muscles of the larynx. When air is forced through, they vibrate and produce sound (the voice).

Voiding   **Quick Reference:** To excrete. To empty.

Advanced Reference: To pass body waste and leave empty. Used in relation to passing of urine. Emptying the bladder.

Volatile   **Quick Reference:** Substance that has a tendency to evaporate easily.

Advanced Reference: Term applied to various anaesthetic agents such as halothane, enflurane, sevoflurane, desflurane, all delivered to the patient via a vaporiser. To some extent all are modern-day ethers, although not in a chemistry sense. They have been improved in terms of hepatoxicity, cardiovascular effects, uptake and elimination from the body. In many instances they are also condition specific.

Voltarol® **Quick Reference:** Non-steroidal anti-inflammatory drug *(NSAID).* Diclofenac sodium.

Advanced Reference: A non-narcotic analgesic used to treat pain and inflammation. May be administered orally, by injection or as a *suppository.* Has a number of side-effects including nausea, gastrointestinal disturbance and can produce rashes and *asthma* symptoms.

Volvulus **Quick Reference:** (vol-view-lus) Condition in which a loop of bowel twists round itself.

Advanced Reference: This twisting can lead to intestinal obstruction and cutting off of the blood supply to an area of the bowel.

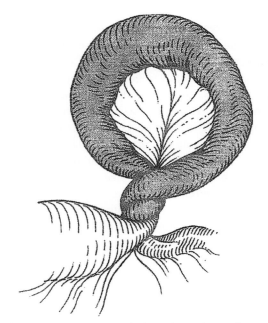

Volvulus – an example of closed-loop obstruction.

Fig. 20. Volvulus. Reprinted with permission from Elsevier.

Vomiting **Quick Reference:** A reflex, protective reaction of the stomach.

Advanced Reference: The expulsion of stomach contents via the oesophagus and mouth. Vomiting is an active process involving muscle, whereas *regurgitation* is a passive action.

Von Recklinghausen's **Quick Reference:** Hereditary disease/disorder involving fibrous swelling of the nerves.

Advanced Reference: Referred to as neurofibromatosis. Patients with this condition may have these growths in their airway, which can cause stridor or upper airway sounds.

Von Willebrand's disease   Quick Reference: Inherited coagulation disorder.

Advanced Reference: Involves the deficiency of a protein involved in platelet adhesion and carriage of *factor VIII*.

Vulva   Quick Reference: The external female genitalia.

Advanced Reference: Includes the mons pubis, labia majora and minora, external urethral orifice and clitoris.

Vulvoplasty   Quick Reference: Surgery performed on the external structures of the vulva.

Advanced Reference: By definition are cosmetic in nature and tend to indicate a number of related procedures, i.e. vulvoplasty, which involves removal of fat from different parts of the vulva; hoodectomy, where tissue surrounding the clitoris is excised; perineoplasty, which tends to be carried out to enhance an *episiotomy* scar. Additionally there is labiaplasty and vulva lipoplasty.

W

Waldeyer's ring **Quick Reference:** (wal-ders) A circle of lymphoid tissue found at the entrance to the *pharynx*.

Advanced Reference: Specialised lymphoid tissue involving tonsils, adenoids and lingual *tonsil*, which acts as a first-line of defence against upper respiratory tract infections.

Wand **Quick Reference:** Generic term for a varied number of pieces of hand-held surgical equipment.

Advanced Reference: Examples are the infrared coagulation wand, the recently introduced radiofrequency device used for detecting missing swabs, plus others utilised in neurosurgery and the intubating wand.

Warfarin **Quick Reference:** A compound that interferes with the clotting of blood.

Advanced Reference: Works by counteracting vitamin K. Usually given orally in the treatment of deep vein thrombosis (DVT), pulmonary embolism, following vascular surgery and the replacement of heart valves. Also used as a rat poison.

Warming blanket **Quick Reference:** A broad term for a range of equipment used to maintain patient's temperature during surgery.

Advanced Reference: Various designs of under- and over-blankets are now used. The original models were water-heated under-blankets placed on the operating table under the patient. Some designs also incorporated a ripple effect as the water circulated, so acting to prevent *pressure sores*. This design could be a problem if intraoperative X-ray was to be used, as the beam had to pass through both the blanket material and the water, or if the patient was to be positioned in a manner that prevented even contact. Therefore, most heating devices are now of the over-blanket type and use warm air as the heating medium.

Wart **Quick Reference:** Hard lump that grows on the skin.

Advanced Reference: Caused by infection with one of the papilloma virus group.

Waterlow scale **Quick Reference:** Pressure sore prevention policy.

Advanced Reference: Basically a risk assessment tool for pressure sore prevention based on risk factors which include: build/height, continence state, neurological deficit, surgery/trauma involved and medications. The patient is given a score for each and when added together this can provide a cumulative risk status.

Water manometer Quick Reference Measuring scale used for *central venous pressure (CVP)*.

Advanced Reference: Involves a drip-set connected to a three-way tap at the junction of the patient-line and the vertical manometer scale which reads in cmH_2O. When no reading is required, the system functions as a standard IV line bypassing the vertical arm of the device, but when the tap is directed appropriately for a reading, back pressure from the patient's circulation brings about a rise of fluid up the measuring column and levels out at the pressure exerted by the patient's CVP. Importantly, the zero (0) on the manometer scale must be at a fixed level (right atrium) at all times for accurate and consistent readings, remembering to make necessary adjustments if the operating table height or tilt is changed.

Waters Quick Reference: Collection of various anaesthetic-related equipment named after or devised by the American anaesthetist R. M. Waters.

Advanced Reference: Known most significantly for the Waters breathing circuit, also referred to as the to-and-fro system, which incorporated a *soda-lime* canister for carbon dioxide absorption. Now widely used without the canister but still referred to as a Waters circuit. He was also the designer of the Waters oropharyngeal airway, which was made of metal with a side-arm for attaching a gas supply.

Water soluble Quick Reference: Indicates that a substance can be washed away with water or will dissolve in water.

Advanced Reference: There are a number of substances and agents which fall into this category, e.g. water-soluble lubricants and certain contrast media used during *angiography*.

Watt Quick Reference: SI unit of power.

Advanced Reference: Equal to 1 *joule* per second.

Weal Quick Reference: Localised area of *oedema*.

Advanced Reference: Commonly found on the skin and produces itching.

Weaning Quick Reference: To wean. To reduce reliance upon.

Advanced Reference: Term used with regard to minimising the patient's reliance on artificial ventilation. Another example is to wean a baby off breast milk and introduce them to normal feeding.

Wedge pressure Quick Reference: Refers to pressure measured within the pulmonary arterial system.

Advanced Reference: Carried out with a CVP-type catheter (*Swann-Ganz*/floatation catheter) inserted via a central vein and guided through the right atrium to the ventricle and onwards to eventually wedge in a branch of the pulmonary artery. The pressure recorded represents left atrial filling pressure, and so left ventricular end-diastolic pressure.

Wedge resection Quick Reference: Surgical excision of part of an organ.

Advanced Reference: An example is resection of an ovary containing a cyst or a wedge. Also termed wedge *excision*.

Welt   **Quick Reference:** Raised ridge of skin.

Advanced Reference: Commonly caused by a blow or impact.

Wenckebach phenomenon   **Quick Reference:** Abnormal heart rhythm.

Advanced Reference: It involves the gradual increase in PR interval until a beat is missed.

Wertheim's procedure   **Quick Reference:** (vert-imes) Type of hysterectomy.

Advanced Reference: Indicates a total hysterectomy involving removal of the uterus, Fallopian tubes, ovaries, *lymph* glands and top portion of the *vagina*.

Whiplash   **Quick Reference:** Neck injury commonly associated with automobile accidents.

Advanced Reference: Happens during sudden acceleration or deceleration when the head may be jerked forwards and/or backwards, flexing and extending the neck which causes injury to the cervical spine and related muscles.

Whipple's   **Quick Reference:** Pancreaticoduodenectomy carried out due to *carcinoma* of the head of the pancreas.

Advanced Reference: Involves removal of the tumour located at the head of the pancreas, which also necessitates removal of the *duodenum*, part of the pyloric end of the stomach and part of the *common bile duct*. The free ends of these structures are then anastomosed separately to a loop of jejunum. If the tumour is inoperable and causing obstructive jaundice, this can be relieved by bypassing the site of obstruction, i.e. *anastomosis* between the gallbladder and jejunum or duodenum.

White matter   **Quick Reference:** Medullated and fibrous part of the brain and spinal column.

Advanced Reference: Parts of the brain and spinal cord composed mainly of nerve fibres.

Whole blood   **Quick Reference:** Term used to indicate a unit of blood that is complete in volume as when removed from the donor (plus anti-clotting agents).

Advanced Reference: The term indicates the alternative to blood that has had volume (plasma) removed, i.e. packed cells or plasma-reduced blood, which is useful when volume replacement is not as critical or the entire objective.

Willis (Circle of)   **Quick Reference:** Circular system of arteries at the base of the brain.

Advanced Reference: Blood is carried to the skull by the left and right carotid and basilar arteries. The communicating branches form a ring and this arrangement provides an alternative supply if one artery fails, but the main function of the circle is to balance the pressure of blood delivered to the brain.

Wilms' tumour   Quick Reference: Malignant tumour of the kidney.

Advanced Reference: A nephroblastoma which occurs in children.

Wiring   Quick Reference: Term used in relation to orthopaedic surgery regarding bone fixation.

Advanced Reference: Usually made of *stainless steel* and used to fixate bone fragments. Also refers to wiring of jaw (mandible) fractures.

Wolff–Parkinson–White syndrome   Quick Reference: A cardiac conduction abnormality.

Advanced Reference: Involves impulses short-cutting to the ventricles and bypassing the atrioventricular (AV) node due to an abnormal conduction pathway between the atria and the ventricles. The electrocardiograph (ECG) reveals a short PR interval that is often incorporated within the QRS complex. Sufferers can sometimes spontaneously go into *supraventricular* tachycardia or atrial fibrillation.

Womb   Quick Reference: The uterus.

Advanced Reference: Lay term for the female uterus.

Wound drain   Quick Reference: An item or piece of equipment used to drain fluids from a body cavity, usually following surgery.

Advanced Reference: Can be of passive or active design. Examples are corrugated drain, sump drain, suction drain and underwater seal drain.

Wright respirometer   Quick Reference: Device used to measure tidal (TV) and minute volume (MV).

Advanced Reference: Both electronic and mechanical versions are available and are usually sited within the expiratory side of the breathing system. For accuracy, the respirometer requires a minimum flow of usually 2 litres per minute.

Wrong site   Quick Reference: Relates to surgical procedures being carried out on the wrong limb or organ.

Advanced Reference: Numerous established and on-going systems are in evidence, all with the aim of preventing operations being carried out on the wrong site.

X

Xenograft   **Quick Reference:** (zen-o-graft) A type of organ or tissue graft.

Advanced Reference: A graft carried out between different species.

Xenon   **Quick Reference:** (ze-nan) Chemical symbol = Xe. An *inert* gas with anaesthetic properties. One of the noble gases, present in the atmosphere.

Advanced Reference: Considered to be a suitable replacement for *nitrous oxide*, as it is more potent, has a low solubility and fast onset and is environmentally friendly, i.e. not a greenhouse gas.

Xiphoid   **Quick Reference:** (zie-foid) Sword-shaped.

Advanced Reference: The xiphoid process is the smallest of the three parts of the sternum. It articulates with the inferior end of the *sternum* and the seventh rib. Also referred to as the *xiphisternum*.

Xiphisternum   **Quick Reference:** (ziffy-stir-num) Notch at the lower end of the sternum.

Advanced Reference: Point where the sternum meets the ribs. Also termed the *xiphoid* process.

X-rays   **Quick Reference:** Also known as Roentgen rays.

Advanced Reference: Electromagnetic radiation of shorter wavelength than *ultraviolet* rays, capable of penetrating many substances as well as producing changes in living matter. Due to this ability to affect matter, protection from X-rays is a vital part of theatre safety which takes the form of *lead aprons*, thyroid protectors, screens and, of great value, the facility to put distance between oneself and the radiation source. This distance should not just involve a direct line from the beam as X-rays have a degree of scatter (*inverse square law* – double your distance, quarter the dose). Monitoring badges which record exposure and absorption should be worn by those in regular contact with X-rays.

Xylocaine   **Quick Reference:** (zie-lo-cane) *Local anaesthetic* (LA) agent. Lignocaine.

Advanced Reference: Most commonly used LA drug. Can be utilised for *infiltration,* intravenously, topically and in epidural and spinal blocks. It has a rapid onset with average duration of 1.5–2 h, which is extended when mixed with *adrenaline.* Produces toxic effects if the maximum dose is exceeded. Also used as an *antiarrhythmic.*

Xylocard®   **Quick Reference:** (zie-lo-card) Proprietary antiarrhythmic drug.

Advanced Reference: Used to treat heartbeat irregularities such as ventricular ectopics and following various forms of heart attack. Available in a pre-loaded syringe for infusion or slow injection. It is a preparation of anhydrous *lignocaine.*

Y

Yankauer **Quick Reference:** (yan-ker) Type of suction catheter.

Advanced Reference: A rigid plastic or metal suction device with a handle and fixed curve, used in both surgery and anaesthesia.

Y-Can™ **Quick Reference:** Trade name of a Y-shaped intravenous (IV) cannula.

Advanced Reference: Designed to have a main arm/channel and side injection/infusion port. Two versions are available, a one-way and a two-way, both available in a full adult and paediatric range. The one-way version has a main channel and flexible remote side-arm through which injections are given, while the two-way allows for both main channel and side-arm to be used simultaneously for injections and infusion.

Y-drip-set **Quick Reference:** Bifurcated intravenous giving-set.

Advanced Reference: An IV drip-set which allows for two infusion lines, e.g. blood and saline, to be run simultaneously.

Y-piece **Quick Reference:** Bifurcated tubing connector.

Advanced Reference: Usually refers to a Y-shaped connector in anaesthetic circuits as well as a small plastic adaptor for joining the likes of suction tubing and can also be used as a straight joint while leaving one arm open in order to reduce vacuum.

Y-Plasty **Quick Reference:** Surgical revision of a scar.

Advanced Reference: Utilises a Y-shaped incision to reduce scar contracture.

Yeast **Quick Reference:** A *fungus.*

Advanced Reference: They produce *fermentation.*

Z

Zadik's operation Quick Reference: Radical excision of the nail bed, commonly of the big toe.

Advanced Reference: Radical excision involves the permanent **ablation** of the nail and nail bed. Other procedures of the big toe include **wedge resection.**

Zantac® Quick Reference: *H2 receptor-blocking* agent.

Advanced Reference: Alternative name is ranitidine. It works by inhibiting gastric secretions. When used, often included as part of the **premedication**, administered approximately one hour before induction of anaesthesia.

Zinacef® Quick reference: (zin-a-sef) A proprietary broad-spectrum antibiotic.

Advanced Reference: A preparation of **cefuroxime** and produced in the form of a powder for reconstitution.

Zinc oxide Quick Reference: Mild astringent used to treat skin rashes.

Advanced Reference: Also used to impregnate bandages and sticking tape/plaster (zinc-oxide tape). In some patients can produce allergic reaction, mainly localised to the skin around the application site.

Zip Quick Reference: Refers to a surgical zip used to close incisions of the abdominal cavity.

Advanced Reference: Following abdominal surgery when the two edges of the incision cannot be approximated due to enlargement of the abdominal contents, a surgical zip can be used. The outer edges of the zip can be cut to the required shape and then stapled or sutured to the skin. It is a temporary measure used until swelling is reduced and the skin edges can be brought together and closed.

Zirconium Quick Reference: Chemical element (Zr) used in the manufacture of prosthetic implants.

Advanced Reference: Grey-white metal that resembles titanium, obtained from zircon (hard translucent mineral). It is lighter than steel and corrosion resistant.

Zoster Quick Reference: refers to Herpes zoster, shingles.

Advanced Reference: Virus responsible for shingles and chickenpox. After initial infection (usually chickenpox as a child), the virus may lay dormant in the nerve root and later in life can reappear and produce Herpes zoster.

Z-plasty Quick Reference: Term used to describe a type of surgical incision which takes the form of a Z.

Advanced Reference: Used for removing scar tissue and lesions of the skin where a broad excision may prove difficult to approximate and close and leave an unsightly scar.

Zygoma   **Quick Reference:** Or zygomatic bone of the face which gives shape to the cheek.

Advanced Reference: The zygomatic arch is an extension of the skull that connects to the zygoma, giving form to the cheek. Often injured during trauma, such as direct impact and requires surgical elevation.

Zygote   **Quick Reference:** (zie-goat) A single fertilised cell.

Advanced Reference: The fertilised ovum. Formed from the fusion of male and female germ cells.

Appendix 1

Signs, symbols and formulae

Acrylic acid:	$C_3H_4O_2$
Aluminium:	Al
Ammonia:	NH_3
Amyl:	C_5H_{11}
Argon:	Ar
Arsenic:	As
Barbituric acid:	$C_4H_4N_2O_3$
Barium:	Ba
Benzene:	C_6H_6
Benzoic acid:	C_6H_5COOH
Bicarbonate:	HCO_3
Boron:	B
Caesium:	Cs
Calcium:	Ca
Calcium carbonate:	$CaCO_3$
Calcium hydroxide:	$Ca(OH)_2$
Calcium oxalate:	CaC_2O_4
Calcium oxide:	CaO
Calcium phosphate:	$Ca_3(PO_4)_2$
Calcium sulphate (gypsum):	$CaSO_4$
Carbohydrate:	$(C \cdot H_2O)_n$
Carbolic acid:	C_6H_5OH
Carbon:	C
Carbon dioxide:	CO_2
Carbon monoxide:	CO
Carbonic acid:	H_2CO_3
Chlorine:	Cl
Chlorine dioxide:	ClO_2
Chromium:	Cr
Cobalt:	Co
Copper:	Cu
Cyanide:	CN
Ethylene:	C_2H_4
Fluorine:	F
Folic acid:	$C_{19}H_{19}N_7O_6$
Gadolinium:	Gd

Gamma-aminobutyric acid:	$C_4H_9NO_2$
Glucose:	$C_6H_{12}O_6$
Glycerin:	$C_3H_8O_3$
Gold:	Au
Helium:	He
Hydrochloric acid:	HCl
Hydrochlorous acid:	HOCl
Hydrocyanic acid:	HCN
Hydrofluoric acid:	HF
Hydrogen:	H_2
Hydrogen cyanide:	HCN
Hydrogen disulphide:	H_2S_2
Hydrogen peroxide:	H_2O_2
Hydrogen sulphide:	H_2S
Iodine:	I
Iron:	Fe
Lactic acid:	$C_3H_6O_3$
Lead:	Pb
Lithium:	Li
Magnesium:	Mg
Manganese:	Mn
Methane:	CH_4
Mercury:	Hg
Molybdenum:	Mo
Neon:	Ne
Nickel:	Ni
Nitric acid:	HNO_3
Nitric oxide:	NO
Nitrogen:	N_2
Nitrous oxide:	N_2O
Oxygen:	O_2
Peracetic acid:	$C_2H_4O_3$
Perfluorohexane:	C_6F_{14}
Phenol:	C_6H_5OH
Phenyl:	Ph
Phosgene:	$COCl_2$
Phosphate:	PO_4^{3-}
Phosphoric acid:	H_3PO_4
Phosphorous acid:	H_3PO_3
Phosphorus:	P
Phytic acid:	$C_6H_{18}P_6O_{24}$
Platinum:	Pt

Plutonium:	Pu
Polyethylene:	PE
Potassium:	K
Potassium cyanide:	KCN
Potassium hydroxide:	KOH
Potassium permanganate:	$KMnO_4$
Propane:	C_3H_8
Prussic acid:	HCN
Radium:	Ra
Radon:	Rn
Selenium:	Se
Silica (silicon dioxide):	SiO_2
Silicon:	Si
Silver:	Ag
Silver nitrate:	$AgNO_3$
Sodium:	Na
Sodium bicarbonate:	$NaHCO_3$
Sodium chloride:	NaCl
Sodium cyanide:	NaCN
Sodium fluoride:	NaF
Sodium hydroxide (caustic soda):	NaOH
Sodium lauryl sulphate:	$CH_3(CH_2)_{11}OSO_3Na$
Sodium nitrate:	$NaNO_3$
Sodium nitrite:	$NaNO_2$
Sodium permanganate:	$NaMnO_4$
Sulphonic acid:	RSO_3H
Sulphur:	S
Sulphur dioxide:	SO_2
Sulphuric acid:	H_2SO_4
Sulphurous acid:	H_2SO_3
Technetium:	Tc
Thallium:	Tl
Tin:	Sn
Titanium:	Ti
TNT:	$CH_3C_6H_2(NO_2)_3$
Trifluoroacetic acid (TFA):	$C_2HF_3O_2$
Tungsten (wolfram):	W
Uranium:	U
Uric acid (lithic acid):	$C_5H_4N_4O_3$
Water:	H_2O
Xenon:	Xe
Zinc:	Zn

Zircon:	$ZrSiO_4$
Zirconium:	Zr
Acetylcholinesterases:	AChE
Acidity/Alkalinity:	pH
Cyanmethaemoglobin:	HiCN
Haematocrit:	Hct
Haemoglobin:	Hb
Hepatitis A:	HepA
Hepatitis B:	HepB
Hepatitis B surface antigen:	HBsAg
Hepatitis C:	HepC
Immunoglobulin E:	IgE
Methaemoglobinazide:	HiN_3
Sickle-cell anaemia:	HbS
Sickle-cell disease:	HbSS
Sickle-cell trait:	HbAS
Arterial carbon dioxide (partial pressure):	PCO_2
Arterial oxygen (partial pressure):	PO_2
Oxygen delivery:	DO_2
Oxygen saturation:	SpO_2
Oxygen uptake:	$\dot{V}O_2$
Vacuum pressure:	VP
Ventilation perfusion:	$\dot{V}/Q$
Centimetres of water:	cmH_2O
Micrometres of mercury:	μmHg
Millimetres of mercury:	mmHg
Absolute zero:	0 K
Celsius:	C
Fahrenheit:	F
Kelvin:	K
Weight:	Wt
Kilogram:	kg
Gram:	g
Milligrams:	mg
Micrograms:	μg
International Units:	i.u.
Metric Tonne:	t

Mole (amount of substance):	mol
Millimole:	mmol
Osmole	osmol
Milliosmole:	mosmol (one-thousandth of $1\,osmol, \times 10^{-3}$)
Milliequivalent:	mEq (one-thousandth, $\times 10^{-3}$)
Cubic capacity:	CC
Millilitres:	ml
Litre:	l
Cubic centimetre:	cm^3
Square meter:	m^2
Cubic millimetre:	mm^3
Centilitre:	cl
Decilitre:	dl
Milli (one-thousandth part):	m (10^{-3})
Micro (one-millionth part):	μ (10^{-6})
Mega (a million):	M (10^6)
Deci:	one-tenth (0.1) (10^{-1})
Centi:	one-hundreth (0.01) (10^{-2})
Nano:	one-billionth (10^{-9})
Atomic weight:	at.Wt.
Gray:	Gy
Roentgen:	R
Sievert:	Sv
Volt:	V
Megavolt:	MV
Watt (power):	W
Ampere (current):	A
Ohm:	Ω
Resistance:	R
Frequency:	f
Hertz:	Hz
Alternating current:	AC
Direct current:	DC
Candela (light):	cd
Joule (energy):	J
Kelvin (temperature):	K
Kilopascal (1000 Pa):	kPa

Newton (force):	N
Pascal (pressure):	Pa
Second:	s
Hour:	h
Minute:	min
Bel:	B
Decibel:	dB
American wire gauge:	AWG
French gauge:	FG
Standard wire gauge:	SWG
Percentage:	%
Plus/minus:	±
Fracture:	#
Female:	♀
Male:	♂
Greater than:	>
Lesser than:	<
Increased or raised:	↑
Decreased or lowered:	↓
Three days:	3/7
One week:	1/52
One month:	1/12
At once:	Stat
Whenever necessary:	p.r.n.
If necessary:	s.o.s.
Every day:	q.d.
To the desired amount:	ad. lib.
Twice a day:	b.i.d.
Three times a day:	t.d.s.
Four times a day:	q.i.d.

Appendix 2

Normal values

Conversion factors

Solutions

1% solution $= 1\,g$ in $100\,ml$

Drug ratios

$1 : 1000 =$
> $= 1\,g$ in $1000\,ml$
> $= 1000\,mg$ in $1000\,ml$
> $= 1\,mg/ml$

To calculate mg/ml of a solution $=$ multiply by 10, e.g.

  $2\% \times 10 = 20\,mg/ml$
$0.5\% \times 10 = 5\,mg/ml$

Fluid conversion

Pints to litres $=$ multiply by 0.568
Litre to pints $=$ multiply by 1.760
1 pint $= 568\,ml = 20$ fluid ounces
$1\,l = 1\,kg$

Weight

Pounds to kilograms $=$ multiply by 0.454
Kilograms to pounds $=$ multiply by 2.205
1 stone $= 6\,kg$ (approximately)

Temperature

Centigrade to Fahrenheit: $F = \left(\frac{9}{5}\,°C\right) + 32$
Fahrenheit to Centigrade: $C = \frac{5}{9}\left(°F - 32\right)$
   (normal body temperature $= 36.8\,°C$ and $98.4\,°F$)

Pressure

$100\,kPa = 1\,bar = 1$ atmosphere $= 15\,lb/in^2 = 760\,mmHg$

Flow

$$Flow = \frac{Pressure}{Resistance}$$

French gauge

FG or (Ch) $= 5\,FG = 1.6\,mm = 0.66\,in$

British horse power

b.h.p. $= 550$ foot-pounds of work per second
$\qquad = 33000$ foot-pounds per minute
$\qquad = 745.7$ watts

Physiological variables

Respiratory values

Adult – based approximately on body weight of 70 kg
Tidal volume (TV) $= 600\,ml$
Respiratory rate (RR) $= 12$–15 breaths per minute
Minute volume (MV) $= TV \times RR$
Anatomical dead space $= 2\,ml/kg$
Vital capacity (VC) $= 5000\,ml$
Total lung capacity $= 6000$–$7000\,ml$
Carbon dioxide production at rest $= 200\,ml/min$

Oxygen carriage in blood

1 g of Hb will combine with 1.31 ml of O_2, therefore: with a Hb of 14 g per 100 ml, approx. 20 ml of O_2 will be carried in combination with Hb in 100 ml of blood.

O_2 consumption (at rest)

125 ml of O_2 per minute per square metre of body surface area.

O_2 delivery to tissue

$$DO_2 = \text{cardiac output (CO)} \times Hb \times O_2 \text{ saturation}$$

or

$$CO\ (l/min) \times Hb \text{ concentration } (g/l) = 1.31\ (ml\ O_2/g\ Hb) \times \%\text{ saturation}$$

Respiratory quotient

$RQ = CO_2$ produced/O_2 consumed

Composition of air

Oxygen $= 21\%$
Carbon dioxide $= 0.03\%$
Nitrogen $= 78\%$

Blood gas/acid–base values

$pH = 7.36–7.42$
$PCO_2 = 35–45\,mmHg$
$PO_2 = 80–100\,mmHg$
O_2 saturation $= 85\%–100\%$
Standard bicarbonate $= 22–26\,mmol/l$
Base excess $= \pm\,3\,mmol/l$

Body water

	Male	Female
Fluid intake (24 h)	3000 ml	2500 ml
Fluid output (24 h)	3000 ml	2500 ml
Total body water	45 l	30 l
Intracellular	30 l	20 l
Extracellular	15 l	12 l

* (+ intravascular and interstitial)

Haematological values

	Male	Female
Haemoglobin (Hb)	14–18 g/100 ml	12–16 g/100 ml
Haematocrit	42%–52%	37%–47%
Erythrocyte sedimentation rate (ESR)	1–13 mm/h	17–20 mm/h
White cells	4000–10 000 cells/mm^3	
Platelets	150 000–400 000/mm^3	

Blood

Circulating volume (adult):	5 l
Blood is suspension of 55% plasma and 45% cells	
Red blood cell count:	5 million per cubic millimetre
Bleeding time:	2–9 min
Blood supply to tissues:	$=$ Cardiac output (CO) $\times$ Hb $\times$ saturation
Blood volumes:	Neonate $=$ 85–90 ml/kg body weight
	Child $=$ 80 ml/kg body weight
	Adult $=$ 70 ml/kg body weight
Blood groups: (% of the population)	O $=$ 46%
	A $=$ 42%
	B $=$ 9%
	AB $=$ 3%
	Rhesus $+$ (D) Factor $=$ 85%
Universal donor:	O Rhesus-negative
Blood replacement guide (approx):	Loss:
	500 ml – replace with crystalloids
	1000 ml – replace/consider with colloids
	1000 ml $+$ $-$ replace with blood

1 unit of blood raises the Hb – 1 g/dl

Measurement of blood loss

Swab weighing: 1 ml of blood weighs 1 g (approx)
Weight of blood loss $=$ weight of used swab minus weight of dry swab

Biochemical values (mmol/l)

Sodium $=$ 133–144
Potassium $=$ 3.2–5.1
Chloride $=$ 96–109
Bicarbonate $=$ 18–29
Calcium $=$ 2.1–2.65
Fasting sugar $=$ 3.4–6.2

Normal values

Cardiovascular

Cardiac output (CO):	Volume of blood pumped by a ventricle in 1 min = heart rate (HR) × stroke volume (SV)
Pulse pressure:	$= \dfrac{\text{Stroke volume}}{\text{Compliance}}$
Stroke volume:	Volume of blood ejected from a ventricle with each heart beat.
Mean arterial pressure:	$= (CO \times SVR) + CVP$ CO = cardiac output. SVR = systemic vascular resistance
Central venous pressure (CVP):	$= 0\text{--}10 \text{ cmH}_2\text{O}$
Pulmonary wedge pressure (PWP):	Approx: 8 mmHg
Cardiac index (CI):	Normal $= 2.5 - 4.5 \text{ l.min}^{-1}.\text{m}^{-2}$ $CI = \dfrac{\text{Cardiac output}}{\text{Body surface area}}$
Ejection fraction (EF):	Normal value $= 65\%\text{--}75\%$ $EF = \dfrac{\text{Stroke volume}}{\text{End diastolic pressure}}$

Diet

(1 calorie = 4.182 kilojoules, kj)
Approximate calorific intake (daily): Male, 2500; female, 2000
Parenteral (TPN):   Approx: 3000 calories in 3 l/24 h (1 cal/ml)
1 teaspoonful = 5 ml
1 tablespoonful = 15 ml

Body mass index

$$BMI = \frac{\text{mass (kg)}}{\text{height (m}^2)}$$

Body surface area calculator: $\dfrac{[\text{weight (kg)} \times 0.425] \times \text{height (cm)} \times 0.725}{139.315}$

Digestion

pH values:
Saliva $= 5.4\text{--}7.5$
Gastric juice $= 1.5\text{--}3.5$
Bile $= 6.0\text{--}8.5$

Normal blood sugar

$$3.88\text{--}5.55 \, \text{mmol/l}$$
$$\text{or}$$
$$70\text{--}100 \, \text{mg/dl}$$

Cholesterol levels

Desired level $= 3 \, \text{mmol/l}$ (USA $= 225 \, \text{mg/dl}$)
Average UK level $= 5.5\text{--}6 \, \text{mmol/l}$

Alcohol consumption

Recommended maximum daily intake:
  Men 3–4 units
  Women 2–3 units
1 unit of alcohol is equivalent to 10 ml or 8 g of pure ethanol;
One 750-ml bottle of 12% contains approx 10 units.
Number of units of alcohol in a drink can be determined by multiplying the volume in millilitres by the % then dividing by 1000:

$$\text{i.e. 1 pint of beer at } 4\% = \frac{568 \times 4}{1000} = 2.3 \, \text{units}$$

ABV = alcohol by volume.

Drug bioavailability

$$\text{Oral bioavailability} = \frac{\text{Amount of drug in the circulation after an oral dose} \times 100}{\text{Amount of drug in the circulation after an intravenous drug}}$$

Urine

Specific gravity:	1.020–1.030
Normal pH range:	4.5–7.8
Bladder filling rate:	Approx: 1 ml per min = 60 ml per hour
Bladder capacity (adult)	Approx: 500 ml

CSF pressure

$10 \, \text{cmH}_2\text{O}$

Intraocular pressure

1.3–2.6 kPa (10–20 cmH_2O)

Inverse square law

Double the distance quarter the dose.

Appendix 3

Assessment/classification systems

Apgar scoring system

Sign	0	1	2
Heart rate	Absent	Slow(<100)	>100
Respiratory effort	Absent	Slow, irregular	Good crying
Muscle tone	Flaccid	Some flexion of extremities	Active motion
Reflex irritability	No response	Grimace	Vigorous cry
Colour	Blue, pale	Body pink, extremities blue	Completely pink

ASA physical status[a] classification

1 Normal healthy patient
2 Patient with mild systemic disease
3 Patient with severe systemic disease
4 Patient with severe systemic disease that is a constant threat to life
5 Moribund patient who is not expected to survive without an operation
6 A deceased brain-dead patient whose organs are being removed for donation

[a] If surgery is emergency physical status is followed by E.

Bispectral index values

Score	State
100	Awake
65–85	Sedation
46–65	General anaesthesia
<40	Burst suppression
0	No electrical activity

Calculating blood loss*a* in theatres

- Weigh dry swab
- Weigh blood-soaked swabs when immediately discharged then subtract dryweight
- Suction bottles:
  Subtract weight of empty containers from used ones or
  Take measurement from graduations on suction vessel
- Estimate loss into drapes + any spilt or pooled blood
- Subtract any irrigation fluid volumes from the measured total to give overall blood loss estimation

a 1 ml of blood weighs approx 1g.

Blood volumes

Neonate	85–90 ml/kg body weight
Child	80 ml/kg body weight
Adult	70 ml/kg body weight

Classification of diabetes mellitus

	Type 1 (insulin dependent)	Type 2 (non-insulin dependent)
Age of onset	Infancy to 20s	60s upwards (sometimes younger)
Pathology	Pancreas unable to produce insulin	Body unable to use insulin properly
Treatment	Insulin	Diet and oral hypoglycaemics

Degree of burn

Degree	Cause	Surface appearance	Colour	Pain level	Healing time
First-degree, superficial	Sunburn, scald, flash flame	Dry, no blisters	Pink	Painful	2–5 days with peeling with no scarring but may discolour
Second-degree, partial thickness	Contact with hot liquids or solids, chemical, flash flame	Moist, blisters	Pink to cherry red	Painful	5–21 days, no grafting, no infection but 21–35 days if infected and may convert to full thickness
Third-degree, full thickness	Contact with hot liquids or solids, flame, chemical or electrical	Dry and leathery until removed, with charred blood vessels visible through charred skin	Mixed white, waxy, pearly or dark mahogany	No pain as nerve endings dead	Large areas, may take months combined with skin grafting but small areas may heal with grafting within weeks

Five predictors of difficult bag/mask ventilation and oxygenation (OBESE)

1 The obese (body mass index >26 kg/m^2)
2 The bearded
3 The elderly
4 The snorers
5 The edentulous

Fluid imbalance (signs)

Fluid deficit	Fluid excess
• Postural hypotension	• Hypertension
• Low or absent JVP	• Raised JVP
• Tachycardia	• Galloping irregular rhythm
• Dry mucosa	• Tachycardia
• Oliguria	• Oedema
• Low supine BP	• Pleural effusion
• Peripheral shutdown	• Ascites
• Shock with possible organ failure	• Pulmonary oedema

Fluid therapy in hypovolaemic shock

Estimated blood loss (ml)	Crystalloid (ml 0.9% NaCl)	Colloid (ml)	Blood/ blood products
1000	500	1000	/
2000	500	1000	4 units whole blood
3000	500	1500	>6 units whole blood

Four Ds of difficult airway

1. Dentition	Prominent incisors, receding chin
2. Distortion	Oedema, blood, vomit, tumour, infection
3. Disproportion	Short, bull neck, large tongue, small mouth
4. Dysmobility	TMJ, cervical spine

Assessment/classification systems

Glasgow coma scale

Eye opening (E)	Verbal response (V)	Motor response (M)
4 = spontaneous	5 = normal orientation	6 = obeys commands
3 = to command	4 = confused	5 = localises to pain
2 = to pain	3 = in appropriate words	4 = withdraws to pain
1 = none	2 = no words, only sounds	3 = flexing response to pain
	1 = none	2 = extends to pain
		1 = none
		Total = E+V+M

Goldman cardiac risk index

Factor	Points
Third heart sound/elevated JVP	11
MI within 6 months	10
Ventricular ectopic beats >5/min	7
Age >70 years	5
Emergency operation	4
Severe aortic stenosis	3
Poor medical condition	3
Abdominal or thoracic operation	3

Score	Incidence of death (%)	Incidence of severe CVS complications (%)
<6	0.2	0.7
<26	4	17
>25	56	22

Intraoperative fluid therapy

Grade	Type of surgery	IV Fluid/rate
Minor operation	ENT, Ophthalmic, etc.	5% Dextrose, 0.9% sodium chloride 6 ml· kg^{-1}· h^{-1}
Intermediate operation	Abdominal (appendix), intrathoracic, etc.	Hartmann's solution 8 ml· kg^{-1}· h^{-1}
Major operation	Major intra-abdominal, fractured femur, etc.	Hartmann's solution 10 ml· kg^{-1}· h^{-1}

Mallampati's airway assessment classification

Class	View
1 (Easy)	Entire tonsil clearly visible
2	Upper half of tonsil fossa visible
3	Soft and hard palate clearly visible
4 (Difficult)	Only hard palate visible

Ramsay sedation scale (ICU)

1. Anxious and agitated
2. Cooperative, orientated and tranquil
3. Responds to verbal commands only
4. Asleep but brisk responses to loud auditory stimulus/light glabellar tap
5. Asleep but sluggish response to loud auditory stimulus/light glabellar tap
6. Asleep, no response

Sliding scale (diabetes/insulin)

Capillary blood glucose (mmol/l)	Insulin infusion rate (units/h[a])
<4	0
4.1–6.5	1
6.6–8.9	2
9.0–11.0	4
11.1–17.0	5
17.1–28.0	6
>28	8

[a] Adjust to suit required blood glucose level.

Surgery-related haemorrhage

Stage	Reaction/cause
Primary haemorrhage	When haemostasis has not been achieved during or at end of surgical procedure
Reactionary haemorrhage	Within 48 h of surgery. Causes include rise in BP as compared to readings at completion of surgery
Secondary haemorrhage	Occurs approximately 7–10 days following surgery. Usually due to wound infection

Appendix 4

Useful websites

www.aagbi.org   Association of Anaesthetists of Great Britain & Ireland
www.afpp.org.uk   Association for Perioperative Practice
www.alfanaes.org   Association of Low-Flow Anaesthesia
www.americanheart.org   American Heart Association
www.amershamhealth.com   GE Imaging site
www.anesthesia-analgesia.org   Anesthesia & Analgesia
www.answers.com   Answers.Com
www.aorn.org   Association of Perioperative Registered Nurses
www.askapatient.com   Ask a Patient, medicine ratings and health-care opinion
www.ast.org   Association of Surgical Technologists
www.bbc.co.uk/health   BBC on-line health page
www.bhf.org.uk   British Heart Foundation
www.bma.org.uk   British Medical Association
www.bnf.org   British National Formulary
www.britishpainsociety.org   the British Pain Society
http://clinicalevidence.bmj.com/ceweb/conditions/index.jsp   BMJ Clinical
   Evidence site
www.ccmtutorials.com   Critical Care Medicine tutorials
www.cochrane.org   Cochrane Collaboration
www.dh.gov.uk   Department of Health
www.doctors.net.uk   Doctors Information website
www.druginfozone.nhs.uk   National Electronic Library for Medicines
www.drugs.com   Drugs.Com
www.emedicine.com   eMedicine(webMD)
www.erc.edu   European Resuscitation Council
www.euroanesthesia.org   European Society of Anaesthesiology
www.fieldmedics.com   Field Medics
www.findarticles.com   Find Articles
www.frca.co.uk   Anaesthesia UK
www.gasmanweb.com   Gas Man
www.gdc-uk.org   General Dental Council
www.health.auckland.ac.nz   Centre for Evidence Based Nursing –
   Auckland Univ.
www.healthatoz.com   Health A to Z
www.healthcarecommission.org.uk   Healthcare Commission

http://health.groups.yahoo.com/group/theatrepractitioners/ Theatre Practitioners chat-site

www.healthguidance.org Ask About Medicine

www.hepc.nhs.uk Hepatitis C website

www.hfea.gov.uk Human Fertilisation & Embryology Authority

www.hpc-uk.org Health Professionals Council

www.hse.gov.uk Health & Safety Executive

www.hse.gov.uk/latex H&S Executive Latex Allergy Awareness Toolkit

www.hsj.co.uk Health Service Journal

www.hta.gov.uk Human Tissue Authority

www.iarc.fr/epic/ European Prospective Investigation into Cancer and Nutrition

www.idsc-uk.org Institute of Decontamination Services

www.joannabriggs.edu.au Joanna Briggs Institute, Adelaide University

www.lasg.co.uk Latex Allergy Support Group

www.library.nhs.uk National Library for Health

www.mhaus.org Malignant Hyperthermia Association of the United States

www.the-mdu.com Medical Defence Union

www.medterms.com Medicine Net

www.mercksource.com Dorlands Medical Dictionary

www.mhra.gov.uk Medicines and Healthcare Products Regulatory Agency

www.mps.org.uk Medical Protection Society

www.My.webmd.com Web MD Health

www.naasp.org.uk National Association of Assistants in Surgical Practice

www.nda.ox.ac.uk Nuffield Department of Anaesthetics

www.nice.org.uk National Institute for Health and Clinical Excellence

www.nmc-uk.org Nursing & Midwifery Council

www.npi.gov.au National Pollutant Inventory

www.npsa.nhs.uk/home National Patient Support (Safety) Agency

www.nursingtimes.net Nursing Times Journal

www.nzats.co.nz New Zealand Anaesthetic Technicians Society

www.oaa-anaes.ac.uk Obstetric Anaesthetists' Association

www.opps.co.uk Opportunities online

www.OTJonline.com The Operating Theatre Journal

www.paramedic.org.uk Ambulance UK/Paramedic UK

www.patient.co.uk Medline/Patient UK

www.ppa.org.uk Prescription and Pricing Authority

www.prodigy.nhs.uk NHS Library for Drugs

www.pubmedcentral.nih.gov PubMed Central

www.qaa.ac.uk Quality Assurance Agency

www.rcn.org.uk Royal College of Nursing

www.rcoa.ac.uk   Royal College of Anaesthetists
www.rcseng.ac.uk   Royal College of Surgeons
www.resus.org.uk   UK Resuscitation Council
www.roysocmed.ac.uk   Royal Society of Medicine
www.sambahq.org   Society of Ambulatory Anaesthesia
www.shotuk.org   Serious Hazards of Transfusion
www.sicklecellsociety.org   Sickle Cell Anaemia Society
www.skillsforhealth.org.uk   Skills Council for Health
www.skillstat.com   ECG tutor
www.smtl.co.uk   Surgical Materials Testing Laboratory
www.soap.org   Society for Obstetric Anaesthesia and Perinatology
www.stands4.com   Abbreviations.com
www.stryker.co.uk   Stryker website
www.surgical-tutor.org.uk   Surgery website
www.trentrdsu.org.uk   Trent research information access gateway
www.uktransplant.org.uk   UK Transplant Organisation
www.vh.org   Virtual Hospital
www.virtual-anaesthesia-textbook.com   Virtual Anaesthesia Textbook
www.vlib.org/Medicine.html   Virtual Library. Medicine & Health
www.worldwidewounds.com   Worldwide Wounds
www.yoursurgery.com   Surgical information site

Appendix 5

Professional bodies and health-related organisations

Action on Smoking and Health (ASH)   www.ash.org.uk
Adverse Psychiatric Reactions Information Link (APRIL)   www.ukppg.org.uk
Arthritis Research Campaign (ARC)   www.arc.org.uk
Association of the British Pharmaceutical Industry (ABPI)   www.abpi.org.uk
Association of Directors of Public Health (ADPH)   www.adsph.org.uk
Association of Operating Department Assistants   www.aodp.org
Association of Professional Ambulance Personnel (APAP)   www.apap.org.uk
Association for Professionals in Infection Control (APIC)   www.apic.org
Blood Pressure Association (BPA)   www.bpassoc.org.uk
British Association of Day Surgery (BADS)   www.bads.co.uk
British Association of Plastic, Reconstructive and Aesthetic Surgeons (BAPRAS)   www.bapras.org.uk
British Association of Sexual Health and HIV (BASHH)   www.bashh.org
British Burn Association (BBA)   http://www.britishburnsassociation.co.uk
British Congenital Cardiac Association (BCCA)   www.congenitalheart.co.uk
British Fertility Society (BFS)   www.britishfertilitysociety.org.uk
British Hypertension Society (BHS)   www.bhsoc.org
British Lung Foundation (BLF)   www.lunguk.org
British Medical Association (BMA)   www.bma.org
British Skin Foundation (BSF)   www.britishskinfoundation.org
British Society of Gastroenterology (BSG)   www.bsg.org.uk
British Thoracic Society (BTS)   www.brit-thoracic.org.uk
British Transplantation Society   www.bts.org.uk
Cardiac Risk in the Young (CRY)   www.c-r-y.org.uk
Centers for Disease Control (CDC)   www.cdc.gov
Centre for Healthcare Associated Infections   http://hcai.nottingham.ac.uk
Centre for Science in the Public Interest   www.cspinet.org
Chartered Society of Physiotheraphy (CSP)   www.csp.org.uk
Chief Medical Officer (CMO)   www.dh.gov.uk
Comment on Reproductive Ethics (CORE)   www.sourcehealth.org
Committee on Carcinogenicity (COC)   www.advisorybodies.doh.org
Consumer Protection Act (CPA)   www.e-laws.gov
Council for Healthcare Regulatory Excellence (CHRE)   www.chre.org.uk
Department of Health (DoH)   www.dh.gov.uk

Developing Patient Partnerships (DPP) www.dpp.org.uk

Diabetes Research & Wellness Foundation (DRWF) www.diabeteswellness.nets

Dignity in Dying (DID) www.dignityindying.org.uk

European Food Safety Authority (EFSA) www.efsa.europa.eu

European Medicines Agency [EM(E)A] www.emea.eu.int

European Society for Human Reproduction and Embryology (ESHRE) www.eshre.com

Food and Drink Federation (FDF) www.fdf.org.uk

General Medical Council (GMC) www.gmc-uk.org

Health Protection Agency (HPA) www.hpa.org.uk

Health Quality Service (HQS) www.hqs.org.uk

Human Genetics Commission (HGAC) www.hgc.gov.uk

Institute of Public Policy Research (IPPR) www.ippr.org.uk

Intensive Care National Audit & Research Centre (ICNARC) www.icnarc.org

International Narcotics Control Board (INCB) www.incb.org

International Osteoporosis Foundation (IOF) www.osteofound.org

Joint Committee on Vaccination & Immunisation (JCVI) www.advisorybodies.doh.gov.uk/jcvi/

Medical Research Council (MRC) www.mrc.ac.uk

Medicines and Healthcare Regulatory Agency (MHRA) www.mhra.gov.uk

Mental Health Foundation (MHF) www.mentalhealth.org.uk

Minimally Invasive Robotic Association (MIRA) www.websurg.com

National Aids Manual (NAM) www.nam.org.uk

National Association of Assistants in Surgical Practice (NAASP) www.naasp.org.uk

National Association of Orthopaedic Nurses (NAON) www.orthonurse.org

National Audit Office (NAO) www.nao.org.uk

National Blood Transfusion Service (NBTS) www.blood.co.uk

National Childbirth Trust (NCT) www.nct.org.uk

National Council for Radiation Protection & Measurements (NCRP) www.ncrponline.org

National Heart, Lung and Blood Institute www.nhlbi.nih.gov

National Infertility Awareness Campaign (NIAC) www.repromed.co.uk

National Institute of Allergy and Infectious Diseases (NIAID) www.niaid.nih.gov

National Institute on Drug Abuse (NIDA) www.nida.nih.gov

National Institute of Environmental Health Sciences (NIEHS) www.niehs.nih.gov

National Institute for Health (NIH) www.nih.gov

National Patient Safety Agency (NPSA) www.surgerydoor.co.uk

National Prescribing Centre (NPC) www.npc.co.uk

National Reporting and Learning System (NRLS) www.pjonline.com

National Research Council (NRC)   www.nationalacademics.org/nrc/
National Screening Committee (NSC)   www.nsc.nhs.uk
Office for National Statistics (ONS)   www.statistics.gov.uk
Paediatric Cardiac Nurses Association (PCNA)   www.pcna.co.uk
Patients Association (PA)   www.patients-association.org.uk
Proprietary Association of Great Britain (PAGB)   www.pagb.co.uk
Purchasing and Supply Agency (PASA)   www.pasa.nhs.uk
Registration, Education & Authorisation of Chemicals (REACH)   www.hse.
gov.uk/reach/index.htm
Royal College of General Practitioners (RCGP)   www.rcgp.org.uk
Royal College of Obstetricians and Gynaecologists (RCOG)   www.rcog.org.uk
Royal Pharmaceutical Society (RPS)   www.rpsgb.org.uk
Royal Society for the Prevention of Accidents (RoSPA)   www.rospa.com
Science Committee on Food (SCF)   www.ec.europa.eu/food
Scientific Advisory Committee on Nutrition (SACN)   www.sacn.gov.uk
Sexual Dysfunction Association (SDA)   www.sexualdysfunctionassociation.
com
Spongiform Encephalopathy Advisory Committee (SEAC)   www.seac.gov.uk
UK Transplant Support Service Authority (UKTSSA)   www.uktransplant.org.uk
United Kingdom Central Council for Nursing Midwifery & Health Visiting
(UKCC)   www.nmc-uk.org
United States Pharmacopeia (USP)   www.usp.org
Unrelated Live Transplant Regulatory Authority (ULTRA)   www.advisorybodies.
doh.gov.uk/ultra
World Health Organization (WHO)   www.who.int
World Federation of Societies of Anaesthesiologists (WFSA)
www.anaesthesiologists.org